Fundamentals of Chinese Acupuncture

— Revised Edition —

Andrew Ellis, Nigel Wiseman, Ken Boss

Paradigm Publications • Brookline, Massachusetts

— 1991 —

Fundamentals of Chinese Acupuncture

Andrew Ellis, Nigel Wiseman, Ken Boss

ISBN 0-912111-33-X

Copyright © 1991 Paradigm Publications

Paradigm Publications
44 Linden Street
Brookline, Massachusetts, 02146 U.S.A.

Publisher: Robert L. Felt
Editor: Richard Feit

Distributed by:
Redwing Book Company, 44 Linden St., Brookline, MA 02146 USA

Preface

The Fundamentals of Chinese Acupuncture is a compilation of information from several sources. Selections from modern and classical Chinese texts were translated to create a book that would foster a greater understanding of the changing tradition of Chinese acupuncture. Our intent was to create a clinical text that would reflect not only the school of acupuncture presented in modern texts from the People's Republic of China but also the Chinese tradition that lies at the heart of these modern teachings. In the presentation of material and Chinese concepts, our objective was to take full account of the historical, cultural, and clinical realities of Chinese acupuncture.

Scope and Contents

The sequence and manner of presentation of this book were chosen both to present a culturally valid view of Chinese acupuncture and to meet the needs of those who wish to study the more sophisticated acupuncture practiced in China. Features were selected to address Western needs as expressed by the most common learning problems identified by acupuncture students and clinicians.

At some time in their studies almost every acupuncturist tries to cross reference the acupoint indications available in different texts. The difficulty this presents is widely known. Students who wish to expand their knowledge and clinicians who hope to discover the often subtle clues that bring success in treatment are faced with a variety of approaches and opinions concerning the meaning and value of Chinese concepts.

For example, readers who see *mental restlessness* in one work, *irritability* in another, and *vexation* in our own are likely to take the words at face value, that is, attach to them the meanings they have in common speech. While these three English expressions are by no means exact synonyms, they are all used to render one Chinese idea. They all represent *fán*. Regardless of which English word readers prefer, this confusion of choice leaves them uncertain, unable to recognize the symptom correctly, and unable to understand its relation to other ideas. Because Chinese acupuncture is heavily reliant on qualities and correspondences, such seemingly minor differences can cause clinicians to look for the wrong clues, or to miss clues that could be clinically useful. Our approach to solving this problem is to preserve the traditional meanings of concepts and their relationships as much as is possible. Thus we have tried to present information in a manner that permits readers to recognize the elements of meaning that are available to those who read Chinese. In the example cited above, our readers are provided with the original definition of the term *fán*. In the glossary we inform them that Chinese

i

clinicians see this idea in terms of restlessness and "hot-headedness" as a subjective feeling, in contradistinction to *zào,* which includes exaggerated physical movement (i.e., an objective facet).

Distinction and accuracy are only part of our approach. To date, we have unified the terminology used in this text with a word-for-word translation of a text commonly used to train Chinese medical students (*Fundamentals of Chinese Medicine*), a comprehensive Chinese, Pinyin and English reference (*A Glossary of Chinese Medicine and Acupuncture Points*) and a study of the clinical and cultural meanings carried by acupoint names (*Grasping the Wind*). It is our goal to facilitate cross-referencing among our own works, and among the works of other authors who preserve linguistic correspondences to the original Chinese. Thus readers acquire the ability to refine their understanding, improve their clinical investigations, and judge the value of ideas for themselves.

Another commonly reported difficulty stems from the differences of texts based on the classics and those designed for modern Western and Chinese classrooms. Concepts differ, as does the relative importance given to concepts and the extent to which biomedically defined diseases are used as the basis of diagnosis and treatment. We have therefore provided information that students and practitioners, physicians and non-physicians, may compare and contrast. The descriptions found in this text expand a method used in Chinese language texts. Both modern and classical locations, indications and channel descriptions are provided. The concepts presented in the *Supplementary Indications* introduce Western readers to the insights available to Chinese practitioners.

Finally, students and clinicians frequently note that they rarely see patients who clearly present the patterns they have learned in school. Some of this difficulty may be traced to the fact that traditional Chinese diagnoses are based on a synthesis of clinical observations, many of which must be seen, felt or perceived. Thus we have selected Chinese texts with detailed clinical descriptions and have presented those texts in a manner that prioritizes the preservation of the distinctions made by Chinese clinicians. This results in sets of functions, clinical observations and indications that are larger and more complex than those of modern basic texts but provide clinicians with the information necessary for advancing their clinical practice.

Although based entirely on Chinese sources, *Fundamentals of Chinese Acupuncture* is designed to fit the Western approach to learning. Therefore, it differs slightly from Chinese texts in presentation and format.

Part I, *Materials and Methods,* introduces the materials needed for the application of acupuncture and related therapies and the methods for performing these therapies.

Part II, *An Introduction to the Channels and Points,* describes the general channel system and discusses the nature of the points and point groupings.

Part III, *Channels and Points,* outlines the pathways, pathologies and points of each channel. Included in this section is a discussion of the points and the location, functions, indications, needling depths and localized anatomy of each point.

Part IV, *Approaches to Point Selection and Combination,* discusses the various ways of selecting and combining acupuncture points in treatment, and the general principles of treatment by acupuncture and moxibustion.

The glossary at the end of the book will help familiarize the reader with some diseases and symptoms discussed in classical texts. The student wishing an elaboration of such functions as drain, calm, boost or harmonize, or symptoms not included in basic texts such as fright wind, gan, goose foot wind, and saber and pearl-string lumps, will find the glossary an invaluable assistance. There is also an index designed to help clinicians discover treatment options according to the principles detailed in Part IV, a point index and a section new to this revised edition that illustrates the modern simplified pathways. This latter feature was added in response to readers' requests for a more immediate visual reference to contrast the more advanced pathway descriptions given in the text.

We have chosen to remain within the confines of a detailed presentation of Chinese acupuncture. We have not dealt with Japanese or Korean acupuncture or any of the modern derivations such as laser acupuncture, ear acupuncture and electrical stimulation of acupuncture points. We have done this as much to preserve the integrity of these other valid forms of acupuncture as that of Chinese acupuncture.

Changing Approaches to Chinese Medicine

For Chinese medicine, the most important period of transmission to the West began in the 1960's, when acupuncture started to develop as a profession among Occidentals. This period followed one of the greatest changes Chinese medicine had ever undergone: its adaptation to the twentieth century.

Western influence, which finally brought about the collapse of Imperial China in 1911, ushered in a new era for Chinese medicine. Traditional healing was spared by the nationalists after the founding of the Republic, and was again spared by the communists after 1950, in part because of the lack of Western medical practitioners, and in part by the purported similarity of Chinese medical theory to marxist ideology. Although it survived, its name *yī* or *yī xué* (medicine) was changed to *zhōng yī* (Chinese medicine), reflecting its declining status relative to its Western rival. After World War II when it was incorporated into a modern mass health-care system, it underwent a thorough revision. Mass health care demanded unified standards of practice, and a unified method of teaching in colleges. The traditional medley of different schools of thought and heterogeneous practices, many of which bordered on shamanism, were unified into a more coherent system, and superstitious elements were expunged. Traditional transmission by individual healers to their apprentices, with its emphasis on memorization of the classics and mnemonic verses, was replaced by efficient modern classroom methods of mass education.

The question naturally arises as to what criteria were applied to determine the composition of this new Chinese medicine. While in the modern era statistically demonstrated clinical efficacy is the only universally acceptable criterion, the science of statistics never developed in traditional China. There were never large hospitals offering the possibility of broad clinical trials; there were never computers to manage the information. The effectiveness of a method of treatment was judged by how it withstood the test of time. In creating the new Chinese medicine, the Chinese selected theories and methods of treatment that were based on a coherent rationale and that were revered over centuries. Although they began to gather statistical data, there is clear evidence that their choices were, and continue to be, not only technical, but also social and political.

Although much older medical literature is available in China, school curriculum is increasingly based on the new literature created by China's universities to meet the exigencies of the modern period. The new literature, for example, barely mentions the *hun,* the *po,* and other "psychic" aspects of the organs. Presumably these ideas are thought to be clinically invalid, to introduce unnecessary elements of superstition, or to require observational skills requiring experience, not classroom training. The new literature also omits mention of many of the sociopolitical analogies of traditional medicine. Analogies of the liver as the general, or the lung as the assistant, have been omitted or minimized because they are reflections of China's pre-communist society. While the new literature includes the five phases, it judges the shortcomings of this theory by reference to marxist doctrine. The new Chinese medicine also has provided explanations for the etiology of diseases that are contained nowhere in the traditional literature, and has applied traditional drug functions to acupuncture points in an effort to homogenize the two distinct traditions.

The problems Chinese medicine has faced in modern China have affected its transmission to the West. The Chinese have played a larger role in presenting Chinese medicine to the West than might have been the case if the Chinese language were easier and took less time to learn. Given this task, the books they have selected to translate into Western languages represent their new view of acupuncture, their attempt to wed traditional medicine with biomedicine, and their concern that without a strong Western orientation acupuncture would be poorly received in the West. Thus the Chinese have presented their new medicine in the way they imagine the West can best accept it, and labeled it "traditional Chinese medicine."

We have been cognizant of this historical perspective and have striven to present the information essential to learning modern Chinese acupuncture in a holistic fashion, hoping to provide Western readers with an opportunity closer to that enjoyed by their Chinese colleagues. Thus our concern to present a culturally and historically sensitive view of Chinese acupuncture has influenced both the information we have presented and the language in which we have presented it.

Content

The discussion of point locations provided our first opportunity to present the traditional picture of acupuncture alongside the new. In most modern texts intended for Western readerships, the Chinese give information needed to locate acupuncture points in the language of Western anatomy combined with the body inch system, and by reference to other acupuncture points. The Western student may have wondered how the Chinese traditionally found the points without the benefits of Western anatomy. Indeed, in the majority of cases, the descriptions of point locations provided by *The Great Compendium of Acupuncture and Moxibustion, The Systematized Canon of Acupuncture* and *The Golden Mirror of Medicine* are not sufficient in themselves to locate a point without demonstration. However, once it is understood that the channel paths these books describe must be learned before the individual points are located, the classical point locations become very clear in almost all cases. They were certainly sufficient in the traditional learning situation in China, where apprentices were shown the points by their teachers.

We include the classical system alongside the modern system not to satisfy the curiosity of the student about the quaint backwardness of the past, but to bring once again the things of the past to the scrutiny of the present. Many students report that the classical locations are easily remembered and serve their daily purpose better than the modern system. Furthermore, because all attempts to illustrate point location fail to some extent, these practical instructions are a considerable aid to learning.

Disease categories are another gray area requiring clarification. In modern literature, the Chinese have discarded many traditional disease categories in preference for Western medical categories. For example, modern texts will speak of tonsillitis rather than *rǔ é* (throat moth), and of hysteria rather than *zàng zào* (visceral agitation). In Chinese texts, equivalents of this type appear side by side with the traditional Chinese descriptions. However, most English language publications disregard the traditional terms altogether. Many Chinese concepts, especially symptoms and diseases, are rendered as Western medical equivalents, even when the clinical studies Western standards demand for such equivalence have not been performed. In many instances Western terms are used when the symptom and sign equivalents are not exact. In the Western clinic these practices are problematic.

This adoption of the definitions of Western medicine creates clinical inaccuracies because exact clinically demonstrable equivalents are rare. For example, most modern Chinese-English dictionaries translate *dān dú* as "erysipelas," yet traditional Chinese dictionaries tell us the term can include *snake girdle cinnabar* (herpes zoster, shingles). Cinnabar describes things red in color. Herpes zoster is red; erysipelas is red; there the identity ends in Western medicine. Thus where texts translate *dān dú* only with the Western medical term *erysipelas,* all the general cases of *dān dú* conveyed by the original Chinese word, including herpes zoster, are lost. Thus clinicians are misled.

To better reflect the traditional concepts, and to properly qualify the Western equivalents, we have taken a dual approach in the presentation of Part III, *The Channels and Points.* Under the section *Indications,* we have kept to the new approach, while in *Supplementary Indications,* we have expressed disease categories and symptoms in a language as faithful to the original sources as possible. Where applicable, the traditional point associations are also listed as are illustrative point combinations. These combinations are not exclusive clinical options, but selections that reflect the Chinese point of view. Thus through the *Supplementary Indications*, the reader is presented with symptoms and diseases that carry with them the frame of reference found in the Chinese language. English terms such as bowstring and elusive masses, clouding inversion, clove sore, intestinal wind, running piglet and straw shoe wind, largely coined by the authors in the absence of any precedent for standard rendering, are defined in the glossary.

In making terminological choices, we have attempted to preserve the Chinese frames of reference within which the Chinese used the terms. This is particularly important because terms from Chinese medicine were heavily borrowed to express Western medical concepts when Western medicine was translated into the Chinese language. People translating Chinese medicine into English both in the East and West have used the same device in reverse. For example, when Western medicine was first translated into Chinese, the term *fēng shī* was appropriated to render the Western medical concept of rheumatism. When translating the Chinese medical concept into English we have the choice as to whether to use our ready-made word rheumatism, or to preserve the original Chinese meaning by rendering it literally as wind-damp. The latter has the advantage of preserving the Chinese point of view, whereas the former does not.

In presenting the traditional indications of acupuncture points, we have not been too shy to include what a modern Westerner might regard as "culturally determined" or superstitious elements. When listing such things as "dreaming of intercourse with ghosts" and "ghost attacks" among supplementary indications from the classics, we are not asking the reader to believe in ghosts, but are presenting information that may help elucidate China's cultural development and the changes in Chinese medicine that parallel it. Historical questions cannot be ignored if clinical performance is to be preserved. In the abovementioned cases, for example, clinicians who see these terms as expressions of what we now call psychological observations will have the benefit of the relevant clinical information.

Translation Method

The problems posed by different and changing approaches to Chinese medicine are intimately related to the problem of terminological choices when translating Chinese medical literature into English. The accurate rendering of Chinese
medicine and acupuncture in English calls for a method that ensures a clear understanding of individual concepts and their clinical viability, preserves their theoretical context, and fosters an accurate overall conception of the discipline. Concepts
in Chinese acupuncture were used in a specific frame of reference. Functions, patterns, indications and theoretical constructs all shared subtle qualitative relationships expressed through the Chinese language. These ideas were not isolated
labels based on solely objective tests. Each was part of a holistic picture.

Let us take as an example the relationships of a single organ, the liver, in its
correspondence to the wood phase. We are told that wood is the "bending and
straightening." Wood as a material is used for its bending qualities, as well as for
its ability to stay straight. In comparison with metal, it is pliable and easy to cut,
though it also has great strength. We can understand more about the concept when
we see that it includes living wood. In modern Chinese, *mù* means the substance
wood, but in ancient China it was also used to mean *tree*. Trees are immobile, but
have a suppleness that enables them to bend in the wind rather than be broken by
it. The living wood also has the quality of orderly upward and outward reaching.
It therefore symbolizes the growth and expansion of plant life in the spring, and by
analogy the physical agility and vigor associated with youth, the springtime of life.

In the human body, the "bending and straightening" of wood is reflected in
the "bending and stretching" of the sinews *(jīn)*. The sinews hold the bones
together and give the body its agility. They have the "springy" quality associated
with wood. In fact, the meanings of the English word "spring" — the season,
growth, jumping, and resilience — are all part of the notion of wood.

The Inner Canon tells us that the liver holds the office of general. This symbol
perfectly fits the qualitative associations of wood. As plant life stretches upward
in the springtime, so a general leads a strong, youthful nation in asserting its
power and expanding its territory. The general is a symbol for a nation flexing its
muscles and extending its claws (the nails, or claws, being the surplus of the
sinews). Since the strong general must make strategies, the faculty to plan and cal-
culate must relate to wood. Since thwarted expansionism and the inability to
express power results in anger, this emotion is also associated with wood. The
sinews of a strong nation brace for attack; the sinews of a weak nation jerk with
fright. Both these responses are associated with the liver. Thus the image of the
general adds another dimension to the qualitative connections between observable
aspects of being human. *The Inner Canon* presents all these as being governed by
or associated with the liver and the concept of wood.

Liver qi enjoys the freedom to stretch outward as trees stretch their branches,
and does so unobservably in a healthy person. When it fails to do so in sickness,

there are signs of stagnation or "frustration" which the Chinese called depressed liver qi. This manifests as lateral costal pain, swelling of the breasts, or as globus hystericus (plum pit qi). Such conditions are often brought about by anger and emotional frustration, liver-related emotions. Making these associations, it is clear that the ancient Chinese were not talking about functions in strict relationship to a complex morphological entity, but about functions qualitatively associated with wood.

Suppleness is the only defense of trees. Being immobile, they must bend to foil their major enemy, wind. Healthy plants are sufficiently supple to survive a wind. The wood of the body can also be blown by wind, especially internal wind. When a wind arises in the body, it can shake the sinews, causing convulsions (*chōu fēng,* literally "wind tugging"). In wind stroke it can — metaphorically — "snap" the branches (limbs), so that they no longer move at all. One Chinese expression for hemiplegia is *piān kū,* hemilateral "withering," which describes the condition by analogy to the dry deadness of trees. Wind is swift and changeable, and takes its victim by surprise. Wind-stroke, epilepsy, tetanus (*pò shāng fēng,* literally "wound wind") all share this characteristic. In the same way, a sudden fright can make the sinews jerk, so that liver disorders are sometimes characterized by susceptibility to fright.

It is clear that in theorizing about the liver the Chinese recognized all the aspects of the body and psyche that shared the expansive thrust of the living wood. They were not describing a simply mechanical system; they were describing aspects of being human that were related by qualitative analogy. Their words were not simply technical labels, as in Western medicine, but also qualitative symbols and images. All things that have to do with the bending, stretching, tensing qualities of the body were seen as belonging within the wood phase and associated with the liver. Even anatomical names were not isolated words but parts of a useful and coherent image of considerable value to the adept clinician. *Sinew* is not merely an ancient label that can be reduced to a familiar Western label such as *tendon* or *muscle,* but part of a delicate image of qualities associated with wood and the liver. Flesh is distinguished from sinew not solely by anatomical features but by the relationship of sinew to the liver and flesh to the spleen.

In Chinese acupuncture, parts of the body, theoretical constructs, organ functions and pathologies, psychological and physical signs, acupoint names and categories, relationships to pathology, and the indications by which treatment is selected are all linked in a subtle mosaic of correspondences that must be preserved for the full clinical picture to be understood. By preserving these associations in the language chosen to express the classical indications for acupoints, we hope to transmit more of the picture that is available to Chinese practitioners.

The clinical relevance of such points of translation cannot be overlooked. Even without reference to the subtleties of Chinese medical thought, recourse to vernacular words and Western concepts very often eliminates useful clinical information. While *infantile convulsions* can describe a condition, it transmits neither the relationships nor the clinical associations that the Chinese term, *child fright wind,* can convey.

Another example, the Chinese term *lì,* shows how recourse to familiar English words in the interpretation of a character fails to inform readers of its clinical meaning. This term is often translated as *benefit,* presumably because that is its most common use in colloquial Chinese. A glance at the origin of the term and closer scrutiny of its usage in everyday Chinese should suffice to make the real meanings of the word clear. Examination of the specific use in Chinese medicine should demonstrate which of the meanings applies in a technical context.

The character *lì* is composed of grain growing in the fields on the left, and a knife on the right. The two parts together convey the notion of grain being cut at harvest time. This image provides the basis for all its usages: *lì* can be used to mean *sharp* (e.g., *lì dāo,* a sharp knife), since a sharp knife is needed to cut the grain. A sharp knife cuts smoothly, so *lì* describes the *smooth course* of events. When everything goes smoothly with the harvest, there is *benefit* or *advantage* to man. Thus *benefit* is only one small aspect of the meaning of this character.

In Chinese medicine, *lì* occurs almost exclusively in phrases where it denotes restoration of normal movement of a body part, or the normal movement of water, damp, qi, etc., through or out of the body. How can one speak of "benefiting water" or "benefiting the joints" without loss of this clinical intent? The English word *disinhibit,* though a partial neologism, clearly conveys the Chinese idea in nearly all contexts. For example, while *benefiting water* misleadingly suggests the idea of increase, *disinhibiting water* suggests the meaning of release clearly and precisely. Admittedly, *benefit* is a plainer English word than *disinhibit.* However, in the Chinese medical context *benefit* is so imprecise as to be meaningless. The acupuncturist, presented with a case of yin vacuity characterized by such signs as thirst, vexation, upper body heat signs, a fine, rapid pulse, and a dry, red tongue, would do the patient nothing but harm if he or she used points that were said to "benefit water." This mistake is certainly avoided when the term is translated as disinhibit.

We have attempted to transmit a picture of Chinese acupuncture that is sensitive not only to the completeness and accuracy of the data, but to its cultural, historical, and clinical background. It is our hope that in a holistic presentation students and practitioners will find clues and images that will make their learning easier and their clinical practice more profound. We hope that this book achieves the goals we have set forth and that through our chosen approach students and clinicians will acquire some of the broader and more subtle view that is available to those who read Chinese. We hope that the reader gains as much from using the book as we have by producing it.

About the Revised Edition

Most of the changes to this revised edition, other than the correction of typographic errors, concern the illustration of basic information. All the channel pathways were redrawn so that specific points (e.g., connecting-*luo*) could be added. Legends noting the keys used have been appended. All the illustrations were re-reviewed by Western teachers and cross-checked to Chinese texts. Two new sections have been added to help clarify locations and aid in cross referencing to other texts: illustrations of points by body area, and illustrations of the modern simplified channel pathways.

The discussion of translation method that appeared in the first edition has been greatly expanded and is now available in *A Glossary of Chinese Medicine and Acupuncture Points* as are responses to the peer review of our texts. All books of this nature will invariably contain errors of omission and commission and we welcome the corrections and suggestions our readers have provided. We hope that their input will continue.

Acknowledgements

Our special thanks go to Huang Sheng-Jing for her philological backup, Fan Shi-Lei for all the stir-fried delicacies that kept the production team going at the critical hour, Susan Goldbaum and Dr. Ken-shi Tsay for their contribution to the techniques sections, Bev Cubbage for typing and editorial assistance, Jim Stegenga for help with the charts, Jim Cleaver for reviewing the point locations and suggesting improvements, Diane Putt for endless nights of emulation, Tong Shi-Fang for her support in typing and databasing the working glossaries, Tom Riihimaki for the needle illustrations, and not least to Richard Feit, Martha Fielding and Bob Felt, who did much more than publishers normally have to do.

We also thank our teachers Shi Neng-Yun, Chen Jun-Chao, Hsu Fu-Su, Li Cheng-Yu, Chang P'u-t'ao, and Robert Liu without whose guidance we would never have been in a position to write this book.

Table of Contents

Part I: Materials & Methods   1

1. Acupuncture   2
    1.1 The Filiform Needle   4
    1.2 Techniques for Needle Insertion   4
       1.2.1 The four techniques of rotating insertion   4
       1.2.2 Tube insertion   6
       1.2.3 Stabbing   6
       1.2.4 Angle and depth of insertion   6
       1.2.5 Withdrawing the needle   8
       1.2.6 Positioning the patient   8
       1.2.7 Needle insertion practice   10
    1.3 Techniques for Needle Manipulation   11
       1.3.1 Basic stimulation methods   11
       1.3.2 Obtaining and moving qi   12
       1.3.3 Classical methods for supplementation and drainage   13
       1.3.4 Combined methods of supplementation and drainage   15
    1.4 Other Materials & Techniques Related to Acupuncture   18
       1.4.1 The three-edged needle — bloodletting   18
       1.4.2 The cutaneous needle   20
       1.4.3 Use of intradermal needles   21

2. Moxibustion   22
    2.1 Direct Moxibustion   22
       2.1.1 Scarring moxibustion   23
       2.1.2 Non-scarring moxibustion   24
    2.2 Indirect Moxibustion   24
       2.2.1 Moxibustion on an insulating medium   24
       2.2.2 Moxa poles   24
       2.2.3 Warming the needle   25
       2.2.4 Warming instruments   25
    2.3 Moxibustion Precautions and Contraindications   26

Part II: An Introduction to the Channels and Points   29

3. The Channels   29
    3.1 Introduction   29
    3.2 The Twelve Regular Channels   31
       3.2.1 Distribution of the twelve regular channels   31
       3.2.2 Channel direction   31
       3.2.3 Interior-exterior relationships of the twelve channels   35
       3.2.4 Channel communication   36

3.2.5 The diurnal flow of qi through the channels   37
3.2.6 Channel pathways and pathologic signs   38
3.3 The Eight Extraordinary Vessels   38
3.4 Connecting Vessels   39
3.5 Channel Divergences   40
3.6 The Twelve Channel Sinews   41
3.7 The Twelve Cutaneous Regions   42
3.8 General Channel Distribution   43
    3.8.1 Channel distribution in the head & face   43
    3.8.2 Channel distribution in the neck & throat   47
    3.8.3 Channel distribution in the shoulder & scapula   48
    3.8.4 Channel distribution in the trunk   49
    3.8.5 Channel distribution in the abdominal region   52

4. The Points   56
4.1 Point Functions and Indications   56
    4.1.1 Relationship of location to point indications and functions   56
    4.1.2 Relationship of the channels to point indications and functions   56
    4.1.3 Relationship of the special point groupings to point indications   58
    4.1.4 Indications and functions gleaned from clinical experience   58
    4.1.5 A note about modern point functions   59
4.2 Special Point Groupings   60
    4.2.1 Source-yuan points   60
    4.2.2 Connecting-luo points   61
    4.2.3 Cleft-xi points   61
    4.2.4 Eight meeting-hui points   62
    4.2.5 Lower uniting-he points   62
    4.2.6 Confluence-jiaohui points of the eight extraordinary vessels   62
    4.2.7 The four command points   63
    4.2.8 The alarm-mu points   64
    4.2.9 Associated-shu points   64
    4.2.10 The five transporting-shu points   64
    4.2.11 The intersection-jiaohui points   66
    4.2.12 Hua Tuo's paravertebral points   66
    4.2.13 Additional point groupings   66
4.3 Locating Acupuncture Points   67
Endnotes to Chapter 4   70

Part III: The Channels and Points   73

5. A Preface to The Channels and Points   73
Key to the illustrations   76

6. The Lung Channel System (Hand Tai Yin)   77
6.1 The Primary Lung Channel   77
6.2 The Connecting Vessel of the Lung Channel   77

   6.3 The Lung Channel Divergence   78
   6.4 The Lung Channel Sinews   79
   Lung Channel Points   80

7. The Large Intestine Channel System (Hand Yang Ming)   89
   7.1 The Primary Large Intestine Channel   89
   7.2 The Connecting Vessel of the Large Intestine Channel   90
   7.3 The Large Intestine Channel Divergence   91
   7.4 The Large Intestine Channel Sinews   92
   Large Intestine Channel Points   93

8. The Stomach Channel System (Foot Yang Ming)   104
   8.1 The Primary Stomach Channel   109
   8.2 The Connecting Vessel of the Stomach Channel   110
   8.3 The Stomach Channel Divergence   111
   8.4 The Stomach Channel Sinews   112
   Stomach Channel Points   114

9. The Spleen Channel System (Foot Tai Yin)   144
   9.1 The Primary Spleen Channel   144
   9.2 The Connecting Vessel of the Spleen Channel   144
   9.3 The Spleen Channel Divergence   145
   9.4 The Spleen Channel Sinews   146
   9.5 The Great Connecting Vessel of the Spleen   147
   Spleen Channel Points   148

10. The Heart Channel System (Hand Shao Yin)   163
   10.1 The Primary Heart Channel   163
   10.2 The Connecting Vessel of the Heart   163
   10.3 The Heart Channel Divergence   164
   10.4 The Heart Channel Sinews   164
   Heart Channel Points   166

11. The Small Intestine Channel System (Hand Tai Yang)   173
   11.1 The Primary Small Intestine Channel   173
   11.2 The Connecting Vessel of the Small Intestine Channel   174
   11.3 The Small Intestine Channel Divergence   175
   11.4 The Small Intestine Channel Sinews   175
   Small Intestine Channel Points   177

12. The Bladder Channel System (Foot Tai Yang)   191
   12.1 The Primary Bladder Channel   191
   12.2 The Connecting Vessel of the Bladder Channel   192
   12.3 The Bladder Channel Divergence   193
   12.4 The Bladder Channel Sinews   194
   Bladder Channel Points   195

13. The Kidney Channel System (Foot Shao Yin)   243
     13.1   The Primary Kidney Channel   243
     13.2   The Connecting Vessel of the Kidney Channel   243
     13.3   The Kidney Channel Divergence   245
     13.4   The Kidney Channel Sinews   245
     Kidney Channel Points   247

14. The Pericardium Channel System (Hand Jue Yin)   266
     14.1   The Primary Pericardium Channel   266
     14.2   The Connecting Vessel of the Pericardium Channel   266
     14.3   The Pericardium Channel Divergence   267
     14.4   The Pericardium Channel Sinews   267
     Pericardium Channel Points   269

15. The Triple Burner Channel System (Hand Shao Yang)   277
     15.1   The Primary Triple Burner Channel   277
     15.2   The Connecting Vessel of the Triple Burner Channel   278
     15.3   The Triple Burner Channel Divergence   279
     15.4   The Triple Burner Channel Sinews   279
     Triple Burner Channel Points   280

16. The Gallbladder Channel System (Foot Shao Yang)   296
     16.1   The Primary Gallbladder Channel   296
     16.2   The Connecting Vessel of the Gallbladder Channel   298
     16.3   The Gallbladder Channel Divergence   298
     16.4   The Gallbladder Channel Sinews   298
     Gallbladder Channel Points   300

17. The Liver Channel System (Foot Jue Yin)   331
     17.1   The Primary Liver Channel   331
     17.2   The Connecting Vessel of the Liver Channel   331
     17.3   The Liver Channel Divergence   332
     17.4   The Liver Channel Sinews   333
     Liver Channel Points   334

18. The Conception Vessel System   345
     18.1   The Primary Conception Vessel Channel   345
     18.2   The Connecting Vessel of the Conception Vessel   345
     Conception Vessel Points   347

19. The Governing Vessel System   369
     19.1   The Primary Governing Vessel Channel   369
     19.2   The Connecting Vessel of the Governing Vessel   370
     Governing Vessel Points   371

20. The Extraordinary Vessels   393
     20.1   The Penetrating Vessel   393
     20.2   The Girdling Vessel   393

20.3 Yin and Yang Motility Vessels   395
20.4 The Yin and Yang Linking Vessels   396

21. Non-Channel Points   398

Part IV: Approaches to Point Selection and Combination   412

22. Selecting Points   412
22.1 Selection of Local, Adjacent, and Distant Points   412
22.2 Selection of Points According to the Affected Channel   413
22.3 Selection of Points According to Past Clinical Experience   429
22.4 Selection of Points by Employment of Special Point Groups   431
     22.4.1 Application of the source-yuan points   431
     22.4.2 Application of connecting-luo points   432
     22.4.3 Applications of cleft-xi points   433
     22.4.4 Applications of meeting-hui points   433
     22.4.5 Applications of lower uniting-he points   433
     22.4.6 Applications of the command points   434
     22.4.7 Applications of alarm-mu points   434
     22.4.8 Applications of the associated-shu points   434
     22.4.9 Applications of transporting-shu points   434
     22.4.10 Applications of intersection-jiaohui points   439

23. General Principles of Point Combining   443
23.1 Dual Employment of Local and Distant Points   443
23.2 Combination of Points on the Front and the Back   443
23.3 Combination of Points from Yin and Yang Channels   444
23.4 Combination of Upper Body and Lower Body Points   446
23.5 Dual Employment of Cleft-xi Points and Meeting-hui Points   446

24. General Therapeutic Principles   447
24.1 Treatment of Root and Branches   447
     24.1.1 Treatment of the root   447
     24.1.2 Treatment of the branches   447
     24.1.3 Simultaneous treatment of root and branches   448
24.2 Additional Considerations of Point Combining   448
Endnotes to Section IV   449

Glossary   451
Bibliography   465
Treatment Research Index   470
Indications Index   471
Points Index   476
Charts of Simplified Channel Pathways & Points   479

• *Application:* The skin-pinching technique is used on areas where the skin is thin, such as on the face and head.

With all rotating insertion techniques, after the superficial layers of skin have been penetrated, the needle is moved to the correct depth with a slow, slight rotation. The needle rotation is performed either in a single direction, or equally in both directions, and is combined with the continuous downward movement of the needle. Insertion rotation is not intended to provide supplementation or drainage stimulation.

1.2.2 Tube insertion

Tube insertion employs the use of a thin stainless steel, glass, or plastic tubular guide into which a tailess needle (without the end ring) is placed before insertion. Insertion tubes are approximately 4 mm shorter than the needles for which they are intended, thus exposing a consistent length of the needle handle when the tube and the needle tip are allowed to rest on the skin surface. The needle is gently tapped into the skin until the top of the needle handle is level with, or just below, the top of the tube. The guide tube is then removed and the needle inserted to the appropriate depth. This technique is most often used with long and/or thin needles, as well as in the treatment of children and adults who are particularly sensitive.

Practitioners who favor the use of insertion tubes often develop skill in manipulating the tube and the needle with one hand. Such skill allows acupuncture points to be palpated and located with the index finger of the left hand, while the tube and needle are prepared with the right hand. Care must be taken when practicing this technique that clean fields are not compromised. The practitioner must not come in contact with the body of the needle.

1.2.3 Stabbing

Stabbing is the insertion technique used on patients with skin that is particularly sensitive or difficult to penetrate. The right hand holds the needle while the left hand is used to stabilize the skin at the acupuncture point. The needle is quickly inserted with a stabbing motion to a depth of 0.6 to 1.0 cm.

1.2.4 Angle and depth of insertion

The correct angle and depth of insertion is determined in part by the physiology of the area being needled and in part by the intended effect of the treatment.

Angle of Insertion: There are three principal angles of insertion as outlined below. These angles are guidelines that are subject to modification according to the requirements of the particular site and the disorders being treated.

Needle Insertion Angle		
Name	**Angle** *(from tangent at point)*	**Comments**
Perpendicular insertion	90°	The most common insertion.
Oblique insertion	45°	Appropriate where the subcutaneous flesh is thin or where an internal organ lies beneath the point. Commonly used on the chest and back. Also employed for moving qi in a given direction.
Transverse insertion	10 to 20 °	Suited for areas with little flesh beneath the skin. The head, face and neck often require transverse insertion. Also useful when joining points.

Depth of Insertion: Depth of insertion is determined by consideration of the local anatomy, the patient's constitution, the season, and the depth and nature of the pathogen.

The practitioner must be aware of the anatomy at each point and the dangers of an excessively deep insertion. The needling depths recommended with each point in Part III of this text are guidelines that must be fitted to the physique of the patient.

The following chart is a condensation of guidelines set forth in the *Inner Canon* regarding depth of insertion based upon patient constitution.

Needle Insertion Depth				
Relative Depth of Insertion	**Constitutional Aspect**			
	Age	**Gender**	**Body Type**	**Qi & Blood**
Shallow	Older Persons & Infants	Female	Thin	Qi & Blood Debility
Deep	Teen & Middle Years	Male	Portly	Abundance of Qi & Blood

In modern practice the practitioner must weigh the clinical propriety of determining·needle depth by the seasons. The *Classic of Difficult Issues* states:

> In spring and summer yang qi is in the upper regions and a person's qi
> also is in the upper regions, therefore one should needle superficially. In
> autumn and winter yang qi is in the lower regions and a person's qi is also
> in the lower regions, therefore one should needle deeply.

This is consistent with the theory put forth in the *Inner Canon*.

In general, heat and vacuity diseases require shallow insertion, and cold and repletion diseases require deep insertion. Needling depths for repletion heat and vacuity cold diseases are determined by the depth of the pathogen.

The depth of the needle insertion should be in accord with the depth of the disease. The *Inner Canon* states:

> Deep needling applied to a superficial disease results in injury [to deeper
> lying flesh]...[and] superficial needling applied to a deep disease does not
> drain [the pathogen].

Whereas an exogenous pathogenic contraction can be treated with shallow needle insertion, a deeper invasion of the pathogen requires deeper insertion. Diseases affecting the flesh, blood aspect, bones, or organs all require deep insertions.

1.2.5 Withdrawing the needle

The speed of withdrawal and other particulars of needle withdrawal are dependent on whether one wishes to supplement or drain the point in question. The following guidelines hold true regardless of the type of effect desired in treatment of the point.

• The needle should be rotated slightly as it is withdrawn to prevent its adhesion to body tissues.

• The needle should be withdrawn to just below the skin and then retained at this depth for a few seconds before it is fully withdrawn. This procedure will generally prevent bleeding and reduce post-needling pain.

• An alcohol-soaked ball of cotton should be used to swab the point after the needle is withdrawn.

• Needles inserted in the region of the eye should be withdrawn slowly and with special care.

1.2.6 Positioning the patient

The position selected for the patient should be one that allows him to be comfortable enough so that he can remain still for the duration of the treatment. The practitioner must also have access to the necessary points. In general, these two criteria can be met by one of the postures illustrated below, but sometimes the treatment must be divided into two or more sections during which the patient assumes different postures to allow the practitioner access to the points to be needled.

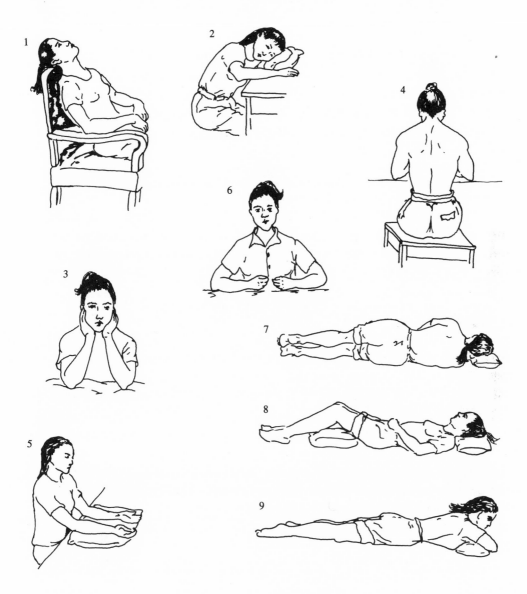

Figure 1.2 Chart of positions and their uses

Note the use of pillows in various positions that allow maximum patient comfort.

Body Positions	
Position	**Areas of Access**
1. Sitting	Head, neck, face and front and sides of body
2. Sitting at a table, leaning to one side	Side of head or neck
3. Supporting the head	Head and face
4. Sitting at a table with the head bowed	Back and lower back (see also prone position)
5. Sitting elbows bent exposing palms	The yin channels of the forearms, face.
6. Sitting elbows bent exposing back of hands	The yang channels of the forearm. If the hands are adjusted, heart and small intestine points will also be available for treatment.
7. Lying on the side	Sides of legs, lateral costal regions; bend the uppermost leg when selecting points in the area of GB-24 or GB-30 and straighten the uppermost leg when selecting points in the area of LV-13 or SP-21.
8. Supine with legs bent	Face, neck, cheek, abdomen, front and sides of lower limbs.
9. Prone	Head, neck, back, lower back, buttocks, back and sides of lower limbs

1.2.7 Needle insertion practice

The student should begin practicing the insertion techniques described herein on a tightly bound pad of paper, a ball of cotton cloth, or a tightly bound piece of sponge rubber. Beginning with a 1 inch-30 gauge needle, the student should gradually progress to longer and thinner needles. After she can easily insert thin needles into the practice material, the student then may begin to practice on her own legs and arms. Points such as LI-11, TB-5, ST-36, and GB-34 are good points for practice. The next step is to practice needle insertion on fellow students. Again, points on the limbs are the safest ones to begin with, followed by points on the body and head. This practice should be supervised by a qualified teacher.

1.3 Techniques for Needle Manipulation

1.3.1 Basic stimulation methods

After the proper depth of insertion has been reached, the point can be stimulated. Stimulation methods vary according to schools of thought, but most methods are variations of the following three.

a) *Lifting and thrusting:* After qi has been obtained, the needle is lifted a short distance (dependent on the depth of the flesh at the point) and then thrust back to the original depth. The direction of insertion should remain constant to avoid localized pain or post-needling pain. The usual distance covered by this motion is 0.3 to 0.5". Care should be taken to avoid raising the needle too far and thus withdrawing the needle or thrusting it too deeply and surpassing the recommended needling depth.

When employing this method strong, quick movements provide a draining stimulation, and slow, light ones are supplementing in nature.

b) *Twirling or rotating:* When the needle has been inserted to the proper depth and qi has been obtained, the practitioner grasps the handle of the needle between his thumb and forefinger and twists the needle first one way and then the other. The arc should not exceed one full turn, or 360°, in order to prevent the needle from adhering to fibrous tissue and causing unnecessary pain.

Rotating the needle rapidly in a wide arc is a draining stimulation, a lesser arc and slower motion provides a supplementing stimulus.

The rotation method can be combined with the lifting and thrusting method described above.

c) *Retaining the needle:* In modern practice needles are often left in place for a period of time ranging from several minutes to two hours depending on the particular condition. This allows for application of other stimulation methods such as warming the needle, electrical stimulation, or intermittent stimulation. Often the needles are retained with little or no additional manipulation.

Needle retention in general can increase the ability of a point to relieve pain and quiet the spirit. Some specific treatments require needle retention to achieve satisfactory results. For example, treatment of appendicitis or asthma generally involves the retention of needles for at least half an hour.

While the needles are in place the patient must be reminded not to move. Should he move slightly, the resulting pain can be relieved by withdrawing the needle to the level just beneath the skin, and then reinserting it to its proper depth.

Needle Manipulation (Cont.)				
Method	**Slow & Quick**	**Lifting & Thrusting**	**According to the Branches**	**Following the Breath**
Description	Refers to the speed of insertion and the speed of withdrawal	Refers to the strength of the lifting and thrusting motion after insertion	Refers to needling according to the hour of the day. Each channel has hours of exuberance and debilitation	Refers to insertion or withdrawal in accordance with the breath
Supplementing	Slow, deliberate insertion and rapid withdrawal (withdraw quickly to just below the surface of the skin, then withdraw completely)	Thrust forcefully and lift gently	Needle when the channel qi is debilitated (the period just following exuberance)	Insert during exhalation and withdraw during inhalation
Draining	Rapid insertion and slow withdrawal	Thrust gently and lift slowly	Needle when the channel is exuberant	Insert during inhalation and withdraw during exhalation
Application	These methods are suitable for harmonizing yin and yang, treating surplus and insufficiency, and treating hot or cold diseases.			

The above methods are not a subject of unanimous agreement. Through the ages different opinions have been proffered. We present them here as an introduction to the subject, realizing that each practitioner must develop his or her own preferences in these matters.

In addition, supplementation and draining can be achieved using mother and child points on the basis of five-phase theory. (See Part IV, the section on the five transporting-shu points, for a further description of this method.)

1.3.4 Combined methods of supplementation and drainage

While there are many methods that combine the above-mentioned techniques, herein we will discuss only the two that are most commonly employed. These methods, one supplementing and one draining, involve manipulating the needle between three depths known as heaven, earth, and human. Heaven is the level just below the skin; earth is the level of deepest insertion; and human is the intermediate level.

燒
山
火
法

a) *Burning mountain fire method:* To perform this technique, insert the needle into the heaven level and then thrust and lift nine times, thrusting forcefully and lifting gently. Then proceed to the human level and repeat this procedure. Finally, enter the earth level and once again repeat the lifting (gently) and thrusting (with force) motion nine times. When this has been done, lift the needle in one slow motion to the heaven level. If a warm, slightly burning sensation has not been achieved, the entire procedure may be repeated three times. If, at that time, the sensation still does not arrive, the practitioner should cease manipulation for a moment and then repeat the above procedure until the appropriate sensation occurs. When removing the needle the point should be covered.

This is a supplementing method that combines the supplementing aspects of the quick and slow, lifting and thrusting, 6 and 9, and opening and covering methods. Further supplementation can be achieved by inserting the needle while the patient exhales and withdrawing it during inhalation. The burning mountain fire method is named for the burning sensation it produces and is useful for supplementing qi of the channels and organs. It can be employed to treat vacuity cold diseases such as the three yin stages of cold damage disease, impotence, incontinence, vaginal protrusion, and swelling and sagging of one testicle.

Step 1:	Determine the depth to which the needle will be inserted. Divide this depth into three equal segments. From the surface of the skin, these depths are called the level of heaven, the level of human, and the level of earth.
Step 2:	Ask the patient to inhale deeply. Steps 2, 3, and 4 are performed during exhalation. Upon exhalation, thrust the needle quickly and lift slowly nine times to the level of heaven.
Step 3:	Thrust the needle quickly and lift slowly nine times in the level of human.
Step 4:	Thrust the needle quickly and lift slowly nine times in the level of earth.

Needle Contraindications	
Point	**Comment**
GV-24	This point is now commonly needled 0.2-0.3".
GV-17	Modern sources needle to 0.3".
BL-9	Currently needled 0.3".
BL-8	Currently needled 0.3-0.5".
GB-18	Currently needled 0.3-0.5".
TB-19	Currently needled 0.1".
TB-20	Currently needled 0.1".
ST-1	Currently needled 0.2-0.3"; it can create a black eye.
GV-11	Some modern sources say a 0.5-1.0 inch insertion is acceptable.
GV-10	See GV-11.
CV-17	Now needled to a depth of 0.3-0.5".
LI-13*	Sight of the radial collateral artery and vein.
HT-2	Currently needled 0.3-0.5".
CV-8*	This is the navel. The *Inner Canon* mentions that needling this point will cause the patient to have a festering navel ulcer, most likely because the navel is susceptible to infection.
KI-11	Currently needled 0.5-0.8".
ST-30	This is the site of a major artery; currently needled 0.3-0.5".
SP-11	Currently needled 0.3-0.5"; it is the site of a major vein and artery.
BL-56	Some modern sources needle this point 1.0-1.5".
CV-9	Currently needled 0.5-1.0". Should not be needled to treat water swelling (employ moxibustion).
CV-1	Currently needled 0.5-0.8".
ST-17*	This is the nipple.
TB-8	Some modern sources needle this point 0.5-1.0".
LV-12*	Site of femoral artery.

1.4 Other Materials & Techniques Related to Acupuncture

1.4.1 The three-edged needle — bloodletting

The three-edged needle (sometimes called the prismatic or ensiform needle) is a thick needle with a sharp, three-edged tip used for letting blood. The use of presterilized, disposable lancets has replaced the three-edged needle for bloodletting in many acupuncture clinics. This procedure employs the three-edged needle to puncture the skin and allow the escape of a few drops of blood. It is performed at the site of a point or at the small veins in the area surrounding a point (such as BL-40). The function of this method is to drain heat or quicken the blood and qi and relieve local congestion (and thus reduce stagnation and swelling).

This procedure is done by first applying pressure to restrict the blood flow of the area, to increase the visibility of the veins and to cause the blood to flow out more easily when the vein is pricked. The point is then swiftly and decisively pricked to a superficial depth of about 0.1 " and a few drops of blood are allowed to escape. Lastly, the point is pressed with sterile cotton until the bleeding ceases.

This method is inappropriate for weak, pregnant, or postpartum patients, hemorrhagic patients, and patients suffering from anemia or low blood pressure. The procedure should be thoroughly explained to the patient before it is performed to allay his or her fears. Furthermore, strict attention must be paid to sterile technique and careful cleaning of the puncture site before and after pricking.

The following chart (continued on the next page) outlines some diseases that respond to bloodletting. Asterisks indicate the situations where this procedure is most commonly employed.

Acupuncture Points Suitable for Bloodletting	
Disease	**Points for Bloodletting**
Wind Strike*	BL-40, LI-4, GB-21
Cholera	BL-40, LU-5, LI-11
Spasm of the Gastrocnemius	SP-1
Cough (with phlegm)	LI-11, LU-5
Headache	ST-8, GV-20
Stomach (Venter) Pain Abdominal pain	BL-38 LV-1
Ingesta damage	GV-20
Jaundice	SP-1, BL-20, BL-21
Spinal pain	BL-38

2. Moxibustion

Moxibustion is the most common method of thermal stimulation of acupuncture points. Dried and sifted leaf particles from the Chinese herb *ài yè* are burned on or above the skin, with the aim of freeing qi and blood, coursing qi, dispersing cold, eliminating damp and warming yang. Moxibustion is also valued for its ability to ward off disease.

Mugwort *(ài yè)* is chosen as the substance to be burnt because of its yang qualities and its use in Chinese herbology for the treatment of cold and damp diseases. In addition, it is of good consistency for forming into cones, burns well, and is a commonly found plant. The English term moxa derives from the Japanese name for this plant — mugusa.

Mugwort is harvested in early summer, after the leaves have developed their characteristic woolly underside. Leaves are dried and aged, and then crushed and sifted to separate the wool from the unwanted leaf and stem material. The amount of sifting and cleaning used in its manufacture (and, to a lesser extent, its age) determines the grade of the moxa. High-grade moxa is ivory to white in color, and is composed nearly entirely of leaf wool. It produces a gentler cauterization, and less smoke and odor when burned, and is thus the preferred moxa for application directly to the skin. High-grade moxa is also more easily shaped, and permits formation of the small, thread-like and sesame size moxa. Moxa that has been cleansed less rigorously, and thus contains higher concentrations of leaf particles, is considered lower grade. Gray or gray-green in color, low-grade (crude) moxa is preferred for indirect moxibustion, a process whereby burning moxa is used to heat, rather than cauterize, the skin. Such applications often require large quantities of moxa wool, while not necessitating the special advantages of the higher grade product.

Moxibustion is divided into two distinct methods; indirect moxibustion and direct moxibustion.

2.1 Direct Moxibustion

Direct moxibustion involves the burning of hand-rolled moxa cones directly on the skin at selected points. This method is again divided into two subcategories: scarring and non-scarring.

2.1.1 Scarring moxibustion

Scarring moxibustion employs a small cone of moxa wool (some less than 1 cm. in diameter) that is placed directly on the skin and completely burned. The area is then wiped clean with a damp cloth and the process is repeated until the prescribed number of cones have been burnt. When this has been done the area should be conscientiously cleaned and dressed.

After one to three days the patient will develop a blister that will eventually leave a small scar. The blister generally takes about a month to heal. During this time, the patient must keep the area clean and frequently change the dressing to prevent infection.

The scarring method is the most potent form of moxibustion. The ancients considered the formation of a blister important in the healing process and thus it is said, "if moxibustion does not form a blister, the disease will not be cured." This method is currently used in China to treat serious vacuity cold or cold-damp diseases.

When performing scarring moxibustion, note the following:

• The pre-burning of a cone or two not quite down to the skin is a gradual way to accustom the patient to the burning pain. These pre-burnt cones, however, should not be counted toward the prescribed number.

• When the moxa is burning, the practitioner can scratch or tap the area around the point to reduce the burning pain.

• The number of recommended cones should be adjusted to the patient's condition. Young and strong patients can withstand more burnings and larger cones than old and weak patients.

• The patient should have the procedure explained to him and be forewarned about the formation of a scar.

• Garlic juice or some other liquid usually is placed on the point being treated in order to secure the moxa cone.

Moxa cones are usually described as large, medium, or small. Large cones are about the size of a broad bean (and are used only in indirect moxibustion); medium cones are the size of a soybean; and small cones are the size of a wheat grain.

2.1.2 Non-scarring moxibustion

Non-scarring moxibustion is the same as the above except that the moxa cone is removed with tweezers when the patient feels pain. Cones are burned until the skin at the point turns red. Care must be taken to avoid accidental scarring when using this technique. This method is less potent than scarring moxibustion and therefore is used for milder vacuity cold patterns. Some sources state that extinguishing the cone by pressing it to the skin provides a supplementing stimulus, and that removing it with tweezers before extinguishing it is draining in nature.

2.3 Moxibustion Precautions and Contraindications

• Moxibustion should not be performed on persons who are hungry, have just overeaten, or are intoxicated.

• Most points that are forbidden to moxibustion are near large blood vessels, on the face, on prominent skin creases, or at or near mucus membranes or sensory organs. These sites are particularly forbidden to direct moxibustion.

• Pregnant women should not receive moxibustion on their abdomen or lower back.

• If small blisters form as a result of moxibustion, they should be protected and allowed to heal without treatment. Large blisters, however, should be punctured and drained, and if infection occurs, appropriate dressing should be applied.

Part II

An Introduction
to the
Channels & Points

Channels

3. The Channels

3.1 Introduction

The channels and connecting vessels are pathways that carry qi, blood, and fluids around the body. They are the communication lines among all parts of the organism. The *Canon of Perplexities* states, "The channels move blood and qi and ensure the free flow of yin and yang, so that the body is properly nourished." The organs, portals, surface skin and body hair, sinews and flesh, bones, and other tissues all rely on communication through the channels, forming an integrated, unified organism.

The channels are described in two main categories: major channels, having clearly defined pathways that penetrate deep into the body, and connecting vessels, which are their branches. *The Gateway to Medicine* states, "The major channels represent the main pathways, and their ramifications are the connecting vessels." There are two types of major channels: the twelve regular channels and the eight extraordinary vessels. Concerning the difference between the regular channels and the extraordinary channels, *The Savior General Compendium* states:

> There are regular channels and extraordinary vessels. The twelve [organ-related] channels are the regular channels. The eight extraordinary vessels are so named because they do not conform to the norm. Qi and blood constantly flow through the twelve regular channels and, when abundant, overflow into the extraordinary vessels.

The connecting vessels are described in four categories: the large ones, of which there are fifteen, are called the fifteen connecting vessels, and serve to connect yin and yang channels; the minute connecting vessels, which are smaller and more widely distributed; and two types of web-like vessels just beneath the skin called superficial connecting vessels and blood connecting vessels.

Twelve divergent channels enhance communication among the organs and the major channels, and among the channels themselves. Finally, twelve sinew channels and twelve cutaneous regions divide the body's musculature and integument into twelve distinct regions corresponding to the twelve regular channels.

Channel theory is of significance in physiology, pathology, pattern identification, and treatment. In physiology, the channels represent the principal pathways by which qi, blood, and the fluids are distributed around the body, providing nourishment and warmth. They also serve as vital links among the organs and other parts of the body. The *Spiritual Axis* explains:

> The channels are the routes by which blood and qi move, and yin and yang circulate, keeping the bones and sinews moistened and the joints lubricated.

3.1.1 Channel function

The blood and fluids are carried through the channels by qi, and in acupuncture the sensation produced when obtaining qi shows that the channel is "live," or has abundant qi. The channels are the transmission lines among the various parts of the body, making the organism a unified whole.

+ The channels respond to dysfunction

3.1.2 Channel pathology

In pathology, exogenous pathogens invade the body through the exterior and penetrate into the interior via the channels in turn, affecting the organs. *Essential Questions* states:

> A pathogen settling in the body must first abide in the surface skin and body hair. If it resists expulsion, it will enter the minute connecting vessels. If it continues to resist, it will enter the larger connecting vessels. If it persists, it will enter the major channels that communicate with the organs in the inner body. When the pathogen spreads to the stomach and intestines, yin and yang are both affected and all the organs suffer damage. This is the sequence by which pathogens penetrating the body through the surface skin and body hair eventually affect the five viscera.

Similarly, organ pathologies may spread to other parts of the body through the channels. A disorder in a given organ may be transmitted through the relevant channel, manifesting as morbidity in regions along the channel's course. An example of this is seen in upflaming of liver fire, which may be characterized not only by reddening of the eyes and pain in the center of the chest, but also by pain in the communicating channel (the hand jue yin pericardium channel) along the inner face of the arm. Disease in one organ can also spread to other organs through the channels. Examples include heart fire, which can pass to the small intestine, and water flood due to kidney vacuity, which intimidates the heart or shoots into the lung. Through channel transference, morbidity in the organs may also be reflected in areas of palpatory tenderness, swellings, indentations, nodules, and hyperemia. These signs are often helpful in diagnosis.

3.1.3 Flow of channel qi

The main significance of channel theory in pattern identification and treatment is found in a series of methods based on the laws governing the flow of channel qi, interorganic connections, pathologic characteristics of the channels, and channel interrelationships. The three most common uses are:

- Determination of channel relevance involves relating the channels to a disorder based on proximity.

- Pattern identification by channels involves analyzing symptoms based on the physiopathologic features of the channels.

• Acupuncture point and drug prescription by channels denotes a method of determining treatment through the physiopathologic features of the channels.

For example, the forehead, cheeks, teeth, lips, and throat are all located on the foot yang ming stomach channel and the hand yang ming large intestine channel. Therefore, disorders such as frontal headache, wind-fire toothache, and sore throat may be treated as yang ming channel disorders. In acumoxatherapy, they are treated by needling the points ST-6, ST-7, ST-36, or ST-44 on the foot yang ming stomach channel; and LI-4 and LI-11 on the hand yang ming large intestine channel.

The channel system is a representation of rivers, streams, reservoirs, and underground springs in the geography of the body. The Chinese names of the points often refer to this metaphor. Springs, streams, seas, pools, marshes, canals, and wells abound in the point names. The channels and their tributaries provide qi and blood and thus warmth and nourishment for the whole body and also serve as lines of communication among the organs and the body. They adjust to the ebb and flow of qi in the body and help maintain a balance of yin and yang, blood and qi, and defense and construction.

3.2 The Twelve Regular Channels

3.2.1 Distribution of the twelve regular channels

The twelve channels are bilaterally symmetrical. They are identified according to the limb along which they flow and according to yin and yang. The yin channels run along the inner surface of the limbs, and across the chest and abdomen. Each is also associated with a viscus. The yang channels run along the outer surfaces of the limbs and over the back and buttocks, and are each associated with a bowel. Yin and yang are each further divided into three subdivisions. In the normal standing position, the tai yin channels run along the anterior medial edge of the limbs; the shao yin channels run along the posterior medial edge, and the jue yin channels run along the midline of the limbs' inner surface. Similarly, the yang ming channels run along the anterior lateral edge of the limbs; the tai yang channels run along the posterior lateral edge of the limbs, and the shao yang channels run along the midline of their outer surface.

3.2.2 Channel direction

Specific laws govern the direction of the twelve regular channels. The three yin channels of the hands all start in the chest and run outward to the hands, where they join with their phase paired hand yang channel. The three yang channels of the hands all start from the hands and ascend to the head and face, where they each meet with the foot channel of the same yang subdivision. The three yang channels of the feet all start from the head and face and descend to the feet, linking with

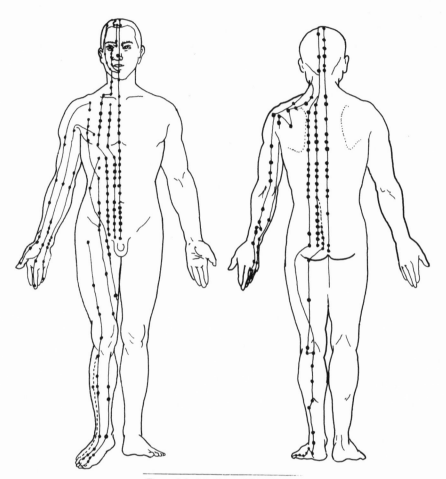

Figure 3.2, 3.3 Channel Distribution

3.2.3 Interior-exterior relationships of the twelve channels

There are two aspects to the interior-exterior relationships of the channels. First, each yang channel is joined to its corresponding yin channel, "interior" being yin and "exterior" being yang. Second, each channel "connects" with the organ that stands in interior-exterior relationship with the organ to which it belongs, or "homes."

The homing and connecting relationships between the channels and organs are as follows:

Channel Relationships		
Channel	**Homing Organ**	**Connecting Organ**
Hand Tai Yin	Lung	Large Intestine
Hand Yang Ming	Large Intestine	Lung
Hand Jue Yin	Pericardium	Triple Burner
Hand Shao Yang	Triple Burner	Pericardium
Hand Shao Yin	Heart	Small Intestine
Hand Tai Yang	Small Intestine	Heart
Foot Tai Yin	Spleen	Stomach
Foot Yang Ming	Stomach	Spleen
Foot Jue Yin	Liver	Gallbladder
Foot Shao Yang	Gallbladder	Liver
Foot Shao Yin	Kidney	Bladder
Foot Tai Yang	Bladder	Kidney

In this way, each channel links both a bowel (exterior) and a viscus (interior), and each yang channel is connected to a yin channel, forming a twofold link between the exterior and the interior.

Flow of Qi in the Channels	
Channel	**Time**
Lung	3:00 am to 5:00 am
Large Intestine	5:00 am to 7:00 am
Stomach	7:00 am to 9:00 am
Spleen	9:00 am to 11:00 am
Heart	11:00 am to 1:00 pm
Small Intestine	1:00 pm to 3:00 pm
Bladder	3:00 pm to 5:00 pm
Kidney	5:00 pm to 7:00 pm
Pericardium	7:00 pm to 9:00 pm
Triple Burner	9:00 pm to 11:00 pm
Gallbladder	11:00 pm to 1:00 am
Liver	1:00 am to 3:00 am

3.2.6 Channel pathways and pathologic signs

The pathways of the regular channels have both internal and external branches. The external aspects of the channels are delineated by the acupuncture points along their course. Their internal branches connect with the home organ (called homing) and with the related organ (called connecting). There are sometimes other internal branches that connect to parts of the body to which the organ pertains. For example, a branch of the large intestine channel descends to the lower leg, specifically ST-37, the lower uniting-he point of the large intestine; and a branch of the kidney channel connects to the root of the tongue, the kidney region in tongue diagnosis.

The internal pathways of the regular channels should not be confused with the channel divergences discussed later. Channel divergences all branch from the main channel on the limbs. After entering the chest and abdomen they either reconnect with the home channel or with the channel divergence of the yin-yang related organ. The internal pathways of the regular channels do not follow this pattern.

3.3 The Eight Extraordinary Vessels

The eight extraordinary vessels are the governing vessel, the conception vessel, the penetrating vessel, the girdling vessel, the yin linking vessel, the yang linking vessel, the yin motility vessel, and the yang motility vessel. They are thus named because they do not fit the pattern of the other major channels: they neither have a continuous, interlinking pattern of circulation, nor are they each associated with a specific major organ. Rather, they serve as reservoirs, filling and emptying in response to the varying conditions of the major channels and exerting a regulating effect on them; hence the designation "vessel."

With the exception of the governing and the conception vessels, the eight extraordinary vessels do not possess their own points, but share points on other channels. Each extraordinary vessel has a specific point (on the limbs) with which it is related. These points and points which are along the pathway of the extraordinary vessels can be used to treat disorders of these vessels. (See Parts II and IV on the confluence-jiaohui points of the eight extraordinary vessels.)

The functions of the eight extraordinary vessels are as follows:

• They provide additional interconnections among the twelve regular channels.

• They regulate the flow of qi and blood in the twelve regular channels. Surplus blood and qi is taken up from the twelve regular channels, and is released when qi and blood in the regular channels is vacuous.

• They are closely related to the liver and the kidney. "The eight extraordinary vessels serve the liver and the kidney."

• They are directly related to the womb, the brain, and other curious organs.

The pathways and associated symptoms of each of the extraordinary vessels are discussed in Part III following.

3.4 Connecting Vessels (LUO)

The connecting vessel system can be divided into two subsystems. The first is that of the fifteen connecting vessels that serve primarily to connect the yin-yang channel pairs, and the second consists of the series of small connecting vessels that help to distribute qi and blood over the entire body.

The fifteen connecting vessels consist of a vessel branching from each of the twelve regular channels, one each from the governing vessel and the conception vessel, and the great connecting vessel of the spleen. The function of the connecting vessels of the twelve regular channels is to connect the channels of the yin-yang organ pairs. The connecting vessel of the governing vessel distributes qi and blood over the back, that of the conception vessel distributes qi and blood over the chest and abdomen, and that of the great connecting vessel of the spleen distributes qi and blood over the trunk.

The fifteen connecting vessels differ from other branches of the fourteen channels. They are mentioned in the *Inner Canon* as having a set of symptoms associated with their disturbance. They are also unique in that each departs from its home channel at an acupuncture point. These points, termed the connecting-luo points, are used to treat diseases involving the yin-yang organ pairs or the disorders associated with the connecting vessel.

The symptoms associated with each connecting vessel are discussed in Part III, and the connecting-luo points are discussed in section 4.2.2 of this chapter.

The other connecting vessels can be pictured as small vessels supplying qi and blood to the tissues that lie between the pathways of the channels. These small vessels are called minute connecting vessels, superficial connecting vessels and blood connecting vessels. Minute connecting vessels are smaller branches than the fifteen connecting vessels. According to classical sources, which offer no further explanation, superficial vessels are observable near to the skin. Vessels termed blood connecting vessels have the appearance of small blood vessels. In practice, the blood connecting vessels are sometimes bled with the aim of moving stagnant qi and blood or clearing blood heat.

3.5 Channel Divergences

A channel divergence branches from each of the twelve regular channels and enters deeply into the body trunk. These are called "channels that diverge from the primary channels," or for convenience, "channel divergences."

The pathways of the channel divergences of the yin and yang channels differ. The divergences of all channels diverge from their home channel on the arms or legs and enter into the trunk of the body and connect with various organs. After that the yang channels (in general) rise to the neck region and re-connect with their home channels. The yin channel divergences, however, connect to the channel divergences of their paired yang bowel and do not rejoin their home channel.

Channel divergences and connecting vessels both serve to connect the yin-yang organ pairs but they differ in important ways. The channel divergences do not have a set of related symptoms whereas the connecting vessels do. The departure of the channel divergences from the home channel is not marked by a specific acupuncture point and the channel divergences traverse the interior of the body while the connecting vessels relate to the exterior of the body.

The importance of the channel divergences is primarily theoretical. Their pathways are used to explain the functions of various acupuncture points and the connection between various organs and parts of the body. For example, points on yin channels that affect the head are said to do so, in part, because the yin channel divergences all connect with yang channel divergences, which then rise to the head. Another example is that of the channel divergence of the bladder channel that diverges from the main channel at the back of the leg and proceeds upward to the anus and thus explains the function of several bladder points on the lower leg with regard to treating hemorrhoids, and other disorders of the anal region.

The pathways of each of the channel divergences are outlined in Part III, *Channels & Points*.

3.6 The Twelve Channel Sinews

The channel sinews are groups of muscles, tendons, and ligaments that follow the paths of the twelve channels. For this reason they are called channel sinews. These channel-like sinews are unique in a number of ways. They have no points associated with them; they do not connect to internal organs, and they all begin at the extremities of one of the four limbs.

The channel sinews generally follow the path of the channel with which they are associated. As they proceed up the four limbs they bind (i.e., link) to the joints, then disperse (spread out) over the chest or back and terminate at the head or on the trunk. Some of the channel sinews enter the chest and abdominal cavities where they disperse at locations specific to their pathway.

The functions of the channel sinews are similar to those ascribed in Western medicine to the musculature. The channel sinews bind the bones and move the joints. For this reason, the set of symptoms associated with them include muscle strains, cramps, spasms, and atrophy.

It can be seen that unlike the regular channels, the channel sinews are not responsible for transportation of qi and blood. They are channel-like sinews, not sinew-like channels.

The four sets of channel sinews grouped by yin and yang and hand and foot are said to unite at the four binding spots. These are as follows:

- The three foot yang channel sinews bind in the region of the cheek.
- The three foot yin channel sinews bind in the genital region.
- The three hand yang channel sinews bind at the corner of the forehead.
- The three hand yin channel sinews bind in the thoracic-abdominal region (near the venter)

The pathways and disorders associated with each channel sinew are listed in Part III, *The Channels & Points*.

3.7 The Twelve Cutaneous Regions

The body's surface is divided into twelve cutaneous regions. Each of these regions is the surface extension of an organ-channel system, served by superficial connecting vessels. Close relationships are observed between the cutaneous regions and their channel systems in pathology, diagnosis, and treatment.

Disease can enter the body through the cutaneous regions and then pass stage-by-stage through the connecting vessels and channels, to the bowels and viscera. Similarly, a disease that has penetrated the interior can be expelled through the exterior.

Discoloration of the skin can be a diagnostic indication of disease in the organ-channel system. Blue-green accompanies pain, a ''dull'' color indicates obstruction, yellow or red indicates heat, while a pale coloration indicates cold or vacuity. The illustration below shows the association of organ-channel systems and skin areas.

In therapy, interior diseases may be treated by applying acumoxatherapy to the associated cutaneous region, just as exterior diseases can be treated by applying acumoxatherapy to the associated organ-channel system.

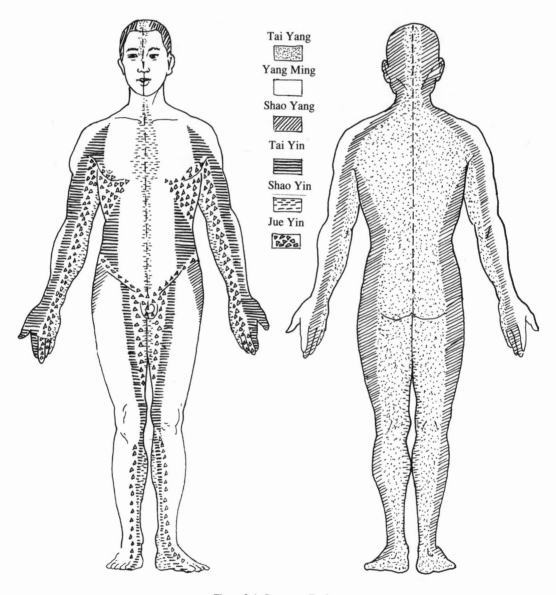

Tai Yang

Yang Ming

Shao Yang

Tai Yin

Shao Yin

Jue Yin

Figure 3.4: Cutaneous Regions

3.8 General Channel Distribution

The channel system covers the entire body. The physiological functions and pathologic changes of each part of the body have specific relationships to the channels and organs to which they are associated. Understanding which channels traverse which parts of the body is essential for diagnosis and treatment. Below is a section by section listing of the channel distribution including the theoretically important relationships among the channels and the body regions.

3.8.1 Channel distribution in the head & face

Vertex

- The bladder channel intersects the vertex.
- The governing vessel crosses the vertex.
- The liver channel meets the governing vessel at the vertex.
- The triple burner channel divergence branches to the vertex.
- The gallbladder channel sinews intersect the vertex.

Brain

- The governing vessel homes to the brain.
- The bladder channel connects with the brain.
- The stomach channel divergence passes through the eyes and enters the brain.

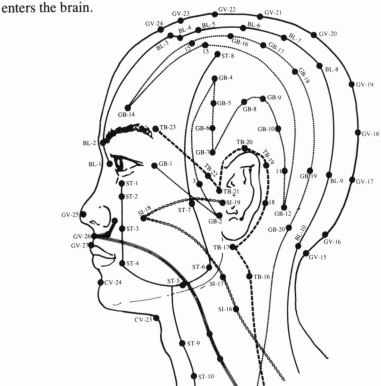

Teeth

- A branch of the large intestine connecting vessel spreads over the teeth.
- The stomach channel enters the upper teeth.
- The large intestine channel spreads through the lower teeth.

Tongue

- The triple burner channel sinews connect with the root of the tongue.
- The bladder channel sinews branch into and bind at the root of the tongue.
- The heart channel opens at the tongue.
- The spleen channel disperses over the inferior surface of the tongue.
- The kidney channel divergence connects to the root of the tongue.

Ear

- The bladder channel goes to the apex of the ear.
- The bladder channel sinews bind behind the ear.
- The gallbladder channel descends behind the ear, enters the ear and travels anterior to the ear.
- The stomach channel rises in front of the ear.
- The small intestine channel enters the ear.
- The triple burner channel goes behind the ear and issues out the apex of the ear. It also enters the ear and travels anterior to the ear.
- The large intestine connecting vessel enters into the ear.
- The gallbladder channel sinews follow behind the ear.
- The stomach channel sinews bind anterior to the ear.
- The small intestine channel sinews bind behind the ear and a branch enters the ear and issues at the apex.
- The pericardium channel divergence issues behind the ear and unites with the triple burner channel divergence.
- The connecting vessels of the kidney, heart, lung, spleen, and stomach all meet in the ear.

Occipital region

- The bladder channel traverses the occipital region.
- The governing vessel channel traverses the occipital region.
- The gallbladder channel traverses the occipital region.
- The bladder channel sinews bind at the occipital bone.
- The kidney channel sinews bind at the occipital bone.

3.8.2 Channel distribution in the neck & throat

Pharynx and upper esophageal opening

- The conception vessel goes to the pharynx and throat.
- The governing vessel enters the throat.
- The penetrating vessel and conception vessel meet at the esophagus.
- The small intestine channel follows the esophagus.
- The heart channel runs up the throat.
- The gallbladder channel divergence runs along both sides of the pharynx.
- The stomach channel divergence follows the esophagus upward.
- The spleen channel divergence unites with the stomach channel divergence at the esophagus.
- The stomach and large intestine channels line the throat.
- The bladder channel connects to the upper esophageal opening.

Trachea

- The stomach and gallbladder channels follow the throat.
- The liver channel follows in back of the throat.
- The heart channel divergence travels along the throat.
- The pericardium channel follows the throat.
- The large intestine channel divergence travels up along the throat.
- The lung channel travels from the trachea to the axilla.

Epiglottal region

- The liver channel enters this area and the penetrating vessel issues from this area.

Larynx

- The kidney channel connects with the root of the tongue and terminates at the larynx.
- The conception vessel connects here.

Nape of neck

- The bladder, governing vessel, small intestine, and gallbladder channels traverse this area.
- The bladder channel divergence issues at the nape of the neck.
- The gallbladder channel divergence issues at the nape of the neck.

- The kidney channel sinews rise along the side of the spine past the nape of the neck, binding at the occipital bone.
- The small intestine and large intestine channel sinews both rise to the back of the neck.

3.8.3 Channel distribution in the shoulder & scapula

- The bladder channel follows the musculature at the scapula region and branches to the scapula.
- The gallbladder channel goes to the shoulder.
- The small intestine channel surrounds the scapula and intersects the shoulder.
- The large intestine channel traverses the shoulder.
- The triple burner channel traverses the upper arm and shoulder.
- The small intestine connecting vessel connects to the top of the shoulder.
- The large intestine connecting vessel connects to the shoulder.
- The bladder channel sinews have a branch that binds at the shoulder.
- The large intestine channel sinews bind at the shoulder and wrap the scapula.
- The lung channel sinews bind at the front of the shoulder.

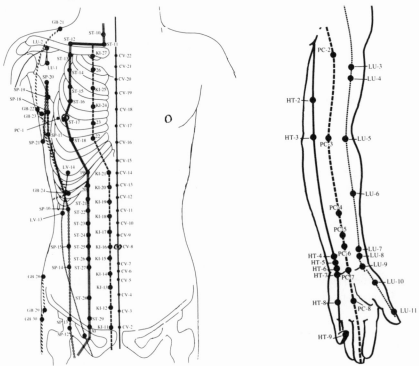

3.8.4 Channel distribution in the trunk

The chest

- The heart channel sinews bind in the chest.
- The lung channel sinews bind in the chest.
- The pericardium channel sinews enter the axilla and disperse in the chest.
- The pericardium channel starts in the chest.
- The pericardium channel divergence enters the chest.
- The triple burner connecting vessel flows into the chest.
- The penetrating channel disperses into the chest.
- The motility vessels rise through the interior of the chest.

Region of CV-17 (center of the chest)

- The triple burner spreads over this region.
- The liver connects at the center of the chest.
- The conception vessel traverses the center of the chest.

Lung

- The lung channel homes to the lung.
- The large intestine channel connects to the lung.
- The heart channel rises to the lung.
- The kidney channel enters the lung.
- The liver channel flows into the lung.

Heart

- The heart channel begins at the heart and homes to the heart.
- The heart connecting vessel enters the heart.
- The small intestine channel connects to the heart.
- The spleen channel flows into the heart.
- The kidney channel connects to the heart.
- The bladder channel divergence disperses over the heart.
- The gallbladder channel divergence binds with the heart.
- The stomach channel divergence penetrates the heart.
- The triple burner connecting vessel connects to the heart.
- The governing vessel links to the heart.

Pericardium

- The pericardium channel homes to the pericardium.
- The triple burner channel connects to the pericardium.
- The kidney connecting vessel travels to below the pericardium.

The breast

- The stomach channel goes through the breast.
- The large intestine channel divergence follows the breast.
- The gallbladder channel sinews connect to the breast.
- The heart channel sinews intersect with the lung channel sinews at the breast.
- The great connecting vessel of the stomach issues from below the left breast.

Spine

- The bladder channel ''pinches'' the spine.
- The kidney channel connects to the spine.
- The stomach channel sinews follow the ribs and home to the spine.
- The bladder channel sinews connect to the spine.
- The kidney channel sinews parallel the spine.
- The large intestine channel sinews ''pinch'' the spine.
- The governing vessel travels through the spine.

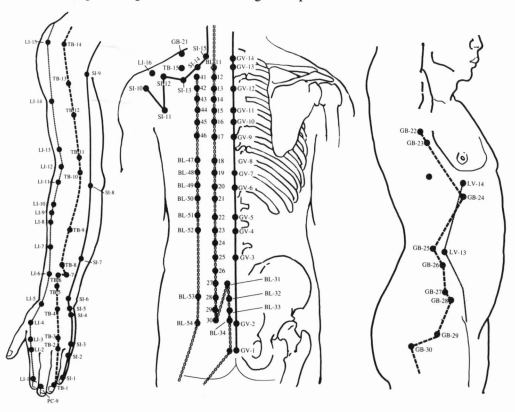

Axilla

- The gallbladder, lung, heart, and pericardium channels pass through the axilla.
- The small intestine channel divergence enters the axilla and travels to the heart.
- The heart channel divergence enters at the axilla.
- The pericardium channel divergence enters at the axilla.
- The lung channel divergence enters the axilla and travels to the lung.
- The bladder channel sinews enter below the axilla.
- The gallbladder channel sinews travel in front of the axilla.
- The small intestine channel sinews enter and bind below the axilla.
- The great connecting vessel of the spleen issues 3″ below the axilla.

Ribs and lateral costal region

- The gallbladder channel follows inside the lateral costal region and traverses the region of the free ribs.
- The pericardium channel issues from the flank.
- The liver channel spreads over the lateral costal region.
- The stomach channel sinews follow the ribs.
- The lung channel sinews go down to the free ribs.
- The pericardium channel sinews disperse out and down over the lateral costal region.
- The spleen channel sinews bind at the lateral costal region.
- The great connecting vessel of the spleen spreads over the chest and lateral costal region.

Liver

- The liver channel homes to the liver.
- The gallbladder channel connects to the liver.
- The gallbladder channel divergence disperses over the liver.

Gallbladder

- The gallbladder channel homes to the gallbladder.
- The liver channel connects to the gallbladder.

Lower back

- The bladder channel traverses the lower back.
- The gallbladder connecting vessel links to the lumbar spine.
- The governing vessel traverses the lower back.

Kidney

- The kidney channel homes to the kidney.
- The bladder channel connects to the kidney.
- The kidney channel divergence goes to the kidney.
- The penetrating vessel begins below the kidney.

Buttocks

- The bladder channel penetrates the buttocks.
- The bladder channel sinews bind at the buttocks.
- The governing vessel diverts into the gluteal region.

Sacrococcyx

- The gallbladder channel sinews bind at the sacrococcyx.
- The bladder channel divergence rises to 5 body inches below the sacrococcyx and enters at the anus.

3.8.5 Channel distribution in the abdominal region

Abdomen

- The stomach channel divergence enters at the abdomen.
- The stomach channel sinews rise through the abdomen.
- The spleen channel enters the abdomen.
- The liver channel goes to the lower abdomen.
- The conception vessel follows the interior of the abdomen.
- The connecting vessel of the conception vessel disperses over the abdomen.
- The kidney, spleen, stomach, and large intestine channels, and the conception vessel traverse the abdomen.

Umbilicus

- The stomach channel "pinches" the umbilicus.
- The spleen channel sinews bind at the umbilicus.
- The heart channel sinews connect to the umbilicus.
- The penetrating vessel "pinches" the umbilicus.
- The governing vessel links to the umbilicus.

Spleen

- The spleen channel homes to the spleen.
- The stomach channel connects to the spleen.

Stomach

- The stomach channel homes to the stomach.
- The spleen channel connects to the stomach.
- The small intestine channel goes to the stomach.
- The liver channel "pinches" the stomach.
- The lung channel follows the upper opening of the stomach.

Intestines

- The large intestine channel homes to the large intestine.
- The lung channel connects to the large intestine.
- The spleen connecting vessel connects with the intestines and stomach.
- The small intestine channel homes to the small intestine.
- The heart channel connects to the small intestine.

Bladder

- The bladder channel homes to the bladder.
- The kidney channel connects to the bladder.
- The triple burner lower uniting-he point is connected to the bladder.

Triple burner

- The triple burner channel homes to the triple burner.
- The pericardium channel connects to the triple burner.
- The lung channel originates in the central burner.

Genital region

- The liver channel passes through the genital region.
- The stomach channel sinews gather at the genital region.
- The spleen channel sinews gather at the genital region.
- The kidney channel sinews gather at the genital region.
- The liver channel sinews gather at the genital region.
- The liver connecting vessel rises to the testicles and binds at the penis. (No mention is made of the female genitals but we can assume a similar pathway.)
- The conception vessel originates above the border of the pubic hair.
- The governing vessel originates in the pelvic cavity (below the lower abdomen) and passes down through the genitals.
- The yin motility vessel enters the genitals.
- The genitals are the sinew gathering.
- The penetrating vessel sinews and the stomach channel sinews unite at the sinew gathering.

3.8.5 Channel distribution in the lower limbs

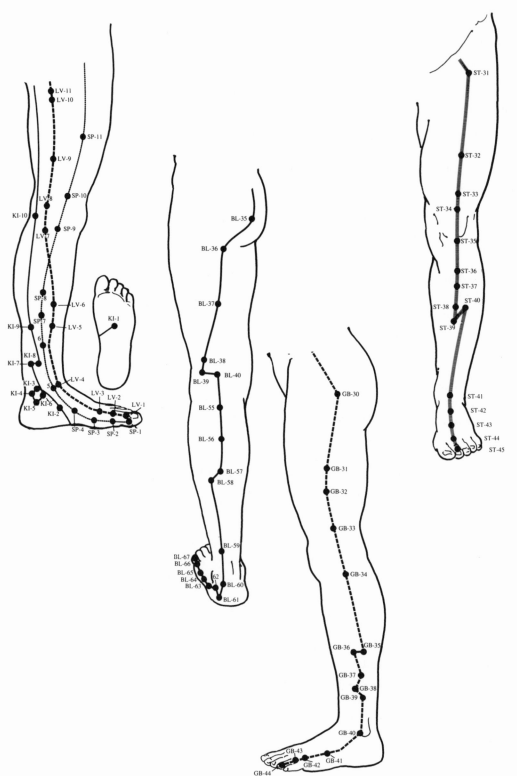

Points

4. The Points

4.1 Point Functions and Indications

Acupuncture points derive their functions from their location, from the channel they belong to, from any special groupings they are part of, and from the clinical observations of generations of practitioners. This section will discuss the various factors that contribute to the functions of acupuncture points.

4.1.1 Relationship of location to point indications and functions

Treatment of disorders by local points. Because stimulation of an acupuncture point moves the qi and blood of the immediate area, each point can treat disorders in its locale. For example, points in the area of the ear can treat ear diseases, those near the eyes can treat eye diseases, and points in the area of a painful joint can treat that joint. This property extends to the internal organs as well. CV-12, which is located near the stomach, can treat stomach diseases. CV-2 treats bladder dysfunction, and BL-23 treats kidney disorders, because of the proximity of these points to particular internal organs.

Regional domain. Some points, because of their prominent location, have the ability to treat an entire region of the body. For example, CV-17 (located in the center of the chest) treats the chest region, and ST-25 (located near the navel) can treat diseases of the stomach and intestines. *Yìn táng* (M-HN-3) treats diseases of the forehead and nose.

Sometimes regional domain is associated with the internal pathway of the channels or the channel divergences. The control over the venter and chest of PC-6 and the ability of BL-57 to treat diseases of the rectal area are examples of this.

4.1.2 Relationship of the channels to point indications and functions

The charts below outline the disease locations and types associated with the fourteen channels.

Channel Indications

Three Yang Channels of the Foot

Channels	Indications		
Foot Yang Ming Stomach	Front of head, mouth, teeth, throat, stomach, and intestines		Spirit-disposition disorders Febrile diseases
Foot Shao Yang Gallbladder	Lateral portion of head, ear, lateral costal region	Eyes	
Foot Tai Yang Bladder	Back of head, back, lower back (associated shu points treat the organs)		

Channel Indications

Three Yin Channels of the Hand

Channels	Indications		
Hand Tai Yin Lung	Lung and throat		Chest Region Disorders
Hand Jue Yin Pericardium	Heart and stomach disorders	Spirit-disposition disorders	
Hand Shao Yin Heart	Heart disorders		

Channel Indications

Three Yang Channels of the Hand

Channels	Indications		
Hand Yang Ming Large Intestine	Front of head, mouth, neck, teeth, nose		Eye, throat, febrile disorders
Hand Shao Yang Triple Burner	Lateral portion of head, lateral costal region	Ear Disorders	
Hand Tai Yang Small Intestine	Back of head, shoulder and scapula, spirit-disposition disorders		

Channel Indications		
Three Yin Channels of the Foot		
Channels	**Indications**	
Foot Tai Yin Spleen	Spleen and stomach and intestines	Genitourinary disorders, menstrual disorders, vaginal discharge, spirit-disposition disorders (especially when combined with the pericardium channel)
Foot Jue Yin Liver	Liver and genitals	
Foot Shao Yin Kidney	Kidney, lung, and throat	

The points on a given channel also affect the organ that is related to that channel. The location of each point, its internal connections, and the special group or groups to which it belongs determine the effect a point has on the internal organs. This explains why points along the same channel can have markedly different functions.

4.1.3 Relationship of the special point groupings to point indications and functions

As a way of dealing with the many points on the body, acupuncturists have, through the centuries, developed point groupings (e.g., ghost points, command points). Points that share certain features have been sorted into groups, thus facilitating memorization and providing the basis for the formation of various systems of treatment. These special point groupings are discussed in the section of that name. (See 4.2 below.) When discussing the function of a point it is necessary to consider the special point groupings to which the point belongs.

4.1.4 Indications and functions gleaned from clinical experience

Many acupuncture points are currently used to treat certain diseases on the basis of the clinical experience of preceding generations of acupuncturists. Most of these "empirical points" are drawn from verses that were the didactic devices of earlier times. For example, according to the *Ode to Elucidate Mysteries*, ST-25 treats incessant dysentery and splenic diarrhea; later books give this point the function of coursing and regulating the large intestines, and supporting earth and transforming damp.

When selecting points for treatment, the factors above must be taken into consideration. The functions mentioned in the Points section of this text were derived by consolidating information about each point in regard to the four factors mentioned above.

4.1.5 A note about modern point functions

Older acupuncture texts generally limited discussion of the clinical application of points to lists of the symptoms treated. Not until the 1950's, when efforts to modernize and standardize the theories of Chinese medicine became social and political imperatives in China, did it become popular to assign functions to the points.

Again, the functions of an acupuncture point were derived from anatomical location, channel location, and the specialized functions of its classical point groupings. To these point characteristics was added the clinical observations of generations of practitioners. Symptomology was also simplified during this time and Western medical terminology was widely substituted for classical descriptions. The chart below compares the symptom list of indications from PC-8 from a sixteenth century acupuncture book, *The Glorious Anthology of Acupuncture,* and that from a modern post-1950's textbook.

Ancient and Contemporary Uses of PC-8	
16th Century	**Current**
Wind strike (stroke), mania and withdrawal, irascibility, happiness, grief and/or laughter without stop, hand bi, heat illnesses that persist several days without perspiration, rib pain that prevents the patient from turning his body, fright, blood in urine or stool, unceasing nosebleed, counterflow qi retching with agitation thirst, inability to eat, fish odor emanating from mouth, mouth sores, fullness in chest and lateral costal region, jaundice (with yellow eyes), infantile gum erosion.	Manic depressive psychosis, cardiac pain, mania and withdrawal, epilepsy, mouth sores, halitosis.

The point functions generally assigned to PC-8 are as follows: clears heart fire, eliminates damp-heat, extinguishes wind, cools blood, quiets the spirit and harmonizes the stomach. When studied with the list of symptoms from which they were derived, the point functions can be useful, but if taken out of context, they are then separated from the hundreds of years of clinical experience that preceded their invention. The functions can then be misleading and even harmful. Knowing that PC-8 eliminates damp-heat is useful information only when combined with the fact that this point treats jaundice or blood in the urine and stool. If a patient has damp-heat but does not present with these particular signs, then PC-8 would not be an appropriate point for stimulation. For this reason, the present text includes enough symptoms from older sources to make the point functions useful.

Point functions are useful guides to point indications and point selection. To aid the student in gaining familiarity with point functions, they are defined in the Glossary.

4.2 Special Point Groupings

Many acupuncture points belong to one or more special groupings, each of which is distinguished by particular treatment actions and special relationships with the channels and connecting vessels. The most commonly employed groupings are the source-yuan points, the connecting-luo points, the associated-shu points, the alarm-mu points, the cleft-xi points, the eight meeting-hui points, and the lower uniting-he points. Thorough knowledge of the functions and usages of special point groupings is essential for appropriate point selection in acumoxatherapy. The special characteristics of frequently encountered groupings are discussed below. See Part IV, *Approaches to Point Selection*, for a discussion of the applications of these point groupings.

4.2.1 Source-yuan points 原穴

As the name implies, source-yuan points are points on each of the twelve regular channels where the source qi resides. The source-yuan points of the six yin channels are the same as the stream-shu points. On the yang channels, the source-yuan point is the point just proximal to the stream-shu point. Source-yuan points are mentioned in the *Inner Canon* as being effective for the treatment of diseases in the five viscera.[1] It also states that the twelve source-yuan points can be palpated to identify repletion or vacuity of source qi in the organ related to the particular channel to which the palpated point belongs.

The source-yuan points are said to be responsible for regulation of source qi and are thus intimately connected to the triple burner, which has the function of moving qi from its source (i.e., from CV-6, "Sea of Qi" to the rest of the body) [q.v. *The Classic of Difficult Issues*]. Because the source-yuan points regulate source qi, they can be used to treat diseases in the viscera and bowels. For example, disease in the liver can be treated by needling the source point of the liver, LV-3, and disease in the lung can be treated by needling LU-9, the source point of the lung.

The Twelve Source-Yuan Points											
Channel	LU	LI	ST	SP	HT	SI	BL	KI	PC	TB	GB	LV
Point	LU-9	LI-4	ST-42	SP-3	HT-7	SI-4	BL-64	KI-3	PC-7	TB-4	GB-40	LV-3

4.2.2 Connecting-luo points 絡穴

The place where the connecting vessel splits from the main channel is termed the connecting-luo point. For example, the connecting vessel of the hand jue yin pericardium channel splits from the pericardium channel at PC-6, the connecting-luo point of the pericardium channel. Each channel that possesses its own points has a connecting-luo point; thus each of the twelve regular channels and the conception and governing vessels has connecting-luo points. Two connecting vessels are associated with the spleen: the spleen connecting vessel, and the great connecting vessel of the spleen. Each of these has a connecting-luo point. In total there are fifteen connecting-luo points.[2]

The Connecting-luo Points														
Channel	LU	LI	ST	SP	HT	SI	BL	KI	PC	TB	GB	LV	CV	GV	GSP
Points	LU-7	LI-6	ST-40	SP-4	HT-5	SI-7	BL-58	KI-4	PC-6	TB-5	GB-37	LV-5	CV-15	GV-1	SP-21

4.2.3 Cleft-xi points 郄穴

The character 郄 has the meaning of cleft or fissure. A small cleft or indentation can be felt at the location of these points. As qi and blood circulate through the channels they accumulate in the cleft points, and for this reason they can reflect repletion or vacuity in the channel on which they are located. Sharp or intense pain on pressure, or redness and swelling, indicates repletion, and dull or mild pain or a depression indicates vacuity.

Each of the twelve regular channels has a cleft-xi point. In addition, these points are found on four of the extraordinary vessels: the yin motility, yang motility, yin linking, and yang linking vessels.

The Cleft-xi Points							
Channel	LU	LI	ST	SP	HT	SI	BL	KI
Points	LU-6	LI-7	ST-34	SP-8	HT-6	SI-6	BL-63	KI-5
Channel	PC	TB	GB	LV	Yang Motility	Yin Motility	Yang Linking	Yin Linking
Points	PC-4	TB-7	GB-36	LV-6	BL-59	KI-8	GB-35	KI-9

4.2.4 Eight meeting-hui points   八會穴

Through centuries of clinical observation the ancient Chinese determined that the eight meeting-hui points have a particular effect on the aspect for which they are named.[3] CV-12, for example, is effective for treating diseases in any of the six bowels, and GB-34 is efficacious for the treatment of diseases that affect the sinews. These points are employed to treat a general category of disease and are combined with others to address specific needs of the patient. For example, BL-17, the meeting-hui point of the blood, can be combined with SP-1 and LV-1 to treat metrorrhagia, and GB-34, the meeting point of the sinews, can be coupled with local points in the treatment of sprains and strains in any part of the body.

The Eight Meeting-hui Points								
Point	LV-13	CV-12	CV-17	BL-17	GB-34	GB-39	BL-11	LU-9
Realm of Treatment	viscera	bowels	qi	blood	sinews	marrow	bones	vessels

4.2.5 Lower uniting-he points   下合穴

The three yang channels of the hand (TB, SI, and LI) intersect with the three yang channels of the foot (GB, BL, and ST) in the upper body. There are three uniting-he points representing the three leg yang channels, and three uniting-he points representing the three arm yang channels. These six points are collectively known as the lower uniting-he points.

The Lower Uniting-he Points					
Stomach	Large Intestine	Small Intestine	Gallbladder	Bladder	Triple Burner
ST-36	ST-37	ST-39	GB-34	BL-40	BL-39

The *Classic of Difficult Issues* explains that the lower uniting-he points for the small and large intestines are located on the stomach channel because these two bowels ''belong'' to the stomach. Furthermore, it implies that the lower uniting point of the triple burner is located on the bladder channel because both these bowels are involved in the movement and transformation of water.

4.2.6 Confluence-jiaohui points of the eight extraordinary vessels 八脈交會穴

The confluence-jiaohui points are located on the four limbs and each is linked, via its home channel, with one of the eight extraordinary vessels. Confluence-jiaohui points are used to treat diseases associated with the extraordinary vessels. The symptomatology of each of these eight vessels is described in Part III, and the clinical applications of the confluence-jiaohui points are discussed in Part IV.[4]

The Confluence-jiaohui Points							
Yin Linking	Penetrating	Yang Linking	Girdling	Conception	Yin Motility	Governing	Yang Motility
PC-6	SP-4	TB-5	GB-41	LU-7	KI-6	SI-3	BL-62

4.2.7 The four command points 四總穴

The command points "command" certain parts of the body and are used to treat ailments that affect those particular sections. For example, LI-4 is the command point of the face and mouth and is useful for treating such disorders as toothache, swollen cheeks, nosebleed and headache. Although these points are first mentioned as a group in a book from the fourteenth century, the basis for choosing them dates from the *Inner Canon*. The *Spiritual Axis* section of that classic states:

> The hand tai yin [lung] and yang ming [large intestine] govern the upper body, and the foot tai yin [spleen] and yang ming [stomach] govern the lower body.
>
> [If there is] pain in the lower back, choose the back of the knee.

The four command points meet these criteria and are employed as outlined in the chart below.

The Four Command Points	
ST-36	Abdomen
BL-40	Back (upper and lower)
LU-7	Head and Back of Neck
LI-4	Face and Mouth

4.2.8 The alarm-mu points 募穴

The Chinese word *mù* actually implies a gathering or collection, because alarm points are spots on the chest and abdomen where the channel qi collects. These points are called "alarm points" in English after their function as diagnostic tools. These points could be called collection points instead of alarm points.[5] They may be palpated for tenderness, lumps, gatherings, depressions, or other aberrant signs. Any abnormal findings indicate that the organ related to the point in question may be suffering from a pathological condition. The alarm points are located directly above (anterior to) or near the organ to which they are related. The alarm point of the stomach, for example, is on the conception vessel, just lateral to the stomach. Clinically, these points are often employed to treat disorders of the six bowels.

The Alarm-mu Points											
LU	LI	ST	SP	HT	SI	BL	KI	PC	TB	GB	LV
LU-1	ST-25	CV-12	LV-13	CV-14	CV-4	CV-3	GB-25	CV-17	CV-5	GB-24	LV-14

4.2.9 Associated-shu points 俞穴

These points are located on the bladder channel 1.5″ lateral to the spine. They are unique in that they are all named for the organ whose qi is said to pass through their locations. The associated-shu point of the heart (BL-15), for example, is named the ''Heart-Shu,'' and the associated-shu point of the lung (BL-13) is called ''Lung-Shu.''

The associated-shu points are used to diagnose and to treat the organ with which they are associated. If the flow of qi in a particular organ is hindered, the qi then collects at the associated-shu point and tenderness or some other abnormality is revealed upon palpation. The *Classic of Difficult Issues* states that yin diseases move to the yang (i.e., the back). Thus the associated-shu points are primarily used to treat diseases of the five viscera (yin) and the tissues and sense organs to which they relate.

The Associated-shu Points											
LU	LI	ST	SP	HT	SI	BL	KI	PC	TB	GB	LV
BL-13	BL-25	BL-21	BL-20	BL-15	BL-27	BL-28	BL-23	BL-14	BL-22	BL-19	BL-18

4.2.10 The five transporting-shu points 五輸穴

Located below the elbows and knees on the pathways of each of the twelve regular channels is a series of five points that are known as the five transporting-shu points. The ancient Chinese likened the flow of qi in the channels to the flow of water from its source in the mountains to its home in the sea. In accordance with this, they named the transporting points at the ends of the fingers and toes well-jing points to represent the shallow and meek nature of qi there. The subsequently more proximal points were named as spring-ying, stream-shu and river-jing points to indicate the gradual change in the nature of qi at the different locations along the extremities. The last of the five transporting-shu points is designated as the uniting-he point in reference to the nature of qi at that point as it enters deeply and unites with its home organ, thus resembling a river as it joins the sea.

Qi at the well points is shallow and small as is the flesh at the base of the fingernails and toenails where most of these points are located. Qi further up the hand or foot, where the spring-ying point is located, is described as slightly larger, like a small spring. At the wrists and ankles qi is described as being like water pouring downward from a shallow place to a deeper one, and the stream-shu points are named for the nature of qi there. Qi that travels along the forearm or calf is free flowing like the water in a river, thus the river-jing points are located in this area. The regions just below the elbows and the knees, where the uniting-he points are located, are fleshy and deep. Qi is said to flow large and deep here as it unites with the organ of the home channel.

There are several aspects involved in proper employment of the five transporting-shu points. For further discussion, see Part IV, *Approaches to Point Selection and Combination.*

Five Transporting Points — Yin Channels (With the Source-Yuan Points)						
	Points / Phase					
Channel	**Well-jing** **Wood**	**Spring-ying** **Fire**	**Stream-shu** **Earth**	**Source-yuan** **Earth**	**River-jing** **Metal**	**Uniting-he** **Water**
Lung	LU-11	LU-10	LU-9	LU-9	LU-8	LU-5
Pericardium	PC-9	PC-8	PC-7	PC-7	PC-5	PC-3
Heart	HT-9	HT-8	HT-7	HT-7	HT-4	HT-3
Spleen	SP-1	SP-2	SP-3	SP-3	SP-5	SP-9
Liver	LV-1	LV-2	LV-3	LV-3	LV-4	LV-8
Kidney	KI-1	KI-2	KI-3	KI-3	KI-7	KI-10

Five Transporting Points — Yang Channels (With the Source-Yuan Points)						
	Points / Phase					
Channel	**Well-jing** **Metal**	**Spring-ying** **Water**	**Stream-shu** **Wood**	**Source-yuan**	**River-jing** **Fire**	**Uniting-he** **Earth**
Large Intestine	LI-1	LI-2	LI-3	LI-4	LI-5	LI-11
Triple Burner	TB-1	TB-2	TB-3	TB-4	TB-6	TB-10
Small Intestine	SI-1	SI-2	SI-3	SI-4	SI-5	SI-8
Stomach	ST-45	ST-44	ST-43	ST-42	ST-41	ST-36
Gallbladder	GB-44	GB-43	GB-41	GB-40	GB-38	GB-34
Bladder	BL-67	BL-66	BL-65	BL-64	BL-60	BL-40

4.2.11 The intersection-jiaohui points   交會穴

Intersection-jiaohui points [6] are those points on the body where two or more channels intersect.

4.2.12 Hua Tuo's paravertebral *(jiá jí)* points   華佗夾脊穴

These points are named after the famous physician of the third century, Hua Tuo. They are situated along both sides of the spine about 0.5″ lateral to the lower end of the spinous process of each vertebra. Their functions are similar to the functions of the governing vessel and associated-shu points between which they are located.

Hua Tuo Paravertebral Points

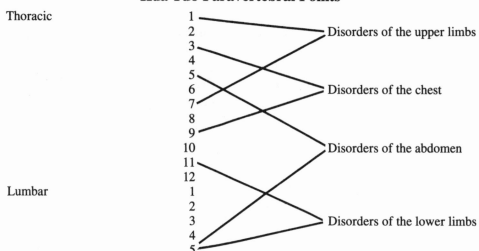

4.2.13 Additional Point Groupings

Acumoxatherapy literature contains many other point groupings that, though they are not as significant as the groupings mentioned above, should be familiar to the student.

回
陽
九
針

The Nine Needles for Returning Yang: This grouping first appeared in an acumoxatherapy "song" in the 16th century. This song lists the following nine points to be used to return yang when yang collapse is present or imminent. Yang collapse is analogous to what Western medicine terms shock, and is characterized by inversion cold in the extremities, aversion to cold, cyan lips, somber white facial color, and a faint pulse verging on expiry. The nine needles for returning yang are GV-15, PC-8, SP-6, KI-1, KI-3, CV-12, GB-30, ST-36, and LI-4.

馬
丹
陽
天
星
穴

Ma Dan-Yang's Twelve Heavenly Star Points: These points are based on the clinical experience of Ma Dan-Yang, a Song Dynasty physician who passed the information on to his students. The points appeared later written in song form. The twelve points are those that he considered the most useful. Ma Dan-Yang's twelve heavenly star points are ST-36, ST-44, LI-11, LI-4, BL-40, BL-57, LV-3, BL-60, GB-30, GB-34, HT-5, and LU-7.

十
三
鬼
穴

The Thirteen Ghost Points: These points originated from the Tang dynasty physician Sun Si Miao's method for treating what we now consider to be severe psychiatric disorders and epileptic conditions. The thirteen ghost points are GV-26, LU-11, SP-1, PC-7, BL-62, GV-16, ST-6, CV-24, PC-8, GV-23, LI-11, CV-1, and M-HN-37.

A-Shi Points: Points that are particularly sensitive to palpation are termed a-shi (literally, "that's it!") points because of the patient's response when the points are pressed. These points are most often used to treat disorders in their immediate vicinity but can treat disorders distant from the point as well. A-shi points are not necessarily on the channels. Because their locations vary and are a reflection of the disease and its relationship to the patient, these points are inherently unchartable.

4.3 Locating Acupuncture Points

Acupuncture points are generally found in depressions in muscles, bones or joints and are often sensitive to pressure. To facilitate location, a system using body landmarks and a relative unit of measurement called a body inch was developed in ancient China and has remained in use. Recent texts have attempted to improve on this method by employing modern Western anatomical terminology in the description of point locations. In order to provide a clear picture of the point locations, included in the points section of this book are locations derived from both modern and ancient texts.

The chart on the following page shows the proportional measurement system used in Part III. It can be seen from this chart that body inches vary in size according to the section of the body that is being measured. For example, the distance between the two nipples is eight body inches and the distance between the two corners of the hairline is nine body inches. It is clear from this that the body inches used for horizontal measure of the forehead are considerably smaller than those used for the horizontal measure of the chest.

The practitioner can use his or her hand to measure body inches. The middle phalangeal bone of the middle finger is considered to be one body inch. The breadth of index and middle finger is 1.5", and the breadth of the four fingers is figured as 3" (see diagram below). The relative size of the fingers of the practitioner and patient must be compensated for when employing this method of measurement.

In truth, the location of acupuncture points requires a sensitivity that is acquired only by practice. In this respect, acupuncture is an art as well as a science.

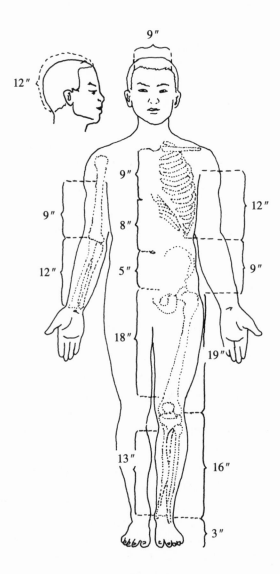

Figure 4.1

Part of Body	Distance	Equal Divis.	Stand. Measure	Remarks
Head	Anterior to posterior hair-line	12″	Vert.	From the point between the eyebrows to GV-14 is 18″, the distance from the point between the eyebrows and the anterior hairline and from GV-14 to the posterior hair-line each being 3″. These measurements apply when the hairline is not distinct.
	From the right to the left mastoid process	9″	Horiz.	Used to measure the horizontal inch of the head. ST-8 to ST-8 is also 9″.
Chest & Abdomen	CV-22 to sternal-xiphoid junction	9″	Vert.	The vertical inch of the chest and rib area is calculated as 1.6″ for each rib and inter-costal space.
	Between the sternal-xiphoid junction and the navel	8″		
	Navel to pubic bone	5″		
	Nipple to nipple	8″	Horiz.	The horizontal inch of the chest and abdomen is calcu-lated by the division between the nipples; in women the dis-tance between right and left ST-12 may be used.
Back	Points on the back are mostly located vertically in relationship to the ver-tebrae. The 7th thoracic vertebrae is level with the interior angle of the scapula.		Vert.	The end of the 12th rib is level with the second lumbar vertebrae and the iliac crest is level with the 4th lumbar ver-tebrae.
Arm	Anterior fold of armpit to elbow crease.	9″	Vert.	Measurement for locating points on the hand channels.
	Elbow crease to wrist crease	12″		
Side of Chest	Armpit to just below the free ribs.	12″	Vert.	
Side of Abdomen	Last rib to hip joint	9″	Vert.	The trochanter is taken to be the hip joint.
Leg	Upper edge of the pubic bone to the medial condyle of the femur	18″	Vert.	Used for measuring the 3 yang channels of the foot. The distance from the gluteal crease to the popliteal crease is calculated as 14″.
	Medial condyle of the tibia to medial malleolus	13″		
	Greater trochanter to center of knee cap	19″		
	Outer eye of the knee to lateral malleolus	16″		
	Tip of the lateral malleolus to sole of foot	3″		

Endnotes

[1] The source points mentioned in this particular section of the *Inner Canon* are the following: LU-9, PC-7, LV-3, SP-3, KI-3, CV-15, and CV-6. These are mentioned as the source-yuan points for the lung, heart, liver, spleen, kidney, gao and huang respectively. (Gao and huang refer to areas in the chest and abdomen.) From this it can be seen that it is the viscera and not the bowels that are represented by source-yuan points. However, another section of the *Inner Canon* mentions the source points of the six bowels, but fails to name them. In modern clinical practice, each of the twelve regular channels is considered to possess source points. The source points for the gao and huang have faded from use in China.

[2] The spleen is primarily associated with the center, but it also is responsible for irrigating the four sides and moving fluids. To accomplish these various tasks the spleen has an extra connecting vessel, called the great connecting vessel, that spreads out over the sides of the body.

[3] The eight meeting-hui points are first mentioned in the *Classic of Difficult Issues* where the text is an expansion of a quote from the *Inner Canon* that mentions that the vessels meet at LU-9.

[4] These connections are as follows:

Connections of the Eight Confluence-Jiaohui Points and the Extraordinary Vessels	
Point	**Connection**
PC-6	PC divergent channel enters the chest area and there connects with the yin linking vessel
SP-4	SP channel intersects with the penetrating vessel at CV-4
TB-5	TB channel connects with the yang linking vessel at TB-15
GB-41	GB channel connects with the girdling vessel after passing the 11th intercostal space
LU-7	LU channel connects with conception vessel at the throat
KI-6	KI channel connects with yin motility vessel in the chest
SI-3	SI channel connects with governing vessel at GV-14
BL-62	BL-62 connects with yang motility vessel directly

[5] Paul Unschuld refers to alarm-mu points as concentration holes.

[6] Consistent translation practices would require that these points be termed confluence-jiaohui points because in Chinese the characters are the same as those that denote the confluence-jiaohui points of the eight extraordinary vessels. To avoid undue confusion we have chosen to denote these points as intersection-jiaohui points.

Part III
The Channels and Points

5. A Preface to The Channels and Points

The descriptions in chapters 6 through 20 of this book begin with a presentation of the channels and channel pathways, including the primary channel, the connecting vessel, the channel divergence and the channel sinews. Illustrations of each are depicted. Following this section is a presentation of individual acupuncture points, with accompanying spot illustrations. Each point is presented with the following detail:

Point Name: Each point may be identified by its alphanumeric code, which places the points in the most widely used order. We have included as well the Chinese name and its pinyin transcription. The English translation of the Chinese name that follows the pinyin may help the student to remember the location or function of the point. These names were chosen to reflect as many of the many meanings of the Chinese characters as possible, though it is important to understand that one single rendering rarely captures the full range of associations of the Chinese. (Readers wishing further elucidation are encouraged to examine our publication on this topic, *Grasping the Wind.*)

Location: The location of points is defined by the modern intepretations of traditional descriptions. These descriptions are expressed in the language of Western anatomy, with measurements in the traditional body inches, the *cun*, and written as ".

We have also included locations from traditional sources such as the *Great Compendium of Acupuncture and Moxibustion* (simply referred to as the *Great Compendium*), the *Golden Mirror of Medicine* (referred to as the *Golden Mirror*), or the *Systematized Canon of Acupuncture* (*The Systematized Canon*). Since acupuncture never developed a precise anatomy, classical point locations often only indicate the precise location once the approximate area is known. Despite this measure of imprecision, they are easier to understand, since they are expressed in a colloquial manner. In the English translation, we have expressed body parts as far as possible in the vernacular, and sometimes have translated the Chinese literally to preserve the simple flavor of the original. Attention should also be paid to the meaning of the following words:

> *midline:* the median line of the head, trunk and limbs
> *upward:* toward the apex above, superior to, or toward the head
> *downward:* away from the apex below, inferior to, or toward the feet
> *inward:* toward the median line, medially
> *outward:* away from the median line, laterally
> *in front of:* anterior to, or distal to
> *behind:* posterior to, or proximal to

Finally, the location section also includes a paragraph describing regional anatomy to help students having a detailed knowledge of anatomy to locate the point accurately and to help all students avoid puncturing important vessels, nerves, or organs.

Functions: These help the student to remember the therapeutic scope of acupoints. As mentioned in Part II, this information should be correlated with indications (listed in the second paragraph of this section) in order to fully understand their meaning. The terms used in this section fall into two basic categories as follows:

Terminology of Point Function	
Supplementation	Boost Fortify Nourish Engender Increase Moisten
Drainage	Dispel Eliminate Expel Clear Resolve Dissipate Disperse

Other terms, which may involve a draining or supplementing stimulus include: quicken, rectify, diffuse, disinhibit, course, soothe, calm, settle, harmonize, regulate, and transform.

While supplementation and drainage represent the two stimuli of acupuncture, the differentiated terms have been drawn from herbal medicine. Students should understand that words such as boost and nourish are largely synonymous with supplementation, though they imply subtle distinctions. Further information is provided on these terms in the glossary at the back of the book, and in the Translator's Foreword to *Fundamentals of Chinese Medicine*.

In the section headed *Indications*, we list the main diseases and patterns the point is most commonly used to treat. In a final paragraph, *Supplementary Indications*, we provide more detailed and additional indications drawn almost exclusively from the classics. The indications in the former section reflect the influence of Western terminology and the indications in the second section are expressed in terminology that reflects their classical origin. For example, the

Chinese term *shàn qì* is rendered as hernia under the main indications, since in modern texts it is used in the meaning it carries in Western medicine; while in the supplementary indications section it is rendered as shàn qì, since the term traditionally had a broader meaning than simply hernia.

In this section, students should realize that the classical Chinese texts were written without punctuation, and the grouping of symptoms was left to the reader's own interpretation. Translation into intelligible English requires some degree of interpretation by the translator. For example, when the Chinese says (literally translated): "cough dyspnea nausea vomiting headache," we render this in the most sensible way possible, e.g.: "cough and dyspnea; nausea and vomiting; headache." Rendering the same string as "cough; dyspnea; nausea; vomiting and headache" presents a different, though less likely interpretation of the information.

Illustrative Point Combinations: These come from mnemonic odes and verses such as *Song of the Jade Dragon*, or *Ode of a Hundred Patterns*. They highlight either special or typical point combinations. An effort has been made to preserve the flavor of the original sources, but not the meter or rhyme.

Stimulation: For acupuncture, we indicate depth of angle and needle insertion. For moxibustion, information includes the number of cones that may be burnt on the point and the number of minutes a warming stimulus may be applied with a moxa pole (moxa cigar). All stimulation information should be taken only as a guideline for treatment and adjusted according to the physiology and condition of the patient.

Point Categories and Associations: This section includes five-phase correspondence of points and indicates special groups to which points belong.

Channel Summary Charts: A chart that describes the current usages of the channel points is included at the end of each chapter. An asterisk indicates the most commonly used points.

Key to the illustrations

The descriptions of the channel pathways in this section are accompanied by illustrations patterned after those used in modern Chinese language acupuncture texts.

In the illustrations of the **primary channels and connecting vessels,** solid lines denote the primary channel pathways, horizontal broken lines represent the internal pathways, slanted broken lines represent channel branch pathways, vertical strips represent secondary pathways. Tightly-spaced broken lines and short arrows represent the pathway of the connecting vessel.

Channel points are marked by solid dots, and intersections with other channels (the intersection-jiaohui points) are indicated by the presence of a hollow triangle. The connecting-luo point is marked by a hollow circle and the lower uniting-he point by a solid square. A solid diamond represents the channel connection with the home organ and a hollow diamond represents the connection with a paired organ. A curved arrow depicts the connecting vessel pathway.

In the illustrations of the **channel divergences** the solid lines are the yang channels and the broken lines are the yin channels. The yin-yang pair is presented together to show the unions of the channel divergence pairs.

The illustrations are intended only as a guide and are not a substitute for the verbal descriptions of the pathways.

Key For Channel Divergences	
————————	Yang Channel
■■■■■■■■■■■■■	Yin Channel

Key to Chart Symbols	
■ ■■ ■	Internal pathway
———	External pathway
▰▰▰	Channel branch pathway
|||||||||||	Secondary pathway
▪▪▪▪▪	Connecting vessel pathway
➴	Connecting vessel pathway
◆	Connection with home organ
◇	Connection with paired organ
◯	Connecting-luo point
△	Intersection-jiaohui point
■	Lower uniting-he Point

6. The Lung Channel System
(Hand Tai Yin) 手太陰肺經

6.1 The Primary Lung Channel

Ren 12

Pathway: The hand tai yin lung channel starts in the region of the stomach in the middle burner and descends to connect with the large intestine. It then returns upward passing the upper opening of the stomach, penetrates the diaphragm, and homes to the lung. Continuing its ascendant path, it passes through the respiratory tract into the throat, then veers downward, following the clavicle to enter the axilla. From here it runs down the anterior aspect of the upper arm, lateral to the heart and pericardium channels, traverses the cubital fossa, and continues along the anterior aspect of the forearm to the radial styloid process of the wrist. It crosses the radial pulse, traverses the thenar eminence, and travels along the radial side of the thumb to its tip.

at LU7

A branch leaves the main pathway proximal to the wrist, passes round to the dorsum of the hand, and then runs down the inside of the index finger to its tip.

Main pathologic signs associated with the external path of the channel: fever and aversion to cold (with or without sweating), nasal congestion, headache, pain in the supraclavicular fossa, chest, shoulders, and back, and cold pain along the channel on the arm.

Main pathologic signs associated with the internal organ: cough, wheezing, and dyspnea, rapid breathing, fullness and oppression in the chest, expectoration of phlegm-drool, dry throat, abnormal urine color, restlessness, spitting of blood, heat in the palms. Other possible symptoms include fullness and distention in the abdomen and thin stool diarrhea.

Exuberance of qi: shoulder and back pain, wind cold contraction with spontaneous sweating, frequent urination, yawning.

Insufficiency of qi: shoulder and back pain accompanied by fear of cold, shortness of breath, distressed rapid breathing and abnormal color of urine.

6.2 The Connecting Vessel of the Lung Channel

Pathway: From the cleft in the flesh one and one-half inches above the wrist (LU-7), the channel branches to the hand yang ming large intestine channel. There is also a branch that breaks from the lung channel at that same point and follows the channel to the inner palm and disperses over the fish border (i.e., the area around LU-10).

Main Pathological Signs:

Repletion: heat in the palm in the region of LU-10.

Vacuity: yawning, frequent urination, urinary incontinence.

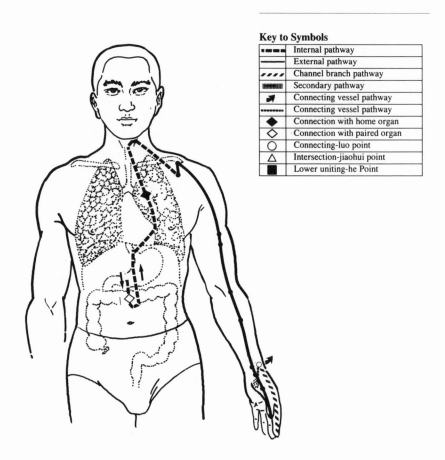

Key to Symbols	
▪▬▬▪	Internal pathway
————	External pathway
⁄⁄⁄⁄	Channel branch pathway
▮▮▮▮▮▮	Secondary pathway
⬏	Connecting vessel pathway
▪▪▪▪▪▪▪	Connecting vessel pathway
◆	Connection with home organ
◇	Connection with paired organ
○	Connecting-luo point
△	Intersection-jiaohui point
■	Lower uniting-he Point

Figure 6.1 - 6.2 Primary channel and connecting vessel of the lung.

6.3 The Lung Channel Divergence

Pathway: After diverging from the primary channel the divergence enters the region below the axilla near GB-22 and from there travels in front of the channel divergence of the heart, enters the lung and proceeds downward to disperse over the large intestine. A branch also rises up to the supraclavicular fossa and follows along the throat where it then unites with the hand yang ming large intestine channel divergence.

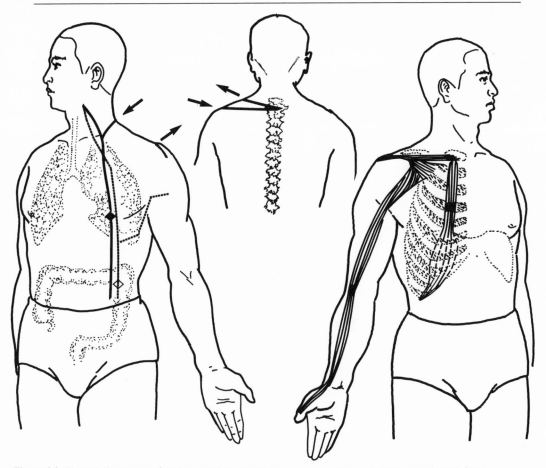

Figure 6.3 Channel divergences of the lung and large intestine.

Figure 6.4 The lung channel sinews.

6.4 The Lung Channel Sinew

Pathway: The hand tai yin channel sinew originates at the thumb and follows along the inside of the thumb to below the wrist where it binds. The sinews then follow the forearm to the elbow where they bind once again and then rise along the inner aspect of the upper arm and enter the axilla. The channel sinew proceeds to the supraclavicular fossa and binds near LI-15. There is also a branch that binds above at the supraclavicular fossa and penetrates and disperses over the diaphragm and then proceeds below the diaphragm and unites at the region of the twelfth rib.

Symptoms associated with the channel: cramping and pain along the course of the sinews that if severe results in accumulation lumps below the ribs, qi counterflow, tension along the ribs and spitting of blood.

LU-1
中府
zhōng fǔ

"Central Treasury"

LU-2

LU-1

Figure 6.5

Location: On the chest, at the level of the first intercostal space, below the lateral extremity of the clavicle, 6″ lateral to the anterior midline (conception vessel).

Classical Location: Six inches lateral from CV-20, three intercostal spaces above the nipple, where a pulsating vessel can be felt. *(The Great Compendium)*

Local Anatomy: Superolaterally, the axillary artery and vein, the thoracoacromial artery and vein. The intermediate supraclavicular nerve, the branches of the anterior thoracic nerve, and the lateral cutaneous branch of the 1st intercostal nerve.

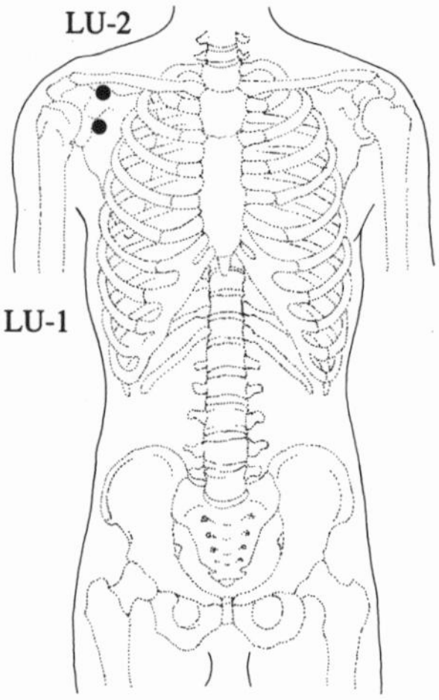

Functions: Clears and diffuses the upper burner and courses lung qi.

Indications: Cough; asthma; pain in the chest, shoulder and back; fullness in the chest.

Supplementary Indications: Coughing or vomiting of pus and blood; pulmonary distention and fullness; sweating; facial swelling; abdominal distention; somnolence; throat bi; fever and vomiting; difficult ingestion; diminished qi with inability to lie flat; aversion to cold; generalized heat vexation; pain in the skin and bone; running piglet; nasal congestion; turbid snivel; goiters and tumors of the neck.

Illustrative Point Combinations & Applications: Thoracic fullness with upper esophageal blockage, combine LU-1 with BL-49. *(Ode of a Hundred Patterns)*

Stimulation: 0.3-0.5″ perpendicular insertion. Moxa: 3-5 cones; pole 5-15 min.

Point Categories & Associations: Alarm-mu point of the lung; intersection-jiaohui point of the hand tai yin lung and foot tai yin spleen channels.

LU-2
雲門
yún mén

"Cloud Gate"

Location: On the chest, in the depression immediately below the lateral extremity of the clavicle, 6″ lateral to the conception vessel.

Classical Location: Below the clavicle, in the depression two inches to the side of ST-13, six inches from the midline of the chest, where a pulsating vessel can be felt. The point is located with the arm raised. *(The Great Compendium)*

Local Anatomy: The cephalic vein, the thoracoacromial artery and vein; inferiorly, the axillary artery. The intermediate and lateral supraclavicular nerve, the branches of the anterior thoracic nerve, and the lateral cord of the brachial plexus.

Functions: Clears lung heat and eliminates vexation; drains heat in the limbs and disinhibits the joints.

Indications: Cough; asthma; pain in the chest, shoulder, and arm; thoracic fullness.

Supplementary Indications: Throat bi; vexation and fullness in the chest; cold damage with persistent heat in the limbs; goiter; counterflow cold in the limbs; a regularly interrupted pulse that is not felt at the inch position.

Stimulation: 0.3-0.5″ perpendicular insertion. Moxa: 3-7 cones; pole 5-15 min.

LU-3
天府
tiān fǔ

"Celestial Storehouse"

Location: On the upper arm, 3″ below the end of the axillary fold, on the radial side of the biceps muscle (m. biceps brachii), 6″ above LU-5.

Classical Location: Located at a pulse three inches below the armpit and five inches above the elbow. The tip of the nose can just reach this point; dab the nose with ink to mark the spot. *(The Great Compendium)*

Local Anatomy: The cephalic vein and muscular branches of the brachial artery and vein. The lateral brachial cutaneous nerve at the place where the musculocutaneous nerve passes through.

Functions: Clears lung heat and regulates lung qi.

Indications: Asthma; nosebleed; pain in the medial aspect of the arm.

Supplementary Indications: Cough qi ascent; dyspnea with inability to catch the breath; sudden thirst; bleeding from nose and mouth; generalized swelling; wind sweating; abstraction and poor memory; lying down with inability to sleep; wailing and ghost talk; goiter; dizziness; tearing.

Stimulation: 0.3-0.5″ perpendicular insertion.
Moxa: direct moxa contraindicated; pole 5 min.

Needle Sensation: Localized numbness and distention spreading upward and downwards.

Contraindications: The *Systematized Canon of Acupuncture* says that moxibustion is contraindicated here because it causes qi counterflow.

LU-4
俠白
xiá bái

"Guarding White"

Location: On the upper arm, 1″ below LU-3, on the radial side of the m. biceps brachii.

Classical Location: Below LU-3 at a pulsating vessel five inches from the elbow. *(The Great Compendium)*

Local Anatomy: See LU-3.

Functions: Regulates qi and blood; relieves pain.

Indications: Cough; thoracic fullness; pain in the medial aspect of the arm.

Supplementary Indications: Qi ascent cough; cardiac pain and shortness of breath; dry retching; red and white sweat macules; vexation and fullness.

Stimulation: 0.3-0.5″ perpendicular insertion.
Moxa: 3-5 cones; pole 10-15 min.

Illustrative Point Combinations & Applications: Needling this point together with PC-6 can relieve thoracic fullness. It is highly effective for neurological palpitations and for intracostal neuralgia.

LU-5
尺澤
chǐ zé

"Cubit Marsh"

water point

Location: At the cubital crease, on the radial side of the tendon of the m. biceps brachii. The point is best located with the elbow slightly flexed.

Classical Location: Where a pulsating vessel can be felt on the elbow crease, in the depression between the sinew and bone, felt with the elbow flexed. *(The Great Compendium)*

Local Anatomy: The branches of the radial recurrent artery and vein, the cephalic vein. The lateral antebrachial cutaneous nerve and the radial nerve.

Functions: Discharges lung fire; downbears counterflow qi; clears upper-burner heat.

Indications: Cough; coughing of blood; tidal fever; asthma; thoracic fullness; sore throat; hypertonicity and pain in the elbow and arm.

Supplementary Indications: Shivering; clonic spasm; pain and hypertonicity of the elbow and arm preventing normal stretching; counterflow cough and dyspnea with fullness; throat bi; aching body and vexation; distention and fullness in the chest and lateral costal region; child fright wind; ejection of blood; nosebleed; enuresis; dry tongue; sudden swelling of the limbs; cold in the arm; shortness of breath; vomiting; cardiac pain.

spasmotic pain in elbow + arm

mastitis

Illustrative Point Combinations & Applications: LU-5 is combined with LI-11 for hypertonicity and aching of the elbow. LU-5 eliminates elbow pain and sinew tension when combined with LI-4.
(Wo Yan's Efficacious Point Applications)

Stimulation: 0.3-0.5 ″ perpendicular insertion.
Moxa: 3-5 cones. pole 5-10 min.

Needle Sensation: Localized needle stimulus sensation and distention, or an electric numbing sensation traveling down the forearm.

Point Categories & Associations: Uniting-he (water) point.

Location: On the palmar aspect of the forearm, on the line joining LU-9 and LU-5, 7 ″ above LU-9, 5 ″ below LU-5.

Classical Location: Below LU-5, seven inches from the crease of the wrist, in the space between the two bones.
(The Golden Mirror)

Local Anatomy: The cephalic vein, the radial artery and vein. The lateral antebrachial cutaneous nerve and the superficial ramus of the radial nerve.

Functions: Moistens the lung and staunches bleeding; clears heat and resolves the exterior.

Indications: Cough; asthma; sore throat; pain in the elbow and arm with difficulty in bending and stretching.

Supplementary Indications: Inversion headache; inversion cold in the arms; absence of sweating; expectoration of blood; loss of voice; sore pharynx; counterflow cough.

Stimulation: 0.3-0.5 ″ perpendicular insertion.
Moxa: 3-5 cones; pole 5-15 min.

Needle Sensation: Localized distention, sometimes spreading distally.

LU-6
孔最
kǒng zuì
"Collection Hole"

Point Categories & Associations: Cleft-xi point of the lung channel.

LU-7
列缺
liè quē

"Broken Sequence"

Location: In the crevice on the most lateral aspect of the radius, just proximal to the styloid process, 1.5″ above the wrist crease. When the thumb and index finger of each hand are interlocked, with the index finger of one hand resting on the styloid process of the other, the point is in the depression just under the tip of the index finger.

Classical Location: One and a half inches from the wrist. When the thumb and index finger of one hand are interlocked with those of the other, the point lies to the edge of the index finger, in a depression between the sinew and bone. *(The Great Compendium)*

Local Anatomy: The cephalic vein, branches of the radial artery and vein. The lateral antebrachial cutaneous nerve and the superficial ramus of the radial nerve.

Functions: Diffuses the lung and dispels cold; courses the channels and frees the connecting vessels. *Clears Obstructed Qi + Blood*

Indications: Headache and stiffness of the neck; cough and asthma; sore throat; facial paralysis; wryness of the eyes and mouth; clenched jaws; weakness of the wrist.

Supplementary Indications: Headache; hemiplegia; enuresis and frequent voidings; pain in the arm and elbow; infantile fright epilepsy; penile pain; bloody urine; seminal loss; restless sleep; generalized wind bi numbness; fever and chills; tension in the chest and back; throat bi; heat in the palms; inversion counterflow in the limbs; toothache; malarial disease; heat and pain in the shoulder and back.

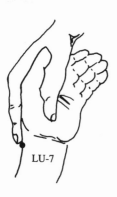

Figure 6.6

Illustrative Point Combinations & Applications: For dyspnea with rapid breathing, use LU-7 and ST-36.
(Song of Point Applications for Miscellaneous Disease)

Stimulation: 0.2-0.4″ oblique insertion toward elbow.
Moxa: 3-5 cones; pole 5-10 min.

Needle Sensation: Localized needle stimulus sensation and distention.

Location: At the palmar wrist crease, in the depression on the radial side of the radial artery.

Classical Location: In the depression of the radial styloid pulse. *(The Great Compendium)*

Local Anatomy: Laterally, the radial artery and vein. The lateral antebrachial cutaneous nerve and the superficial ramus of the radial nerve.

LU-8
經渠
jīng qú
"Channel Ditch"

Functions: Diffuses the lung and downbears qi; courses wind and resolves the exterior.

Indications: Cough; asthma; sore throat; pain in the chest and wrist.

Supplementary Indications: Fever and chills; pain in the chest and back; absence of sweating in heat diseases; cardiac pain, retching and vomiting; throat bi; heat in the palms; pain on the inner face of the arm; pain in the wrist; inflated feeling in the chest; frequent yawning.

Stimulation: 0.1.-0.2″ perpendicular insertion. *avoid radial artery* Moxa: pole 5-10 min. (Traditionally contraindicated for moxibustion.)

Point Categories & Associations: River-jing (metal) point.

Location: At the transverse crease of the wrist, in the depression of the radial side of the radial artery.

Classical Location: At the pulsating vessel, at the inside extremity of the crease behind the hand. *(The Golden Mirror)*

Local Anatomy: The radial artery and vein. The lateral antebrachial cutaneous nerve and the superficial ramus of the radial nerve.

LU-9
太淵
tài yuān
"Great Abyss"

Functions: Dispels wind and transforms phlegm; rectifies the lung and suppresses cough; clears and depurates upper-burner and lung qi.

Indications: Asthma; cough; expectoration of blood; sore throat; palpitations; pain in the chest and medial aspect of the forearm.

Supplementary Indications: Dyspnea and fullness in the chest; eye pain and screens; throat bi; toothache; headache; pain in the clavicle; pain along the inner face of the forearm; cardiac pain; thoracic bi; cold inversion; retching; quivering with cold; dry pharynx; manic raving; pain or lack of strength in the wrist; body fever and sweating in thermic disease; cold in the palms; lack of radial pulse.

Stimulation: 0.2-0.3 ″ perpendicular insertion.
Moxa: 1-3 cones; pole 3-5 min.
Needle Sensation: Localized needle stimulus sensation and distention.

Point Categories & Associations: Meeting-hui point of the vessels; stream-shu (earth) point; source-yuan point of the lung.

LU-10
魚際
yú jì

"Fish Border"

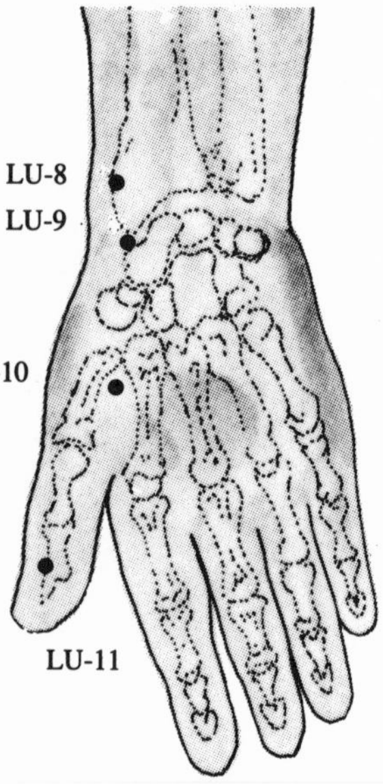

LU-8
LU-9

LU-10

LU-11

Figure 6.7

Location: On the thenar eminence, midway along the first metacarpal bone, on the border of the red and white skin.

Classical Location: Behind the base joint of the thumb, in the depression on the inside border of the red and white flesh. *(The Great Compendium)*

Local Anatomy: Venules of the thumb draining to the cephalic vein. The superficial ramus of the radial nerve.

Functions: Courses the lung and harmonizes the stomach; disinhibits the throat; clears blood heat; abates fever.

Indications: Cough; expectoration of blood; sore throat; fever.

Supplementary Indications: Loss of voice; dizziness and headache; cardiac bi pain; sorrow and fear; pain in the chest and back; aversion to cold; genital damp itch; abdominal pain with inability to eat; hypertonicity of the elbow and fullness in the limbs; body fever with sweating; mania; yellow tongue fur; tetany; qi ascent; tearing; malarial disease; vexation and diminished qi; dry throat and thirst; cough with pain in the sacrum; gastric counterflow; cholera.

Illustrative Point Combinations & Applications: For sore throat, use TB-2 and LU-10. *(Ode of a Hundred Patterns)*

Stimulation: 0.5-0.7 ″ perpendicular insertion. Moxa: 3 cones; pole 1-3 min.
Needle Sensation: Localized needle stimulus sensation and distention.

Point Categories & Associations: Spring-ying (fire) point.

Location: On the radial side of the thumb, about 0.1 ″ proximal to the corner of the nail.
Classical Location: On the inside of the thumb, about the width of a Chinese leek leaf from the corner of the nail.
(The Great Compendium)

LU-11
少商
shào shāng
"Lesser Shang"

Note: This leaf can be presumed to have been considerably smaller in the past than it is today. This may explain why some translators render it as chive.
Local Anatomy: The arterial and venous network formed by the palmar digital proprial artery and veins. The terminal nerve network formed by the mixed branches of the lateral antebrachial cutaneous nerve and the superficial ramus of the radial nerve as well as the palmar digital proprial nerve of the median nerve.

Functions: Frees channel qi; revives inversion patients; clears lung counterflow; disinhibits the throat; courses and discharges surging counterflow qi fire in the twelve channels.
Indications: Cough counterflow and asthma; sore, swollen throat; nosebleed; pain and hypertonicity of the fingers; heat diseases; clouding inversion; mania and withdrawal.
Supplementary Indications: Sweating and aversion to cold; swelling of the neck and throat bi; throat moth in children; persistent nosebleed; bowstring and elusive masses in males; mumps; toothache.
Illustrative Point Combinations & Applications: Combine LU-11 with LI-3 for blood-vacuity thirst. *(Ode of a Hundred Patterns)*.

For infantile fright wind, needle LU-11 and mildly drain GV-26 and KI-1. *(Song of Point Applications for Miscellaneous Disease)*

Stimulation: 0.1 ″ upward oblique insertion; bleed with a three-edged needle for wind strike inversion or severe sore, swollen throat.
Needle Sensation: Localized pain.

Point Categories & Associations: Well-jing (wood) point.

Hand Tai Yang Lung Channel			
Point	**Location**	Indications	
		Primary	**Secondary**
*LU-1	Chest	Cough dyspnea chest pain	
LU-2		Cough dyspnea chest pain	
Chest: Disorders of the chest and lung			
LU-3	Upper arm	Dyspnea nosebleed	
LU-4		Cough	
*LU-5	Elbow	Cough coughing blood dyspnea fullness in the chest	Tidal fever child fright wind
*LU-6	Forearm	Cough coughing blood	
*LU-7		Cough pain and swelling of the throat	Headache wry mouth
LU-8		Cough pain and swelling of the throat	
*LU-9	Wrist	Cough pain and swelling of the throat	Lack of pulse
*LU-10	Palm	Coughing blood pain and swelling of the throat	Fever loss of voice
*LU-11	Thumb	Pain and swelling of the throat cough	Fever stupor mania and withdrawal
Hand and arm: Disorders of the throat, chest and lung			

7. The Large Intestine Channel System (Hand Yang Ming) 手陽明大腸經

7.1 The Primary Large Intestine Channel

Pathway: The hand yang ming large intestine channel begins at the radial side of the tip of the index finger and proceeds upward between the first and second metacarpal bones of the hand and between the tendons of the extensor pollicis longus and brevis muscles at the wrist. It continues along the radial margin of the forearm to the radial margin of the lateral aspect of the elbow, then up the lateral aspect of the upper arm and over the shoulder joint. After intersecting the hand tai yang small intestine channel at SI-12, it rises to just below the spinous process of the seventh cervical vertebra, and intersects with the governing vessel at GV-14, where all six yang regular channels meet. It then travels straight into the supraclavicular fossa to ST-12, from where it connects through to the lung, passes through the diaphragm, and homes to the large intestine.

A branch separates from the main channel at ST-12 in the supraclavicular fossa, passes up the neck, and traverses the cheek before entering the lower gum. From here it skirts around the lips, passes the foot yang ming channel at ST-4, and then meets the same channel coming from the other side of the body at the philtrum. It then continues around the nostril of the opposite side to terminate at the side of the nose. In other words, the right and left channels cross over at the philtrum and run for the last short stretch on the opposite side of the body from which they originated.

The *Spiritual Axis* describes yet another branch that separates from the main channel at ST-12, descends past ST-13 and penetrates the lung, passes through the diaphragm, homes to the large intestine, and descends to the lower limb to emerge at ST-37, which is the lower uniting-he point of the large intestine.

Main pathologic signs associated with the external course of the channel: fever, parched, dry mouth and thirst, sore throat, nosebleed, toothache, pain and reddening of the eyes, swelling of the neck, palpable red swelling and inhibited bending and stretching of the fingers. There may also be pain, sensation of cold, or painful and palpably hot, red swelling in the region of the shoulder and upper arm.

Main pathologic signs associated with the internal organ: lower abdominal pain, migratory abdominal pain, borborygmi, thin stool, and excretion of thick, slimy yellow matter. There may also be rapid breathing and dyspnea.

Exuberance of qi: Distention swelling and heat along the course of the channel.

Insufficiency of qi: Cold and shivering with an inability to regain warmth.

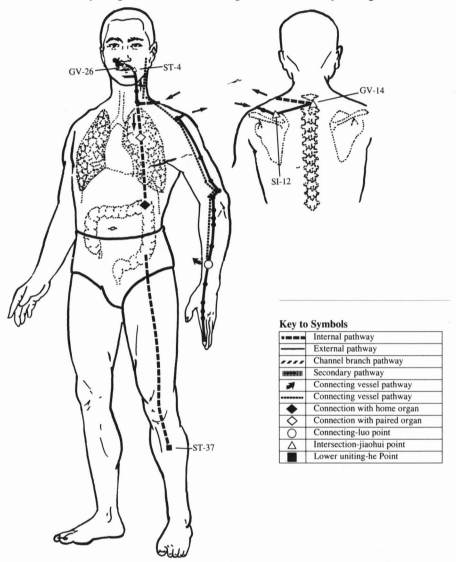

Key to Symbols

▪▬▬▪	Internal pathway
———	External pathway
⁄⁄⁄⁄	Channel branch pathway
‖‖‖‖‖	Secondary pathway
➹	Connecting vessel pathway
▪▪▪▪▪▪	Connecting vessel pathway
◆	Connection with home organ
◇	Connection with paired organ
○	Connecting-luo point
△	Intersection-jiaohui point
■	Lower uniting-he Point

7.2 The Connecting Vessel of the Large Intestine Channel

Pathway: This vessel separates from the primary channel 3 ″ proximal to the wrist at LI-6 and branches to the lung channel. Another branch separates from the primary channel at the same point and rises up the arm, passes through the shoulder region and proceeds to the corner of the jaw, from where it separates into two branches. One branch spreads over the teeth and another enters the ear to unite with the channels of the gallbladder, triple burner, small intestine, and stomach.

Main pathologic signs:

Symptoms of repletion: Tooth decay; deafness.

Symptoms of vacuity: Tooth sensitivity to cold; bi.

7.3 The Large Intestine Channel Divergence

Pathway: After leaving the primary channel at the shoulder near LI-15 and crossing over to the 7th cervical vertebrae this divergence then enters the body cavity and proceeds downward to the large intestine. It also homes to the lung from where it rises along the throat and surfaces again to join its primary channel, the hand yang ming (LI).

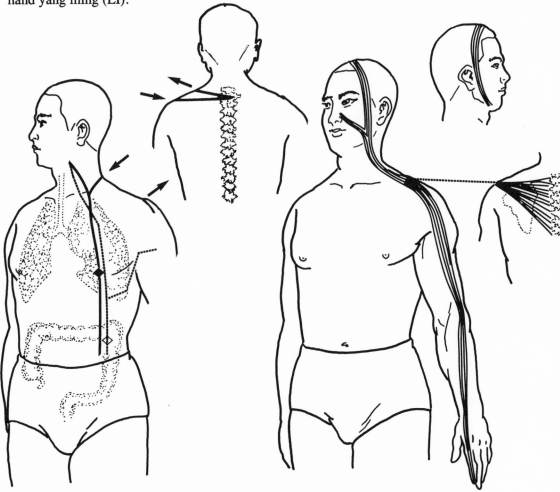

Figure 7.3 Channel divergences of the large intestine and lung.   **Figure 7.4** The large intestine channel sinews.

7.4 The Large Intestine Channel Sinews

Pathway: The sinew begins at the tip of the index finger and binds at the dorsal aspect of the wrist. It then proceeds up the forearm and binds at the lateral aspect of the elbow, and continues upward along the lateral aspect of the upper arm and binds at the shoulder.

One branch breaks from the shoulder, wraps the scapula and clasps to the spine. Another branch separates from the shoulder and proceeds upward along the neck. This branch splits at the jaw and one fork binds at the side of the nose while the other follows anterior to the small intestine channel sinew up over the head to bind at the submandibular region on the opposite side of the head.

Main pathologic signs: Spasms, stiffness, pain or strain along the course of the channel sinew; inability to raise the arm; inability to turn the neck to the left or right.

Location: On the radial side of the index finger, about 0.1″ proximal to the corner of the nail.

Classical Location: On the inside of the index finger, the width of a Chinese leek leaf from the corner of the nail.
(The Great Compendium)

Local Anatomy: The arterial and venous network formed by the dorsal and digital arteries and veins. The palmar digital proprial nerve derived from the median nerve.

Functions: Resolves the exterior and abates heat; clears the lung and disinhibits the throat; courses and discharges yang ming pathogenic heat; opens the portals and revives the spirit.

Indications: Toothache; sore, swollen throat; swelling of the submandibular region; numbness of the fingers; heat diseases; clouding inversion.

Supplementary Indications: Heat disease with sweating; blindness; deafness and tinnitus; throat bi preventing speech; shoulder and back pain reaching into the clavicle; cold and heat malaria; thoracic qi fullness.

Illustrative Point Combinations & Applications: A principal use of LI-1 is in treating sudden wind strike and fulminant clouding with phlegm congestion. *(The Golden Mirror of Medicine)*

Stimulation: 0.1″ upward oblique insertion; bleed as for LU-11. Moxa: 1-3 cones; pole 5 min.

Point Categories & Associations: Well-jing (metal) point.

LI-1
商陽
shāng yáng
"Shang Yang"

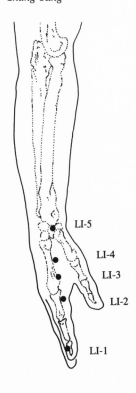

Figure 7.5

Location: On the radial side of the index finger, distal to the metacarpophalangeal joint, at the border of the red and white skin. The point is located with the finger slightly flexed.

Classical Location: On the inner side of the index finger, in the depression at the base joint. *(The Great Compendium)*

Local Anatomy: The dorsal digital and palmar digital proprial arteries and veins derived from the radial artery and vein. The dorsal digital nerve of the radial nerve and the palmar digital proprial nerve of the median nerve.

LI-2
二間
èr jiān
"Second Space"

Functions: Dissipates pathogenic heat; disinhibits the throat.

Indications: Clouded vision; nosebleed; toothache; sore, swollen throat; heat diseases.

Supplementary Indications: Severe clouding of vision; throat bi; submandibular swelling; shoulder and back pain; wryness of mouth and eyes; headache.

Illustrative Point Combinations & Applications: Dong Shi Jing Chang uses this point contralaterally to treat low back pain.

Note: Dong Shi Jing Chang was a well known acupuncturist (1916-1975) who used points in a non-traditional fashion. His treatments were known to be quite effective and for this reason some are included in this book.

Stimulation: 0.2-0.3″ perpendicular insertion.
Moxa: 3 cones; pole 5 min.

Point Categories & Associations: Spring-ying (water) point.

LI-3
三間
sān jiān

"Third Space"

Location: On the radial side of the index finger proximal to the head of the 2nd metacarpal bone. Easily located when a loose fist is formed.

Classical Location: In the depression behind the base joint of the index finger, on the inner side. *(The Great Compendium)*

Local Anatomy: The dorsal venous network of the hand and the branch of the 1st dorsal metacarpal artery. The superficial ramus of the radial nerve.

Functions: Discharges pathogenic heat; disinhibits the throat; regulates bowel qi.

Indications: Eye pain; toothache; sore, swollen throat; redness and swelling of the fingers and backs of the hands.

Supplementary Indications: Acute eye pain; aching among the lower teeth; throat bi; blockage of the pharynx; fever and chills; abdominal fullness and rumbling intestines; shoulder pain; dryness of the mouth and lips; body fever; dyspnea; fecal stoppage.

Illustrative Point Combinations & Applications: There is the wonder of LI-3, and BL-23, which are good for treating wind taxation in the shoulder and back. *(Ode of Xi Hong)*

Stimulation: 0.5-1.0″ perpendicular insertion.
Moxa: 3 cones; pole 5-10 min.

Point Categories & Associations: Stream-shu (wood) point.

Location: In the center of the flesh between the 1st and 2nd meta-carpal bones, slightly closer to the 2nd metacarpal bone. If the transverse crease of the interphalangeal joint of the thumb of one hand is lined up with the margin of the web between the thumb and the index finger of the other hand, the point is where the tip of the thumb touches.

Classical Location: In the depression where the index finger and thumb bones part. *(The Great Compendium)*

Local Anatomy: The venous network of the dorsum of the hand; proximally, exactly on the radial artery piercing from the dorsum to the palm of the hand. The superficial ramus of the radial nerve; deeper, the palmar digital proprial nerve derived from the median nerve.

Functions: Frees the channels and quickens the connecting vessels; courses wind and resolves the exterior; clears and discharges lung heat; frees gastrointestinal downbearing; relieves pain and quiets the spirit.

Indications: Headache; painful swelling and reddening of the eyes; nosebleed; swelling of the face; sore, swollen throat; hypertonicity of the fingers; pain in the arm; wryness of the eyes and mouth; sweating or absence of it in heat diseases; menstrual block; pro-longed labor; dysentery.

Supplementary Indications: Wind strike trismus; malaria with fever and chills; mania; loss of voice; wind papules; cardiac pain; unilateral or ambilateral headache; great thirst, fever and aversion to cold in cold damage; headache and rigid spine; child throat moth.

Stimulation: 0.5-0.8″ perpendicular insertion.
Moxa: 3 cones; pole 5-15 min.

Needle Sensation: Distention and numbness, spreading down to the fingers or up to the elbow, sometimes radiating into the shoulder or even the face.

Contraindications: This point is contraindicated for pregnant women.

LI-4
合谷
hé gǔ
"Union Valley"

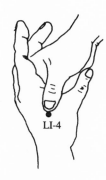

Figure 7.6

Point Categories & Associations: Source-yuan point; LI-4 is the command point of the face and mouth.

LI-5
陽溪 (陽谿)
yáng xi

"Yang Ravine"

Location: On the radial side of the wrist. When the thumb is extended, it is in the depression between the tendons of the long and short extensor muscles of the thumb (m. extensor pollicis longus and m. extensor pollicis brevis).

Classical Location: In the depression between the two sinews on the upper face of the wrist. *(The Great Compendium)*

Local Anatomy: The cephalic vein, the radial artery and its dorsal carpal branch. The superficial ramus of the radial nerve.

Functions: Dispels wind and drains fire; dissipates yang ming pathogenic heat.

Indications: Headache; painful swelling and reddening of the eyes; toothache; sore, swollen throat; pain in the wrist.

Supplementary Indications: Deafness; tinnitus; throat bi; inability to lift the arm; heat in the palm; pain at the root of the tongue; vexation; protrusion of the tongue.

Illustrative Point Combinations & Applications: With LI-2, it treats toothache, lumbar pain, and throat bi. *(Ode of Xi Hong)*

LI-15 and LI-5 disperse extreme heat related to skin rashes. *(Ode of a Hundred Patterns)*

Stimulation: 0.3-0.5″ perpendicular insertion.
Moxa: 3 cones; pole 5-15 min.

Needle Sensation: Localized needle stimulus sensation and distention.

Point Categories & Associations: River-jing (fire) point.

LI-6
偏歷
piān lì

"Veering Passage"

Location: One quarter of the way (i.e., 3″) along the line that runs from LI-5 to LI-11.

Classical Location: Moving upward from LI-5, it is three inches behind the wrist. *(The Golden Mirror)*

Local Anatomy: The cephalic vein; on the radial side the lateral antebrachial cutaneous nerve and the superficial ramus of the radial nerve. On the ulnar side, the posterior antebrachial cutaneous nerve and the posterior antebrachial interosseous nerve.

Functions: Regulates the waterways; frees the vessels and connecting vessels.

Indications: Nosebleed; deafness; aching of the hand and arm; water swelling.

Supplementary Indications: Loss of visual acuity; tinnitus; throat bi; aching shoulder and upper arm; inhibited urination; water gu; dry retching; swelling of the lateral region of the cheek; madness with continual talking.

Stimulation: 0.3-0.5 ″ perpendicular insertion.
Moxa: 3-5 cones; pole 5-10 min.

Point Categories & Associations: Connecting-luo point of the large intestine channel connecting to the lung channel.

Location: With the ulna facing down and the elbow flexed, this point is 5 ″ above LI-5. Locate the point while making a fist.
Classical Location: Three inches up from LI-6.
(The Golden Mirror)

LI-7
溫溜
wēn liū

"Warm Flow"

Note: *The Great Compendium* lists LI-7 as being between 5 ″ and 6 ″ up from the wrist, relative to the size of the patient.

Local Anatomy: The muscular branch of the radial artery, the cephalic vein. The posterior antebrachial cutaneous nerve and the deep ramus of the radial nerve.

Functions: Clears pathogenic heat; rectifies the stomach and intestines.

Indications: Headache; facial swelling; sore, swollen throat; borborygmi and abdominal pain; aching of the shoulder and arm.

Supplementary Indications: Toothache and pain in the mouth and tongue; throat bi; inability to lift the shoulder; eructation; rumbling intestines and abdominal pain; clove sores and yong; epilepsy; red, swollen face; swelling of the limbs; vomiting of drool; intestinal qi block.

Illustrative Point Combinations & Applications: Stiffness in the neck in cold damage is treated by LI-7 and LV-14.
(Ode of a Hundred Patterns)

Stimulation: 0.5-0.8 ″ perpendicular insertion.
Moxa 3-5 cones; 5-10 min.

Point Categories & Associations: Cleft-xi point of the hand yang ming large intestine channel.

LI-8
下廉
xià lián

"Lower Ridge"

Location: 4″ below LI-11.
Classical Location: Under the radius, one inch from LI-9, at the border of the protuberant flesh of the radius.
(The Great Compendium)
Local Anatomy: See LI-7.

Functions: Dissipates wind and clears heat; frees the channels and relieves pain.
Indications: Pain in the elbow and arm; abdominal pain.
Supplementary Indications: Headache or head wind; dizziness; eye pain; pain in the umbilical region; untransformed digestate; abdominal fullness; swill diarrhea; dyspnea; bloody urine; manic raving.

Stimulation: 0.5-0.7″ perpendicular insertion.
Moxa: 3 cones; pole 2-5 min.

LI-9
上廉
shàng lián

"Upper Ridge"

Location: 1″ above LI-8 and 3″ below LI-11 on the line running from LI-5 to LI-11.
Classical Location: Three inches below LI-11.
(The Great Compendium)
Local Anatomy: See LI-7.

Functions: Courses the channels and quickens the connecting vessels; frees bowel qi.
Indications: Aching shoulder and arm; paralysis of the upper limbs; numbness of the hand and arm; rumbling intestines and abdominal pain.
Supplementary Indications: Brain wind and headache; numbness of the feet; wind-water knee swelling; difficult urination with dark-colored urine; hemiplegia.

Stimulation: 0.7-1.0″ perpendicular insertion.
Moxa: 3-7 cones; pole 5-10 min.

Location: 2″ below LI-11 on the line drawn from LI-5.

Classical Location: Two inches below LI-11; the flesh bulges
when pressure is applied. *(The Great Compendium)*

Local Anatomy: The branches of the radial recurrent artery and
vein. For nerves, see LI-7.

LI-10
手千里
shǒu sān lǐ

"Arm Three Li"

Functions: Dispels wind and frees the connecting vessels; harmonizes the stomach and disinhibits the intestines.

Indications: Abdominal pain, vomiting and diarrhea; aching in the
shoulder and upper arm; paralysis of the upper limbs.

Supplementary Indications: Toothache; pain in the cheek and submandibular region; stubborn numbness of the hand and arm; wind
strike wryness of the mouth; hemiplegia; cholera; fecal incontinence; scrofulous lumps; periodic cold in the intestines; pain in
the back and lumbar region; vacuity weakness due to the
five taxations.

Illustrative Point Combinations & Applications: LI-10 and ST-36
are needled to treat digestate aggregation and qi lumps.
(Ode of Xi Hong)

Head wind, visual dizziness, and stiffness of the neck can be
treated with BL-62, BL-63 and LI-10.
(Song of Point Applications for Miscellaneous Disease)

Stimulation: 1- 2 ″ perpendicular insertion.
Moxa: 3-7 cones; pole 5-10 min.

Location: When the elbow is flexed the point is in the depression
at the lateral end of the transverse cubital crease, midway between
LU-5 and the lateral epicondyle of the humerus.

Classical Location: At the outer side of the radius at the elbow.
When the hand is placed on the chest, the point is in the depression
at the end of the elbow crease. *(The Great Compendium)*

Local Anatomy: The branches of the radial recurrent artery and
vein. The posterior antebrachial cutaneous nerve; deeper, on the
medial side, the radial nerve.

LI-11
曲池
qū chí

"Pool at the Bend"

Functions: Courses pathogenic heat; disinhibits the joints; eliminates water-damp; courses wind and resolves the exterior; harmonizes qi and blood.

Indications: Pain in the elbow and arm; paralysis of the upper limbs; scrofulous lumps; wind papules; abdominal pain; vomiting; dysentery; heat diseases; sore, swollen throat.

Supplementary Indications: Non-abatement of residual fever in cold damage; painful reddening of the eyes; toothache and throat bi; pain in the elbow with difficulty in bending and stretching; thin, weak elbows; hemiplegia; amenorrhea; dormant papules; vexation and fullness in the chest; dry skin; lax sinews; swelling of the head; headache.

Illustrative Point Combinations & Applications: HT-9 and LI-11 relieve fevers [of all types]. *(Ode of a Hundred Patterns)*

LI-11 and GB-21 are used to relieve pain in the upper arm. Soon the patient will again pull back the bow [and shoot]. *(Ode to Elucidate Mysteries)*

LI-11 and LI-4 are the main points for diseases of the head, face, ears, eyes, mouth and nose. *(Song of Point Applications for Miscellaneous Disease)*

Stimulation: 1.0-1.5 " perpendicular insertion.
Moxa 3-7 cones; pole 10-30 min.

Needle Sensation: Distention and numbness, sometimes extending to the wrist and hand, or to the shoulder.

Point Categories & Associations: Uniting-he (earth) point; 12th ghost point.

LI-12
肘髎
zhǒu liáo

"Elbow Bone-Hole"

Location: When the elbow is flexed, the point is superior to the epicondyle of the humerus, about 1 " superolateral to LI-11.

Classical Location: In the depression on the outer side of the large elbow bone. *(The Great Compendium)*

Local Anatomy: The radial collateral artery and vein. The posterior antebrachial cutaneous nerve; deeper, on the medial side, the radial nerve.

Functions: Courses the channels and quickens the connecting vessels; disinhibits the joints.

Indications: Pain, hypertonicity, and numbness of the elbow and arm.

Supplementary Indications: Wind bi of the elbow.

Stimulation: 0.3-0.5 ″ perpendicular insertion.
Moxa: 3 cones; pole 5-10 min.
Needle Sensation: Localized needle stimulus sensation and distention.

LI-13
手五里
(shǒu) wǔ lǐ
"Five Li (arm)"

Location: 3 ″ above LI-11 on the line joining LI-11 and LI-15.
Classical Location: At the pulsating vessel, three inches above the elbow and slightly inward. *(The Great Compendium)*
Local Anatomy: The radial collateral artery and vein. The posterior antebrachial cutaneous nerve; deeper, the radial nerve.

Functions: Courses the channels and quickens the connecting vessels; disinhibits the joints.
Indications: Hypertonicity and pain in the elbow and arm; scrofula.
Supplementary Indications: Distention, fullness and pain below the heart; qi ascent; wind taxation; fright and fear; blood ejection; cough; blurry vision.
Illustrative Point Combinations & Applications: LI-13 and LI-14 treat scrofula and sores. *(Ode of a Hundred Patterns)*

Stimulation: 0.3-0.7 ″ perpendicular insertion.
Moxa 7-15 cones; pole 5-20 min.

Note: The ancient contraindication of this point is no longer recognized, and is tentatively ascribed to the thick needles used at the time, which probably caused damage to the artery or radial nerve. The finer needles now available enable the point to be used to great effect, provided adequate care is taken to avoid the nerve.

LI-14
臂臑
bì nào
"Upper Arm"

Location: On the upper arm, slightly superior to the insertion of the deltoid muscle (m. deltoideus), on the line connecting LI-11 and LI-15.
Classical Location: Up four body inches from LI-13, in the depression between the two sinews and bone, felt when the arm is raised and the hand held flat. *(The Great Compendium)*
Local Anatomy: The branches of the posterior circumflex humeral artery and vein, the deep brachial artery and vein. The posterior brachial cutaneous nerve; deeper, the radial nerve.

Functions: Courses and frees the channels and connecting vessels; relieves pain.

Indications: Pain in the shoulder and arm; scrofula.

Supplementary Indications: Fever and chills; hypertonicity of the neck; pain in the back and shoulder preventing the arm from being lifted; thin weak arms.

Illustrative Point Combinations & Applications: LI-13 and LI-14 are combined to treat scrofulous lumps.
(Ode of a Hundred Patterns)

Stimulation: 0.5-0.7″ perpendicular or upward oblique insertion. Moxa 3-7 cones; pole 5-10 min.

Point Categories & Associations: Intersection-jiaohui point of the hand yang ming large intestine channel with the foot yang ming stomach channel and the yang linking vessel.

LI-15
肩髃
jiān yú

"Shoulder Bone"

Location: Inferior to the acromion, and slightly anterior to the middle of the upper portion of the deltoid muscle (m. deltoideus). When the arm is in full abduction, the point is in the anterior of the two depressions appearing at the border of the acromiohumeral junction.

Classical Location: In the depression between the sinew and bone at the end of the humerus where it meets the shoulder bone.
A hollow appears at the point when the arm is lifted.
(The Great Compendium)

Local Anatomy: The posterior circumflex artery and vein. The lateral supraclavicular nerve and axillary nerve.

Functions: Courses wind and quickens the connecting vessels; harmonizes qi and blood; disinhibits the joints; dispels pathogens and resolves heat.

Indications: Pain in the shoulder and arm; paralysis of the upper limbs; wind papules; scrofulous lumps.

Supplementary Indications: Heat in the shoulder; bi of the fingers; hemilateral wind and hemiplegia; thin, weak arms; shoulder wind; toothache; wind and damp contending in both shoulders; seminal discharge due to taxation.

Illustrative Point Combinations & Applications: Stimulation of LI-15 and LI-5 disperses extreme heat related to skin rashes. *(Ode of a Hundred Patterns)*

Aching of the hands making it difficult to grasp things can be treated with LI-11, LI-4 and LI-15. *(Song More Precious than Jade)*

Stimulation: 0.6-1.2″ downward oblique insertion.
Moxa: 7-14 cones; pole 5-10 min.

Needle Sensation: Distention and numbness, sometimes extending to the elbow.

Point Categories & Associations: Intersection-jiaohui point of the hand tai yang small intestine channel with the hand yang ming large intestine channel and the yang motility vessel.

Location: On the superior aspect of the shoulder, in the depression between acromial extremity of the clavicle and the scapular spine.

Classical Location: Up from the tip of the shoulder, in the depression that lies between the two forking bones. *(The Great Compendium)*

Local Anatomy: The jugular vein. Superficially, the lateral supraclavicular nerve, the branch of the accessory nerve; deeper, the suprascapular artery and vein, and the suprascapular nerve.

LI-16
巨骨
jù gǔ
"Great Bone"

Functions: Courses and quickens the connecting vessels; disinhibits the joints.

Indications: Shoulder pain; pain in the arm preventing bending and stretching.

Supplementary Indications: Static blood in the chest; fright epilepsy; scrofulous lumps; goiter.

Stimulation: 0.5-0.7″ perpendicular insertion.
Moxa 3-7 cones; pole 5-20 min.

Needle Sensation: Localized needle stimulus sensation and distention.

Point Categories & Associations: Intersection-jiaohui point of the hand yang ming large intestine channel and the yang motility vessel.

Point Categories & Associations: Intersection-jiaohui point of the hand yang ming large intestine channel and the yang motility vessel.

LI-17
天鼎
tiān dǐng

"*Celestial Tripod*"

Location: On the anterior lateral aspect of the neck, superior to the midpoint of the supraclavicular fossa, on the posterior border of the sternocleidomastoid muscle (m. sternocleidomastoideus).

Classical Location: Above the supraclavicular fossa, one inch below LI-18. *(The Great Compendium)*

Local Anatomy: The external jugular vein; Superficially, the supraclavicular nerve on the posterior border of sternocleidomastoid muscle (m. sternocleidomastoideus) just where the cutaneous cervical nerve emerges; deeper, the phrenic nerve.

Functions: Disinhibits the throat and clears lung qi.

Indications: Sore, swollen throat; loss of voice; scrofulous lumps; qi goiter.

Supplementary Indications: Fulminant loss of voice and qi blockage; throat bi; throat rattle.

Stimulation: 0.3-0.5" perpendicular insertion.
Moxa: 3-7 cones; pole 5-10 min.

LI-18
扶突
fú tú

"*Protuberance Assistant*"

Location: On the lateral aspect of the neck, level with the tip of the Adam's apple, between the sternal head and clavicular head of the sternocleidomastoid muscle (m. sternocleidomastoideus).

Classical Location: Going up from LI-17, it is one inch below the angle of the mandible, and one inch and five fen behind ST-9. The point is found in supine posture. *(The Golden Mirror)*

Local Anatomy: Deeper on the medial side, the ascending cervical artery and vein. The great auricular nerve, the cutaneous cervical nerve, lesser occipital nerve and accessory nerve.

Functions: Regulates qi and blood; disinhibits the throat.

Indications: Cough, asthma; sore, swollen throat; loss of voice; scrofulous lumps; qi goiter.

Supplementary Indications: Frog rattle in the throat; inhibited throat.

Stimulation: 0.3″ perpendicular insertion;
Moxa: 4 cones; pole 5-10 min.

Location: Directly below the lateral margin of the nostril, level with GV-26.

Classical Location: Below the nostril, five fen from the philtrum. *(The Great Compendium)*

Local Anatomy: The superior labial branches of the facial artery and vein. The anastomotic branch of the facial nerve and the infraorbital nerve.

Functions: Diffuses lung qi and clears lung heat; clears the nose and rouses the spirit.

Indications: Nosebleed; nasal congestion; wryness of the mouth.

Supplementary Indications: Nasal sores and polyps; runny nose with clear snivel; clenched jaws; death-like inversion.

Illustrative Point Combinations & Applications: For nosebleed, use GV-23 and LI-19.
(Song of Point Applications for Miscellaneous Disease)

Stimulation: 0.2-0.3″ inward oblique insertion.
Moxa: contraindicated.

Needle Sensation: Localized distention and pain.

LI-19

口禾髎

hé liáo

"Grain Bone-Hole"

LI-20
迎香
yíng xiāng
"Welcome Fragrance"

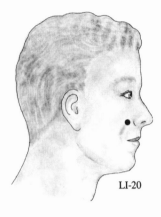

LI-20

Figure 7.7

Location: In the nasolabial groove, at the level of the midpoint of the lateral border of ala nasi.

Classical Location: Up one inch from LI-19, five fen to the side of the nostril. *(The Great Compendium)*

Local Anatomy: The facial artery and vein, the branches of the infraorbital artery and vein. The anastomotic branch of the facial and infraorbital nerves.

Functions: Unblocks the nose; dissipates the wind pathogen; clears qi fire.

Indications: Nasal congestion; nosebleed; wryness of the mouth; facial itching; facial swelling.

Supplementary Indications: Nasal polyps; heat and redness of the eye.

Illustrative Point Combinations & Applications: LI-20, when bled, provides marvelous treatment for heat and reddening of the eyes; it can be combined with GB-15, LV-3, and LI-4.
(Song of Point Applications for Miscellaneous Disease)

Nasal congestion impeding the sense of smell can be treated with LI-20, combined with GV-23.
(Wo Yan's Efficacious Point Applications)

Stimulation: 0.3 " downward or oblique insertion. Can also be needled medially or upward.
Moxa: contraindicated.

Point Categories & Associations: Intersection-jiaohui point of the hand yang ming large intestine and foot yang ming stomach channels.

Point	Location	Indications	
		Primary	**Secondary**
*LI-1	Index finger	Deafness toothache swelling of the jaw pain and swelling of the throat	Stupor heat disease
LI-2		Visual dizziness nosebleed toothache wry mouth	
*LI-3		Lower toothache pain and swelling of the throat	
*LI-4	Back of hand	Headache nosebleed deafness toothache wry mouth pain and swelling of the throat	Heat disease copious perspiration
*LI-5	Wrist	Headache red eyes deafness toothache	
*LI-6	Forearm	Nosebleed	Edema
LI-7		Headache facial swelling pain and swelling of the throat	Intestinal rumbling abdominal pain
LI-8		Arm and elbow pain	Abdominal pain
LI-9		Paralysis of the upper limbs	Intestinal rumbling abdominal pain
*LI-10		Toothache swelling of the cheeks paralysis of the upper limbs	Abdominal pain diarrhea
*LI-11	Elbow	Pain and swelling of the throat paralysis of the upper limbs	Heat disease dormant papules abdominal pain ejection drainage
Hand to Elbow: Disorders of the head, face, eyes, nose, mouth and teeth; heat disease			

Hand Yang Ming Large Intestine Channel

Hand to Elbow: Disorders of the head, face, eyes, nose, mouth and teeth; heat disease

Hand Yang Ming Large Intestine Channel (continued)			
Point	Location	Indications	
		Primary	**Secondary**
LI-12		Upper arm and elbow pain	
LI-13	Upper arm	Upper arm and elbow pain	
*LI-14		Upper arm pain	
*LI-15		Shoulder and upper arm pain paralysis of the upper limbs	
LI-16	Shoulder	Shoulder and upper arm pain	
Upper arm and shoulder: Localized disorders			
LI-17	Neck	Sudden loss of voice pain and swelling of the throat	
*LI-18		Sudden loss of voice pain and swelling of the throat	
Neck: Disorders of the throat			
LI-19	Face	Nasal congestion nosebleed wry mouth	
*LI-20		Nasal congestion deep source nasal congestion nosebleed wry mouth	
Face: Disorders of the nose			

8. The Stomach Channel System (Foot Yang Ming) 足陽明胃經

8.1 The Primary Stomach Channel

Pathway: The foot yang ming stomach channel starts at the side of the nose, and then ascends to the inner canthus of the eye to intersect the foot tai yang bladder channel at BL-1. It then descends parallel to the nose, penetrates the maxilla into the upper gum and joins the governing vessel at GV-26 in the philtrum. It skirts back along the upper and lower lips to join the conception vessel at CV-24 in the mentolabial groove on the chin. From this point it runs along the mandible to the point ST-5 and rounds the angle of the mandible to ST-6. It proceeds upward in front of the ear, intersects with the foot shao yang gallbladder channel at GB-3, and continues along the hairline. It then intersects the foot shao yang channel again at GB-6, crosses to the middle of the forehead and intersects with the governing vessel at GV-24.

A branch separates at ST-5, runs down the throat to ST-9, and then continues down to the supraclavicular fossa. From there it crosses through to the back to intersect the governing vessel at GV-14, and then descends internally, crosses the diaphragm and intersects with the conception vessel internally at CV-13 and CV-12 before homing to the stomach and connecting with the spleen.

Another branch separates at ST-12, runs down the surface of the trunk along the mammillary line, and continues downward, passing beside the umbilicus to enter the qi thoroughfare (the inguinal region) at ST-30.

Yet another branch starts in the area of the pylorus, descends internally to join the branch just described at ST-30 in the inguinal region. It emerges here and runs down to ST-31 on the anterior aspect of the thigh. It then travels down the thigh to the high point above the knee at ST-32, continues to the patella, then proceeds downward along the lateral side of the tibia to ST-42 on the dorsum of the foot and terminates at the lateral side of the tip of the second toe.

A branch separates at ST-36, three body-inches below the knee, and runs down lateral and parallel to the main branch, terminating on the lateral side of the middle toe.

Still another branch breaks off from the main branch on the dorsum of the foot at ST-42, terminating on the medial side of the great toe, where it connects with the spleen channel at SP-1.

Main pathologic signs associated with the external course of the channel: high fever or malaria; flushed face; sweating; clouding of the spirit and delirium; manic agitation; aversion to cold; pain in the eyes; dry nose and nosebleed; lesions of the lips and in the mouth; sore larynx; swelling in the neck; wryness of the mouth; chest pain; cold or pain, redness, and swelling in the lower limbs.

Main pathologic signs associated with the internal organ: pronounced abdominal distention, fullness, and edema; restlessness and discomfort while active or recumbent; or mania and withdrawal. There may also be hyperpepsia and rapid hungering, and yellow urine.

Exuberance of qi: heat in the anterior aspect of the body; persistent hunger; yellow urine.

Insufficiency of qi: cold in the anterior aspect of the body; shivering; stomach cold resulting in distention and fullness.

8.2 The Connecting Vessel of the Stomach Channel

Pathway: This vessel separates from the primary channel at ST-40 and connects to the foot tai yin spleen channel. Another branch begins at the same point (ST-40) and ascends along the lateral aspect of the lower leg and up the upper leg and trunk to the crown of the head where it unites with the other yang channels above, and connects with the throat and the upper opening of the esophagus below.

Main pathologic signs:

Qi counterflow in the vessel; throat bi and sudden loss of voice.

Repletion: mania and withdrawal.

Vacuity: atony of the lower leg muscles.

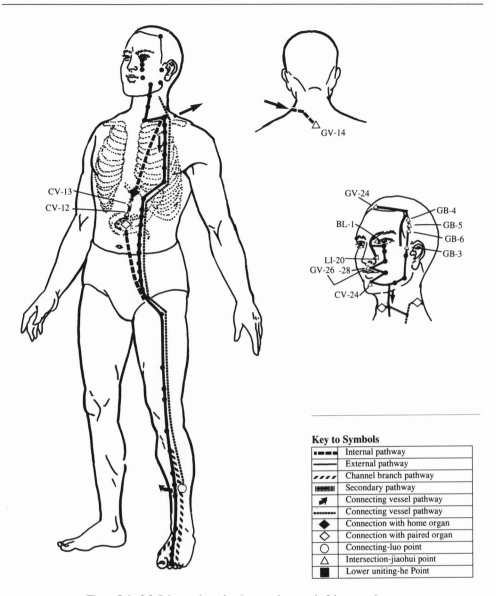

Key to Symbols

▪▬▬▪	Internal pathway
▬▬	External pathway
⁄⁄⁄⁄	Channel branch pathway
⫿⫿⫿⫿	Secondary pathway
➚	Connecting vessel pathway
▪▪▪▪▪▪	Connecting vessel pathway
◆	Connection with home organ
◇	Connection with paired organ
○	Connecting-luo point
△	Intersection-jiaohui point
■	Lower uniting-he Point

Figure 8.1 - 8.2 Primary channel and connecting vessel of the stomach.

8.3 The Stomach Channel Divergence

Pathway: This pathway diverges from the primary channel at the thigh and enters the abdominal cavity where it homes to the stomach and disperses over the spleen. It then rises passing the heart and following the pharynx to issue at the mouth. It then continues upward past the root of the nose to the suborbital region. The divergence then enters inward behind the eye and unites with the primary channel.

111

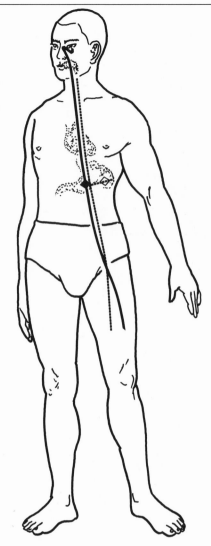

Figure 8.3 Channel divergences of the stomach and spleen.

8.4 The Stomach Channel Sinews

Pathway: These sinews originate at the middle three toes and bind at the top of the dorsum of the foot. The sinews then slant laterally and rise upward along the lateral aspect of the shin and bind at the lateral aspect of the knee. From here, this branch rises to bind at the hip and then follows the ribs and homes to the spine.

Another branch forks from the ankle and follows the tibia upward and binds at the knee. Here a branch binds outward to the lateral side of the fibia and unites with the foot shao yang gallbladder channel. The main branch rises from the knee, crosses the thigh, binds at the inguinal region and gathers at the genitals. The sinews then ascend the abdomen, bind at the supraclavicular fossa and travel up the neck and "pinch" the mouth. They unite at the side of the nose. At this point the sinews unite with those of the foot tai yang bladder channel. The sinews of the foot tai yang channel enmesh above the eye and the sinews of the foot yang ming channel enmesh below the eye. There is another sub-branch that separates at the jaw and binds in front of the ear.

Main pathologic signs: Strained middle toe; spasms of the lower leg; hardened muscles in the foot, pain and spasms of the thigh muscles; swellings in the inguinal region; kui shan; abdominal sinew tension or spasms extending to the neck and jaw; sudden dryness of the mouth; spasms (cold pathogen) with inability to close the eye; heat (pathogen) with inability to open the eye. If the sinews of the jaw receive cold they become tense and pull the mouth to an abnormal position; if these sinews receive heat they become loose and this results in wryness of the mouth.

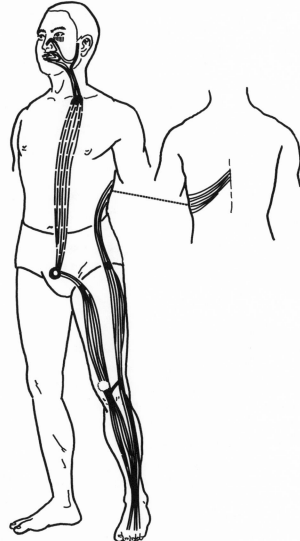

Figure 8.4 The stomach channel sinews.

ST-1
承泣
chéng qì

"Tear Container"

Location: Between the eyeball and the midpoint of the infraorbital ridge.

Classical Location: In the depression in the lower eyelid, seven fen below the eye, level with the pupil when the eye looks straight forward. *(The Great Compendium)*

Local Anatomy: The branches of the infraorbital and ophthalmic arteries and veins. The branch of the intraorbital nerve, the inferior branch of the oculomotor nerve and the muscular branch of the facial nerve.

Functions: Dispels wind and dissipates fire; courses pathogens and brightens the eyes.

Indications: Painful, red eyes; tearing when exposed to wind; night blindness; wryness of the mouth and eyes; twitching of the eyelids.

Supplementary Indications: Nearsightedness.

Stimulation: 0.3-0.7″ perpendicular insertion.

Needle Sensation: Localized needle stimulus sensation and distention.

Contraindications: Deep insertion contraindication.
Moxa: contraindicated.

Point Categories & Associations: Intersection-jiaohui point of the foot yang ming stomach channel and yang motility and conception vessels.

ST-2
四白
sì bái

"Four Whites"

Location: In the depression at the infraorbital foramen.

Classical Location: Three fen below ST-1, in the hollow of the cheekbone, level with the pupil. *(The Golden Mirror)*

Local Anatomy: The branches of the facial artery and vein, the infraorbital artery and vein. The branches of the facial nerve (the point lies exactly on the course of the infraorbital nerve).

Functions: Courses wind and quickens the connecting vessels; soothes the sinews and relieves pain.

Indications: Painful, red eyes; wryness of the eyes and mouth; twitching of the eyelids; facial pain.

Supplementary Indications: Headache; dizziness; itchy eyelid rims.

Stimulation: 0.2-0.3″ perpendicular insertion.
Needle Sensation: Localized needle stimulus sensation and distention that sometimes radiates upwards.

Contraindications: Deep insertion contraindication.
Moxa: contraindicated

Location: Directly below the pupil, at the level of the lower border of ala nasi, on the lateral side of the nasolabial groove.	**ST-3**

Location: Directly below the pupil, at the level of the lower border of ala nasi, on the lateral side of the nasolabial groove.
Classical Location: Down from ST-2, in line with ST-1 and ST-2, eight fen out from the nostrils. *(The Golden Mirror)*
Local Anatomy: The branches of the facial and infraorbital arteries and veins. The branches of the facial and infraorbital nerves.

ST-3
巨髎
jù liáo
"Great Bone-Hole"

Functions: Courses wind and quickens the connecting vessels; disperses swelling and relieves pain.
Indications: Wryness of the eyes and mouth; twitching of the eyelids; nosebleed; toothache; swelling of the lips and cheek.
Supplementary Indications: Nearsightedness; tearing; aversion to wind and cold in the face; eye screens.
Illustrative Point Combinations & Applications: Blood stasis lodged in the diaphragm and chest can be treated with ST-3 and BL-23. *(Ode of a Hundred Patterns)*

Stimulation: 0.3-0.4″ perpendicular insertion.
Moxa: 5 cones; pole 5 min.

Point Categories & Associations: Intersection-jiaohui point of the hand yang ming large intestine and foot yang ming stomach channels and the yang motility vessel.

Location: Lateral to the corner of the mouth, directly below ST-3.
Classical Location: Below ST-3, about four fen out from the corner of the mouth. Close below, a pulsating vessel can be faintly felt. *(The Golden Mirror)*
Local Anatomy: The facial artery and vein. Superficially the branches of the facial and infraorbital nerves; deeper, the terminal branch of the buccal nerve.

ST-4
地倉
dì cāng
"Earth Granary"

Functions: Dispels wind; frees qi stagnation.

Indications: Wryness of the mouth; drooling; twitching of the eyelids.

Supplementary Indications: Loss of speech; loss of voice; fecal stoppage in children; inability to close the eyes; inability to eat.

Illustrative Point Combinations & Applications: ST-4 and ST-6 for wryness of the mouth. *(Ode of the Jade Dragon)*

Stimulation: 0.5-1.0" oblique insertion towards ST-6.
Moxa: 3-7 cones; pole 5 min.

Needle Sensation: Localized needle stimulus sensation and distention.

Point Categories & Associations: Intersection-jiaohui point of the foot yang ming stomach and hand yang ming large intestine channels and the conception and yang motility vessels.

ST-5
大迎
dà yíng
"Great Reception"

Location: Anterior to the angle of the mandible, on the anterior border of masseter muscle (m. masseter), in the groove-like depression appearing when the cheek is bulged.

Classical Location: One inch and two fen from the angle of the mandible, in the depression in the bone in which a pulsation can be felt. *(The Great Compendium)*

Local Anatomy: Anteriorly, the facial artery and vein. The facial and buccal nerves.

Functions: Courses wind and quickens the connecting vessels.

Indications: Clenched jaws; wryness of the mouth; swelling of the cheek; toothache.

Supplementary Indications: Fever; stiff tongue inhibiting speech; scrofulous lumps; fullness in the stomach; counterflow dyspnea; inability to chew; frequent yawning; inability to close the eyes; dislocation of the jaw.

Stimulation: 0.3" oblique insertion towards ST-6. Avoid the artery. Alternatively, 0.5-1.5" transverse insertion joining CV-24 or ST-6.
Moxa: 3 cones; pole 5-10 min.

Location: One finger breadth anterior and superior to the lower angle of the mandible where the masseter muscle (m. masseter) attaches. At the prominence of the muscle when the teeth are clenched.

Classical Location: Eight fen below the ear, in the depression just in front of the angle of the mandible. The point is found in lateral recumbent posture, in the hollow that appears when the mouth is opened. *(The Great Compendium)*

Local Anatomy: The masseteric artery. The great auricular nerve, facial nerve and masseteric nerve.

Functions: Opens the jaw and frees the connecting vessels; dispels wind and regulates qi.

Indications: Wryness of the mouth; swelling of the cheek; toothache; clenched jaws; painful stiffness of the neck; mumps.

Supplementary Indications: Loss of voice; aversion to wind and cold.

Illustrative Point Combinations & Applications: For wryness of the mouth and eyes, use ST-6 and ST-4.
(Song of the Jade Dragon)

Stimulation: 0.3-0.5″ perpendicular insertion, or oblique insertion toward ST-4.
Moxa: 3 cones; pole 15 min.

Point Categories & Associations: The seventh of the thirteen ghost points.

ST-6
頰車
jiá chē
"Jawbone"

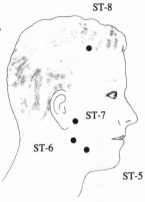

Figure 8.5

Location: In the depression at the lower border of the zygomatic arch, anterior to the condyloid process of the mandible.

Classical Location: Below GB-3, on the lower aspect of the pulsating vessel in front of the ear. A hollow felt when the mouth is closed disappears when the mouth is opened. The point is found with the patient in lateral recumbent posture and mouth closed. *(The Great Compendium)*

Local Anatomy: Superficially, the transverse facial artery and vein; at the deepest level, the maxillary artery and vein. The zygomatic branch of the facial nerve and the branches of the auriculotemporal nerve.

ST-7
下關
xià guān
"Below the Joint"

117

Functions: Courses wind and quickens the connecting vessels; opens the portals and sharpens the hearing.

Indications: Deafness; tinnitus; ear pain with purulent discharge; wryness of the mouth and eyes; toothache; inhibited opening and closing of the jaws.

Supplementary Indications: Trismus; loss of voice; aversion to wind and cold.

Stimulation: 0.3-0.5 " perpendicular insertion; 1.0-1.5 " transverse insertion joining ST-6. Moxa: 3 cones; pole 5-10 min.

Point Categories & Associations: Intersection-jiaohui point of the foot yang ming stomach and foot shao yang gallbladder channels.

ST-8
頭維
tóu wéi

"Head Corner"

Location: 0.5 " within the anterior hairline at the corner of the forehead, 4.5 " lateral to the governing vessel.

Classical Location: At the corners of the forehead within the hair-line, one inch and five fen to the side of GB-13, four inches and five fen from GV-24. *(The Great Compendium)*

Local Anatomy: The frontal branches of the superficial temporal artery and vein. The branch of the auriculotemporal nerve and temporal branch of the facial nerve.

Functions: Dispels wind and discharges fire; relieves pain; clears the head and brightens the eyes.

Indications: Headache; visual dizziness; eye pain; tearing when exposed to wind.

Supplementary Indications: Dyspnea counterflow; vexation and fullness; splitting headache; eyes painful as if fit to burst from their sockets.

Illustrative Point Combinations & Applications: BL-2 and ST-8 treat headache and eye pain. *(Ode of the Jade Dragon)*

Stimulation: 0.5-1.0 " upward or downward transverse insertion. Moxa: pole 5-10 min.

Point Categories & Associations: Intersection-jiaohui point of the foot yang ming stomach and foot shao yang gallbladder channels.

Location: Level with the tip of the Adam's apple, on the course of the common carotid artery, at the anterior border of the sterno-cleidomastoid muscle (m. sternocleidomastoideus).

Classical Location: At the major pulsating vessel of the neck, one inch and five fen to the side of the Adam's apple. *(The Great Compendium)*

Local Anatomy: The superior thyroid artery, the anterior jugular vein; laterally, the internal jugular vein; on the bifurcation of the internal and the external carotid artery. Superficially, the cutaneous cervical nerve, the cervical branch of the facial nerve; deeper, the sympathetic trunk; laterally, the ascending branch of the hypoglossal and vagus nerves.

Functions: Frees the channels and connecting vessels; regulates qi and the blood; clears heat and calms dyspnea.

Indications: Sore, swollen throat; dyspnea; dizziness; red facial complexion.

Supplementary Indications: Cough; pain, fullness, or thoracic oppression; goiter; scrofulous lumps; vomiting and hiccoughing; headache; fever; tinnitus; lumbar pain.

Stimulation: 0.3-0.5″ perpendicular insertion.

To avoid the artery, push it towards the sternocleidomastoid muscle (m. sternocleidomastoideus) with the thumb and index finger of the left hand.

Point Categories & Associations: Intersection-jiaohui point of foot yang ming stomach and foot shao yang gallbladder channels.

ST-9
人迎
rén yíng
"Man's Prognosis"

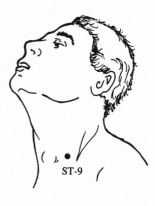

Figure 8.6

Location: At the anterior margin of the sternocleidomastoid muscle (m. sternocleidomastoideus), midway between ST-9 and ST-11.

Classical Location: In front of the major sinew of the neck, directly below ST-9 and above ST-11. *(The Great Compendium)*

Local Anatomy: The common carotid artery. Superficially, the cutaneous cervical nerve; deeper, the superior cardiac nerve that issues from the sympathetic nerve and the sympathetic trunk.

ST-10
水突
shuǐ tú
"Water Prominence"

119

Supplementary Indications: Cough from counterflow qi ascent; spitting of turbid foam, pus, and blood; pain in the chest; branching fullness in the chest and lateral costal region.

Stimulation: 0.3″ downward oblique insertion.
Moxa: 3-5 cones; pole 5-15 min.

ST-15
屋翳
wū yì

"Roof"

Location: In the 2nd intercostal space, on the mammillary line.

Classical Location: One inch and six fen below ST-13, four inches from the median line. The point is found in supine posture.
(The Great Compendium)

Local Anatomy: The pectoral branch of the thoracoacromial artery and vein, second intercostal artery and vein. The anterior cutaneous branches of the thoracic nerves, and the medial pectoral nerve.

Functions: Courses wind and relieves pain.

Indications: Cough, dyspnea; thoracic pain and distention; mammary yong.

Supplementary Indications: Cough from counterflow qi ascent; pain in the breast; generalized wind itching or pain with discomfort exacerbated by clothes; pain and lack of strength in the limbs; infantile dyspnea with distention.

Illustrative Point Combinations & Applications: BL-67 and ST-15 treat itching diseases that are accompanied by pain.
(Ode of a Hundred Patterns)

Stimulation: 0.3″ downward oblique insertion.
Moxa: 3-5 cones; pole 5-15 min.

ST-16
膺窗
yīng chuāng

"Breast Window"

Location: In the third intercostal space, on the mammillary line.

Classical Location: In the depression one inch and six fen below ST-15, four inches either side of the median line.
(The Great Compendium)

Local Anatomy: The lateral thoracic artery and vein. The branch of the anterior thoracic nerve.

Functions: Clears heat and resolves depression; relieves pain and disperses swelling.

Indications: Cough; asthma; thoracic pain and distention; breast yong.

Supplementary Indications: Wheezing and dyspnea; cough counterflow; fever and chills; thoracic fullness and shortness of breath; restless sleep; pain in the ribs; intestinal shan pain; swelling of the lips; rumbling intestines and outpour diarrhea.

Stimulation: 0.3″ downward oblique insertion.
Moxa: 3-5 cones; pole 5-15 min.

Location: In the center of the nipple.
Classical Location: Center of the nipple.
(The Great Compendium)

Note: This point serves primarily to determine points on the chest and abdomen. The distance between the two nipples is measured as 8.0″.
Local Anatomy: The anterior and lateral cutaneous branches of the 4th intercostal nerve.

Contraindications: Acupuncture and moxibustion contraindicated.

ST-17
乳中
rǔ zhōng
"Breast Center"

Location: In the fifth intercostal space, one rib below the nipple.
Classical Location: In the depression one inch and six fen below ST-17, four inches either side of the midline. The point is found in supine posture. *(The Great Compendium)*
Local Anatomy: The branches of the intercostal artery and vein. The branch of the 5th intercostal nerve.

Functions: Diffuses the connecting vessels of the breast; quickens the blood and transforms depression.
Indications: Cough; asthma; breast yong; scant breast milk; thoracic pain.
Supplementary Indications: Cough counterflow and distressed rapid breathing; pain and swelling of the breast; pain and oppression below the chest; esophageal constriction with difficult ingestion; abdominal fullness; shortness of breath; eructation; retention of afterbirth.
Illustrative Point Combinations & Applications: ST-18 with KI-27 treats cough and wheezing. *(Ode of the Jade Dragon)*

Stimulation: 0.3″ upward oblique insertion.
Moxa: 5 cones; pole 5-20 min.

ST-18
乳根
rǔ gēn
"Breast Root"

ST-19
不容

bù róng

"Not Contained"

Location: 6″ above the umbilicus and 2″ lateral to CV-14.

Classical Location: At the end of the fourth rib below ST-18, two inches either side of the center line. *(The Great Compendium)*

Local Anatomy: Branches of the 7th intercostal artery and vein, branches of the superior epigastric artery and vein. Branch of the 7th intercostal nerve.

Functions: Regulates the center and harmonizes the stomach.

Indications: Abdominal distention; vomiting; stomach pain; poor appetite.

Supplementary Indications: Blood ejection; cough and dyspnea; chest and back pain; difficult ingestion; shrugging of the shoulders to facilitate breathing; dry mouth; infantile eye gan; night blindness; vacuity rumbling of the intestines.

Stimulation: 0.5-0.7″ perpendicular insertion.
Moxa: 5 cones; pole 5-20 min.

ST-20
承滿

chéng mǎn

"Assuming Fullness"

Location: 5″ above the umbilicus, 2″ lateral to CV-13, or 1″ below ST-19.

Classical Location: One inch below ST-19, two inches either side of the midline. *(The Golden Mirror)*

Local Anatomy: See ST-19.

Functions: Harmonizes the stomach and rectifies qi.

Indications: Stomach pain; abdominal distention; vomiting; poor appetite.

Supplementary Indications: Rumbling intestines and shan pain; difficult ingestion; diarrhea or dysentery; jaundice; painful hardening beneath the ribs; counterflow qi ascent dyspnea; spitting blood.

Stimulation: 0.7-10″ perpendicular insertion.
Moxa: 5 cones; pole 5-20 min.

Location: 4″ above the umbilicus, 2″ lateral to CV-12.

Classical Location: One inch below ST-20, two inches either side of the midline. *(The Golden Mirror)*

Local Anatomy: Branches of the 8th intercostal and superior epigastric arteries and veins.

ST-21
梁門
liáng mén
"Beam Gate"

Functions: Regulates center qi; harmonizes the stomach and intestines; transforms accumulations and stagnations; fortifies the spleen, strengthening its function of moving and transforming the digestate.

Indications: Stomach pain; vomiting; poor appetite; thin stool.

Supplementary Indications: Qi accumulation beneath the lateral costal region; no thought of food; pain in the venter; efflux diarrhea; shan pain; prolapse of the rectum; painful binding accumulation of qi in the abdomen; untransformed digestate in the stool.

Stimulation: 0.7-1.0″ perpendicular insertion.
Moxa: 5 cones; pole 5-20 min.

Needle Sensation: Localized distention or feeling of heaviness, sometimes spreading downward and outward.

Location: 3″ above the umbilicus, 2″ lateral to CV-11, or 1″ below ST-21.

Classical Location: One inch below ST-21, two inches either side of the midline. *(The Golden Mirror)*

Local Anatomy: See ST-21.

ST-22
關門
guān mén
"Pass Gate"

Functions: Regulates the stomach and intestines.

Indications: Abdominal distention and pain; rumbling intestines and diarrhea; poor appetite; water swelling.

Supplementary Indications: Thoracic fullness and qi accumulation; pain in the venter; acute umbilical pain; enuresis; constipation; no desire to eat; phlegm malaria with quivering from cold; abdominal qi movement.

Stimulation: 0.7-1.0″ perpendicular insertion.
Moxa: 5 cones; pole 5-20 min.

ST-23
太乙
tài yǐ

"Supreme Unity"

Location: 2″ above the umbilicus, 2″ lateral to CV-10.

Classical Location: One inch below ST-22, two inches either side of the midline. *(The Golden Mirror)*

Local Anatomy: Branches of the 8th and 9th intercostal and inferior epigastric arteries and veins. Branches of the 8th and 9th intercostal nerves.

Functions: Clears the heart and quiets the spirit; fortifies the spleen and harmonizes the center.

Indications: Mania and withdrawal; vexation; stomach pain; indigestion.

Supplementary Indications: Intestinal shan; enuresis; protrusion of the tongue; foot qi.

Stimulation: 0.7-1.0″ perpendicular insertion.
Moxa 5 cones; pole 5-20 min.

ST-24
滑肉門
huá ròu mén

*"Slippery
    Flesh Gate"*

Location: 1″ above the umbilicus, 2″ lateral to CV-9.

Classical Location: One inch below ST-23, two inches either side of the midline. *(The Golden Mirror)*

Local Anatomy: Branches of the 9th intercostal and inferior epigastric arteries and veins. Branch of the 9th intercostal nerve.

Functions: Quiets the spirit and stabilizes the disposition; regulates and harmonizes the stomach and intestines.

Indications: Mania and withdrawal; vomiting; stomach pain.

Supplementary Indications: Stiff tongue; vomiting of blood; gastrointestinal disorders; prolapse of the rectum; counterflow retching; protrusion of the tongue.

Stimulation: 0.5-1.0″ perpendicular insertion.
Moxa: 5 cones; pole 5-20 min.

ST-25
天樞
tiān shū

"Celestial Pivot"

Location: 2″ lateral to the center of the umbilicus (CV-8).

Classical Location: One inch below ST-24, in the depression two inches lateral to the center of the navel. *(The Golden Mirror)*

Local Anatomy: Branches of the 10th intercostal and inferior epigastric arteries and veins.

Functions: Courses and regulates the large intestine; supports earth and transforms damp.

Indications: Abdominal pain; diarrhea; dysentery; constipation; borborygmi; abdominal distention; edema; irregular menstruation.

Supplementary Indications: Turbid strangury; infertility; severe heat with raving; umbilical shan with localized pain sometimes surging up into the heart; qi shan; retching; facial swelling; running piglet; untransformed digestate; generalized swelling; uterine pain; inhibited urination; cholera; persistent diarrhea; frequent defecation.

Illustrative Point Combinations & Applications: Persistent dysentery with abdominal pain can be treated with ST-25 and ST-36.

Persistent dysentery can be treated with ST-25, as well as with PC-6 and SP-6. *(Ode to Elucidate Mysteries)*

Stimulation: 0.5-1.2 perpendicular insertion.
Moxa: 7-15 cones; pole 10-20 min.

Point Categories & Associations: Alarm-mu point of the large intestine.

Location: 1″ below the umbilicus, 2″ lateral to CV-7, or 1″ below ST-25.

Classical Location: One inch below ST-25, two inches either side of the midline. *(The Golden Mirror)*

Local Anatomy: See ST-25.

Functions: Dissipates cold; relieves pain; rectifies qi.

Indications: Abdominal pain; hernia.

Supplementary Indications: Menstrual pain.

Stimulation: 0.5-1.2″ perpendicular insertion.
Moxa: 7-15 cones; pole 10-20 min.

ST-26

外陵

wài líng

"Outer Mound"

Location: 2″ below the umbilicus, 2″ lateral to CV-5.

Classical Location: One inch below ST-26, two inches either side of the midline. *(The Golden Mirror)*

Local Anatomy: Branches of the 11th intercostal artery and vein; laterally, the inferior epigastric artery and vein. The 11th intercostal nerve.

ST-27

大巨

dà jù

"Great Gigantic"

Functions: Supplements the kidney and boosts qi; invigorates yang.

Indications: Lower abdominal distention and fullness; inhibited urination; hernia; seminal emission; premature ejaculation.

Supplementary Indications: Kui shan; hemiplegia; fatigued limbs; loss of sleep and susceptibility to fright; vexation thirst.

Stimulation: 0.5-1.2 ″ perpendicular insertion.
Moxa 7-15 cones; pole 10-20 min.

ST-28
水道
shuǐ dào

"Waterway"

Location: 3 ″ below the umbilicus; 2 ″ lateral to CV-4.

Classical Location: One inch below ST-27, two inches either side of CV-4. *(A Concise Acupuncture Text)*

The Great Compendium lists the location of this point as three inches below ST-27.

Local Anatomy: Branches of the subcostal artery and vein; laterally the inferior epigastric artery and vein. Branch of the subcostal nerve.

Functions: Clears damp-heat and disinhibits the lower burner.

Indications: Lower abdominal distention and fullness; hernia; urinary stoppage.

Supplementary Indications: Vulpine shan; cold in the bladder; heat binding in the triple burner; menstrual low back pain; uterine conglomeration.

Illustrative Point Combinations & Applications: For water diseases, which are among the most insufferable, and abdominal fullness and vacuity distention failing to disperse, first apply moxa at CV-9 and ST-28, and then needle ST-36 and CV-7.
(Song of the Jade Dragon)

Stimulation: 0.5-1.2 ″ perpendicular insertion.
Moxa: 7-15 cones; pole 10-30 min.

ST-29
歸來
guī lái

"Return"

Location: 4 ″ below the umbilicus, 2 ″ lateral to CV-3.

Classical Location: Two inches below ST-28, two inches either side of the midline. *(The Great Compendium)*

Local Anatomy: Laterally, the inferior epigastric artery and vein. The iliohypogastric nerve.

Functions: Rectifies the lower burner; warms the womb.

Indications: Abdominal pain; hernia; menstrual block; prolapse of the uterus.

Supplementary Indications: Running piglet; the seven shan; retraction of the testicles; frigidity, swelling and pain of the genitals; vaginal discharge; accumulated frigidity of the blood storehouse (uterus); impotence.

Stimulation: 0.5-1.2″ perpendicular insertion.
Moxa: 7-15 cones; pole 10-20 min.

Location: 5″ below the umbilicus, 2″ lateral to CV-2, superior to the inguinal groove, on the medial side of the femoral artery.

Classical Location: One inch below ST-29, two inches either side of the midline, in the depression where a pulsating vessel — the starting point of the penetrating vessel — can be felt.
(The Great Compendium)

Local Anatomy: Branches of the superficial epigastric artery and vein; laterally the inferior epigastric artery and vein. The pathway of the ilioinguinal nerve.

Functions: Soothes the sinew gathering; dissipates inversion qi; regulates the bladder; harmonizes construction and the blood.

Indications: Pain and swelling of the external genitalia; hernia; menstrual disorders.

Supplementary Indications: Shan pain and sagging; running piglet; non-conception; fullness in the lateral costal region; abdominal pain; fulminant abdominal distention and fullness; prolapse of the rectum; sensation of pain and weakness (in the shins); urinary stoppage; heat strangury; stone water swelling; difficulty in lactation; fetus surging up into the heart causing pain that makes rest difficult; impotence; gastrosplenic vacuity; rumbling intestines.

Stimulation: 0.5-1.0″ perpendicular insertion.
Moxa: 3-7 cones; pole 5-15 min.

ST-30
氣衝
qì chōng
"Surging Qi"

Location: Below the anterior superior iliac spine, nearly level with the perineum, in the depression on the lateral side of the sartorius muscle (m. sartorius) when the thigh is flexed.

Classical Location: In the parting of the flesh behind the crouching rabbit above the knee. *(The Systematized Canon)*

ST-31
髀關
bì guān
"Inferior Joint"

129

Local Anatomy: At the deep level, the branches of the lateral circumflex femoral artery and vein. The lateral femoral cutaneous nerve.

Functions: Warms the channels and quickens the connecting vessels; courses wind and dissipates cold.

Indications: Pain in the thigh; atrophy, bi, and impeded bending and stretching of the lower extremities.

Supplementary Indications: Pain in the lumbus and cold in the knees; abdominal pain; numbness of the lower extremities; jaundice.

Stimulation: 0.5-1.5″ perpendicular insertion.
Moxa: 3 cones; pole 5-15 min.

ST-32
伏兔

fú tù

"Crouching
Rabbit"

Location: 6″ above the laterosuperior border of the patella, on the line connecting the anterior superior iliac spine and lateral border of the patella.

Classical Location: At the prominence of the flesh six inches above the knee. *(The Systematized Canon)*

Local Anatomy: Branches of the lateral circumflex femoral artery and vein. The anterior and lateral femoral cutaneous nerves.

Functions: Warms the channels and dissipates cold; courses wind and quickens the connecting vessels.

Indications: Pain in the lumbar and iliac region; cold knees; paralysis of the lower limbs; beriberi.

Supplementary Indications: Shan; mania evil; diminished qi.

Stimulation: 0.5-1.5″ perpendicular insertion.
Moxa: 3-5 cones; pole 5-15 min.

ST-33
陰市

yīn shì

"Yin Market"

Location: 3″ above the laterosuperior border of the patella.

Classical Location: Three inches above the knee, in the depression below the crouching rabbit. The point is found in a kneeling position. *(The Great Compendium)*

Local Anatomy: The descending branch of the lateral circumflex femoral artery. The anterior and lateral femoral cutaneous nerves.

Functions: Courses wind and dissipates cold; frees the channels and quickens the connecting vessels; disinhibits the joints.

Indications: Paralysis, pain, and inhibited bending and stretching of the lower extremities.

Supplementary Indications: Cold shan pain; abdominal distention and fullness; cold in the knees; hypertonicity of the lower extremities.

Illustrative Point Combinations & Applications: GB-31 and ST-33 eliminate lack of strength in the legs and feet.
(Ode of the Jade Dragon)

Pain in the thighs and knees can be cured with stimulation of ST-33 combined with GB-31.
(Wo Yan's Efficacious Point Applications)

Stimulation: 0.5-1.0″ perpendicular insertion.
Moxa: 3-5 cones; pole 5-15 min.

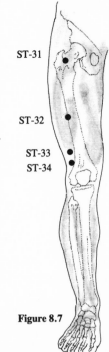

ST-31

ST-32

ST-33

ST-34

Figure 8.7

Location: 2″ above the laterosuperior border of the patella.
Classical Location: Two inches above the knee, one inch below ST-33 in the depression between two sinews.
(The Golden Mirror)
Local Anatomy: See ST-33.

ST-34
梁丘
liáng qiū
"Beam Hill"

Functions: Regulates the stomach and rectifies qi; harmonizes the center and downbears counterflow; frees the channels and quickens the connecting vessels.

Indications: Pain and swelling of the knees; paralysis of the lower extremities; stomach pain; mammary yong.

Supplementary Indications: Low back pain; cold lower limbs.

Stimulation: 0.5-1.0 perpendicular insertion.
Moxa: 3-7 cones; pole 5-15 min.

Point Categories & Associations: The cleft-xi point of the stomach channel.

ST-35
犢鼻
dú bí

"Calf's Nose"

Location: In the depression below the patella and lateral to the patellar ligament when the knee is bent.

Classical Location: Below the kneecap, above the lower leg bone, in the depression lateral to the large sinew that looks like the nose of an ox, hence the name. *(The Great Compendium)*

Local Anatomy: The arterial and venous network around the knee joint. The lateral sural cutaneous nerve and the articular branch of the common peroneal nerve.

Functions: Frees the channels and quickens the connecting vessels; courses wind and dissipates cold; disperses swelling and relieves pain.

Indications: Pain and numbness of the knee; inhibited bending and stretching of the leg.

Supplementary Indications: Swelling of the ox's nose.

Illustrative Point Combinations & Applications: When the knees are swollen like dippers, regardless of cause, apply moxa at ST-35 and ST-36. *(Song More Precious than Jade)*

Stimulation: 0.5-1.0″ oblique insertion slightly toward medial side. Moxa: 5-7 cones; pole 5-15 min.

Needle Sensation: Distention and heat in the knee joint.

ST-36
足三里
zú sān lǐ

"Leg Three Li"

Location: 3″ below ST-35, roughly 1″ lateral to the crest of the tibia. If the palm of the hand is placed over the patella, the point is located at the level where the middle finger ends.

Classical Location: Three body inches below the knee, on the lateral edge of the shinbone, in the fleshy part of the major sinew, at the point where it divides under pressure. The location can be confirmed by applying extreme pressure at the point (with the foot in raised position), whereupon the pulse at ST-41 ceases. *(The Great Compendium)*

Local Anatomy: The anterior tibial artery and vein. Superficially, the lateral sural cutaneous nerve and the cutaneous branch of the saphenous nerve; deeper, the deep peroneal nerve.

Functions: Rectifies the spleen and stomach; regulates central qi; harmonizes the intestines and disperses stagnation; breaks thoracic blood stasis; courses wind and transforms damp; frees and regulates qi and blood of the channels; supports the correct and banks up the origin; dispels pathogens and prevents disease.

Indications: Stomach pain; abdominal distention; indigestion; vomiting; borborygmi; diarrhea; constipation; dysentery; breast yong; dizziness; epilepsy; paralysis due to wind strike; foot qi; water swelling; aching knee and tibia.

Supplementary Indications: Pain, fullness and distention in the venter; abdominal pain; cholera; stoppage of the diaphragm and throat; difficult ingestion; wryness of the mouth; eye disease; pharyngeal bi; fever; enuresis; swelling of the feet; rumbling intestines; heaviness in the head and pain in the forehead at the outset of heat disease; vexation, oppression and generalized fever; inhibited urination; lower abdominal swelling and pain; branching fullness in the chest and lateral costal region; swelling and pain in the extremities; thoracic blood stasis; palpitations with vacuity vexation and agitation.

Illustrative Point Combinations & Applications: For toothache, headache and throat bi, first needle LI-2, then needle ST-36. *(The Celestial Emperor's Secret)*

For accumulations in the stomach, needling ST-36 with CV-21 is effective in a way few people know; ST-36 is effective for treating bowstring and elusive masses in males. *(Ode of Xi Hong)*

For sufferers of liver disease with diminished blood and clouded, flowery vision, supplement BL-18 and drain ST-36. *(Ode of the Jade Dragon)*

Stimulation: 0.5-1.5″ perpendicular insertion.
Moxa: 3-7 cones; pole 5-20 min.

Needle Sensation: Localized distention and numbness, sometimes extending along the channel to the foot or the abdomen.

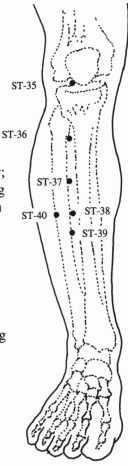

Figure 8.8

Point Categories & Associations: Uniting-he (earth) point; one of the nine needles for returning yang.

ST-37
上巨虚
shàng jù xū

"Upper Great Hollow"

Location: 6″ below ST-35, a finger's breadth lateral to the anterior crest of the tibia.
Classical Location: Three inches below ST-36, in the depression between the sinew and bone. The point is found with the leg raised. *(The Great Compendium)*
Local Anatomy: See ST-36.

Functions: Rectifies the spleen and harmonizes the stomach; frees the intestines and transforms stagnation; courses the channels and regulates qi; clears and disinhibits damp-heat.
Indications: Abdominal pain or distention; dysentery; borborygmi; diarrhea; intestinal yong; hemiplegia; foot qi.
Supplementary Indications: Gastrosplenic vacuity; swill diarrhea; fullness in the chest and lateral costal region; swelling of the knee; pain in the navel; untransformed digestate; vacuity taxation.

Stimulation: 0.5-1.3″ perpendicular insertion.
Moxa: 3-7 cones; pole 5-20 min.

Point Categories & Associations: Lower uniting-he point of the large intestine.

ST-38
條口
tiáo kǒu

"Ribbon Opening"

Location: 2″ below ST-37, 8″ below ST-35, at the midpoint between ST-35 and ST-41, near the edge of the tibia.
Classical Location: 2″ below ST-37, locate with the foot raised. *(The Golden Mirror)*
Local Anatomy: See ST-36.

Functions: Soothes the sinews and quickens the connecting vessels; warms the channels and dissipates cold.
Indications: Atony of the lower leg; shoulder pain.
Supplementary Indications: Pain in the lower leg; pain in the venter; intestinal shan pain; dysentery; sore pharynx; swelling of the knee and thigh; cold pain and swelling.
Illustrative Point Combinations & Applications: Difficulty in moving the legs is treated by first needling GB-39 and then ST-38. *(Song of Point Applications for Miscellaneous Disease)*

Stimulation: 0.5-1.0″ perpendicular insertion.
Moxa: 3-5 cones; pole 5-20 min.

Location: One finger's breadth lateral to the anterior crest of the tibia, 3″ below ST-37.

Classical Location: One inch below ST-38, in the depression between the sinew and bone. *(The Golden Mirror)*

Local Anatomy: The anterior tibial artery and vein. Branches of the superficial peroneal nerve and the deep peroneal nerve.

Functions: Clears heat and disinhibits damp; clears the bowels and transforms stasis.

Indications: Abdominal pain; backache referring to the testicles; mammary yong; atony or bi of the lower extremities.

Supplementary Indications: Stomach heat; abdominal pain; diarrhea and dysentery; mania and withdrawal; swelling and pain in the shin.

Stimulation: 0.5-1.0″ perpendicular insertion.
Moxa: 7-15 cones; pole 5-20 min.

Point Categories & Associations: Lower uniting-he point of the small intestine.

ST-39
下巨虛
xià jù xū
"Lower Great Hollow"

Location: 8″ below ST-35, about one finger's breadth lateral to ST-38.

Classical Location: ST-40 lies upward and outward from ST-39, eight inches above the outer ankle bone, in a depression on the outer face of the lower leg bone. *(The Golden Mirror)*

Local Anatomy: Branches of the anterior tibial artery and vein. The superficial peroneal nerve.

Functions: Harmonizes the stomach; transforms phlegm-damp; clears the spirit-disposition.

Indications: Chest pain; asthma; copious phlegm; sore, swollen throat; loss of locomotive power, pain, and swelling of lower extremities; headache; dizziness; epilepsy.

ST-40
豐隆
fēng lóng
"Bountiful Bulge"

Supplementary Indications: Qi counterflow; throat bi and sudden loss of voice; connecting vessel repletion; mania and withdrawal; connecting vessel vacuity; non-contraction of legs; withering of the calves; vomiting; constipation; foot qi; inversion headache; vexation; swelling of the face; swelling of the limbs; enduring menstrual block; phlegm diseases.

Stimulation: 0.5-1.0″ perpendicular insertion.
Moxa: 7-15 cones; pole 5-20 min.

Point Categories & Associations: Connecting-luo point of the stomach channel, connecting to the spleen channel.

ST-41
解溪（解谿）

jiě xī

"Ravine Divide"

Location: At the junction of the dorsum of the foot and the leg, between the tendons of the long extensor muscle of the toes and the long extensor muscle of the great toe (m. extensor digitorum longus and m. extensor hallucis longus), approximately at the level of the tip of the external malleolus.

Classical Location: One and a half inches back from ST-42, in the depression on the center line in the bend of the ankle.
(The Great Compendium)

Local Anatomy: The anterior tibial artery vein. The superficial and deep peroneal nerves.

Functions: Supports spleen qi; transforms damp and stagnation; clears stomach heat; stabilizes the spirit-disposition.

Indications: Swelling of the head and face; headache; dizziness; abdominal distention; constipation; loss of locomotive ability of the lower limbs; withdrawal patterns.

Supplementary Indications: Eye diseases; pain in the foot or knees; cholera and cramp; eructation; stomach heat; delirious speech; malarial disease; heaviness of the thigh and knee; sinew bi; reddening of the eyes and face; pain in the ankle; fright palpitations; racing of the heart; swelling of the abdomen; vacuity swelling of the shin.

Illustrative Point Combinations & Applications: Fright palpitations and racing of the heart can be treated without error through GB-35 and ST-41. *(Ode of a Hundred Patterns)*

Stimulation: 0.5-0.8 ″ perpendicular insertion.
Moxa: 3-5 cones; pole 5-15 min.

Point Categories & Associations: River-jing (fire) point.

Location: At the highest point of the dorsum of the foot, in the depression between the 2nd and 3rd metatarsal bones and the cuneiform bone.

Classical Location: 5 ″ from the tip of the toes, 2 ″ from ST-43, in the depression on the high point of the instep, where a pulse can be felt. *(The Great Compendium)*

Local Anatomy: The dorsal artery and vein of the foot, the dorsal venous network of the foot. Superficially, the medial dorsal cutaneous nerve of the foot derived from the superficial peroneal nerve; deeper, the deep peroneal nerve.

Functions: Supports earth and transforms damp; harmonizes the stomach and stabilizes the spirit.

Indications: Wryness of the mouth; atony of the lower extremities; redness and swelling of the dorsum of the foot.

Supplementary Indications: Swelling of the head and face; aching among the upper teeth; abdominal swelling; mania and withdrawal; malarial disease; wind heaviness in the head; pain in the forehead; abdominal distention with no desire to eat.

Stimulation: 0.3 ″ oblique or perpendicular insertion. Avoid the artery. Moxa: 3 cones; pole 5-10 min.

Point Categories & Associations: Source-yuan point of the stomach channel.

ST-42
衝陽
chōng yáng
"Surging Yang"

Location: In the depression distal to the junction of the 2nd and 3rd metatarsal bones.

Classical Location: Up from the outer aspect of the second toe, in the depression behind the base joint, two inches up from ST-44. *(The Great Compendium)*

Local Anatomy: The dorsal venous network of the foot. The medial dorsal cutaneous nerve of the foot.

ST-43
陷谷
xiàn gǔ
"Sunken Valley"

Functions: Fortifies the spleen and disinhibits damp; harmonizes the stomach and downbears counterflow.

Indications: Swelling of the face; edema; rumbling intestines and abdominal pain; painful swelling of the dorsum of the foot.

Supplementary Indications: Redness of the face and eyes; abdominal water; night sweating; fever; persistent counterflow cough.

Illustrative Point Combinations & Applications: CV-10 and ST-43 will calm rumbling intestines. *(Ode of a Hundred Patterns)*

Stimulation: 0.3-0.5″ perpendicular insertion.
Moxa: 3-7 cones; pole 2-7 min.

Point Categories & Associations: Stream-shu (wood) point.

ST-44
內庭

nèi tíng

"Inner Court"

Location: Proximal to the web margin between the 2nd and 3rd toes, in the depression distal and lateral to the 2nd metatarsophalangeal joint.

Classical Location: Below ST-43, on the outer side of the second toe, in the depression in front of the base joint.
(The Golden Mirror)

Local Anatomy: The dorsal venous network of the foot. The point where the lateral branch of the medial dorsal cutaneous nerve divides into the dorsal digital nerves.

Functions: Promotes free downbearing of stomach qi; harmonizes the intestines and transforms stagnation.

Indications: Toothache; wryness of the mouth; nosebleed; abdominal pain and distention; diarrhea and dysentery; painful swelling of the dorsum of the foot; heat diseases.

Supplementary Indications: Trismus; throat bi; intestinal shan pain; malaria with no desire to eat; aversion to cold; urinary stoppage; rumbling of the intestines; abdominal distention and fullness; dormant papules.

Illustrative Point Combinations & Applications: ST-36 and ST-44 have a wondrous effect on diseases of the abdomen.
(The Thousand Gold Piece Prescriptions)

ST-44 and GB-41 rectify lower abdominal distention.
(Ode of the Jade Dragon)

Stimulation: 0.3-0.5″ perpendicular insertion.
Moxa: 3-5 cones; pole 5-7 min.

Point Categories & Associations: Spring-ying (water) point.

Location: On the lateral side of the 2nd toe, about 0.1″ proximal to the corner of the nail.

Classical Location: On the outer side of the end of the toe next to the great toe, the breadth of a Chinese leek leaf from the corner of the nail. *(The Great Compendium)*

Local Anatomy: The arterial and venous network formed by the dorsal digital artery and vein of the foot. The dorsal digital nerve derived from the superficial peroneal nerve.

Functions: Frees the channels and resuscitates; harmonizes the stomach and clears the spirit; courses and discharges yang ming pathogenic heat.

Indications: Swelling of the face; wryness of the mouth; toothache; nosebleed; abdominal distention and fullness; cold in the lower leg and foot; heat diseases; increased dreaming; mania and withdrawal.

Supplementary Indications: Trismus; throat bi; fever; copious clear snivel with nosebleed.

Illustrative Point Combinations & Applications: For dreaming with heavy pressure sensation (as if unable to move), combine ST-45 with SP-1. *(Ode of a Hundred Patterns)*

Stimulation: 0.1″ perpendicular insertion.
Moxa: 3 cones; pole 3 min.

Point Categories & Associations: Well-jing (metal) point.

ST-45
厲兌
lì duì

"Severe Mouth"

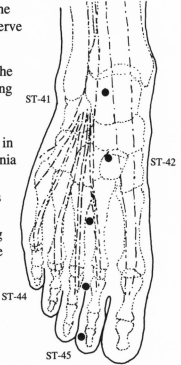

Figure 8.9

139

Foot Yang Ming Stomach Channel			
Point	**Location**	Indications	
		Primary	**Secondary**
*ST-1	Face	Red, swollen, painful eyes	
*ST-2		Red, swollen, painful eyes wry mouth and eyes	
ST-3		Wry mouth and eyes nosebleed toothache	
*ST-4		Wry mouth	
ST-5		Wry mouth swelling of the cheeks toothache	
*ST-6		Wry mouth swelling of the cheeks toothache clenched jaw	
*ST-7		Wry mouth toothache deafness clenched jaw	
*ST-8	Side of head	Headache eye disease	
Head & Face: Disorders of the head, face, eyes, nose, mouth, and teeth			
ST-9	Neck	Pain and swelling 　of the throat dyspnea	
ST-10		Pain and swelling of the throat dyspnea	
ST-11		Pain and swelling 　of the throat	
ST-12	Chest	Cough and dyspnea pain and swelling of the throat	
ST-13		Cough and dyspnea	
ST-14		Cough pain & distention of the 　chest & lateral costal region	
Neck & Chest: Disorders of the throat, chest, and lung			

Foot Yang Ming Stomach Channel (continued)			
Point	**Location**	Indications	
		Primary	**Secondary**
ST-15	Chest	Cough mammary yong	
ST-16		Cough mammary yong pain & distention of the chest & lateral costal region	
ST-17		**Contraindicated for needling and moxibustion**	
ST-18		Cough, chest pain shortage of breast milk	
Neck & Chest: Disorders of the throat, chest, and lung			
ST-19	Upper abdomen	Stomach pain vomiting abdominal distention	
ST-20		Intestinal rumbling abdominal distention stomach pain	
*ST-21		Loss of appetite stomach pain	
ST-22		Intestinal rumbling diarrhea abdominal distension	
ST-23		Stomach pain	Mania and withdrawal
ST-24		Vomiting	Mania and withdrawal
*ST-25		Dysenteric disease intestinal rumbling abdominal distention periumbilical pain	
Upper Abdomen: Gastric and intestinal pain; mental disorders			
ST-26	Lower abdomen	Abdominal pain	Hernia
ST-27		Lower abdominal distention and pain inhibited urination	Hernia

Foot Yang Ming Stomach Channel (continued)			
Point	**Location**	**Indications**	
		Primary	**Secondary**
ST-28	Lower abdomen	Inhibited urination	Hernia
*ST-29		Menstrual disorders	Hernia
ST-30		Menstrual disorders impotence	
Lower abdomen: Genitourinary and gynecologic disorders			
ST-31	Upper leg	Paralysis of the lower limbs	
*ST-32		Paralysis of the lower limbs	
ST-33		Hypertonicity of the legs	Hernia
*ST-34		Stomach pain knee pain	
ST-35	Knee	Pain and numbness of the knee	
Upper leg and knee: Localized disorders			
*ST-36	Lower leg	Stomach pain abdominal distention diarrhea constipation pain & aching of the knee & lower leg	Promotes health and fitness of entire body
*ST-37		Intestinal rumbling diarrhea abdominal distention	Appendicitis
ST-38		Paralysis of the lower limbs	
*ST-39		Lower abdominal pain paralysis of the lower limbs	Mammary yong
*ST-40		Vomiting constipation copious phlegm	cough dizziness mania and withdrawal
Lower leg: Gastric, intestinal and mental disorders			

Foot Yang Ming Stomach Channel (continued)			
Point	**Location**	**Indications**	
		Primary	**Secondary**
*ST-41	Ankle	Headache	Mania and withdrawal
ST-42		Wry mouth and eyes	
ST-43		Red, swollen, painful eyes intestinal rumbling abdominal distention	Heat disease
*ST-44		Wry mouth toothache pain and swelling of the throat abdominal distention dysenteric disease	Heat disease
*ST-45	Toe	Toothache pain and swelling of the throat abdominal distention	Heat disease excessive dreaming mania and withdrawal
Foot: Disorders of the head, face, eyes, nose, mouth, teeth, throat, stomach and intestines; mental disorders; heat disease			

9. The Spleen Channel System
(Foot Tai Yin) 足太陰脾經

9.1 The Primary Spleen Channel

Pathway: The foot tai yin spleen channel starts on the medial tip of the great toe and runs along the border of the light and dark skin on the medial aspect of the foot. It then passes in front of the medial malleolus and up the posterior side of the leg along the posterior margin of the tibia. Here it crosses and runs anterior to the foot jue yin liver channel, passing medial to the knee and running up the anteromedial abdomen and intersecting the conception vessel at CV-3 and CV-4 before homing to the spleen and connecting with the stomach. It then continues upward and passes through the diaphragm to intersect with the foot shao yang gallbladder channel at GB-24 and the foot jue yin liver channel at LV-14. From there it ascends to the side of the esophagus, crosses the hand tai yin lung channel at LU-1, and finally proceeds up to the root of the tongue to disperse over its lower surface.

A branch breaks off in the area of the stomach, crossing the diaphragm to transport qi to the heart.

Main pathologic signs associated with the exterior course of the channel: heaviness in the head or body; fatigue and weakness of the limbs; general fever; pain in the posterior mandibular region and the lower cheek; motor impairment of the tongue; wasting and atony of the muscles of the limbs; cold along the inside of the thigh and knee; edematous swelling of the legs and feet.

Main pathologic signs associated with the internal organ: pain in the venter and thin diarrhea or stool containing undigested food; borborygmi; retching and nausea; abdominal lump glomus; reduced food intake; jaundice; inhibited urination.

Exuberance of qi: spasm, foot pain.

Insufficiency of qi: abdominal fullness; intestinal rumbling; untransformed digestate; swill diarrhea.

9.2 The Connecting Vessel of the Spleen Channel

Pathway: This vessel separates from the primary channel at SP-4 and connects to the foot yang ming stomach channel. A branch ascends to connect to the intestines and stomach.

Main pathologic signs:

Inversion qi rising counterflow; cholera.

Repletion: cutting pain in the abdomen.

Vacuity: drum distention.

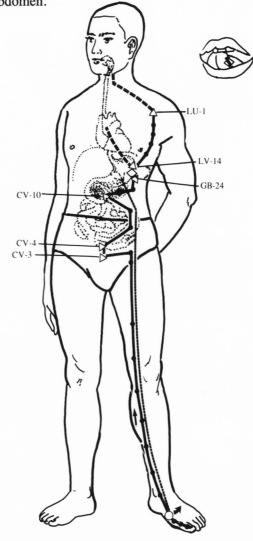

CV-10

LU-1

LV-14

GB-24

CV-4
CV-3

Key to Symbols

▪▪▪▪	Internal pathway
———	External pathway
⁄⁄⁄⁄	Channel branch pathway
▥▥▥	Secondary pathway
➴	Connecting vessel pathway
········	Connecting vessel pathway
◆	Connection with home organ
◇	Connection with paired organ
○	Connecting-luo point
△	Intersection-jiaohui point
■	Lower uniting-he Point

Figure 9.1 - 12.2 Primary channel and connecting vessel of the spleen.

9.3 The Spleen Channel Divergence

Pathway: The divergence leaves the primary channel at the thigh and ascends to the hip where it unites with the foot yang ming stomach channel divergence. It then rises and binds at the pharynx and links with the root of the tongue.

145

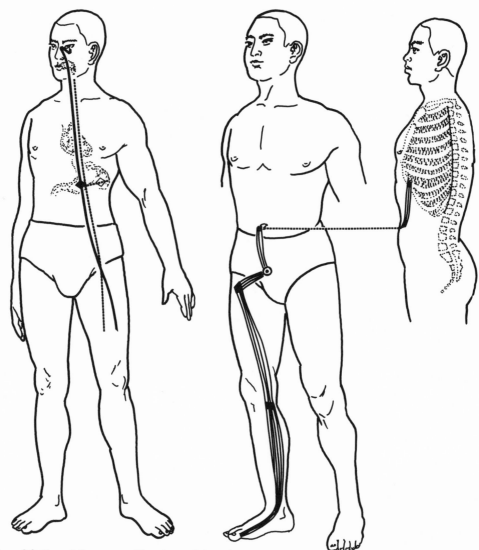

Figure 9.3 Channel divergences of the spleen and stomach.

Figure 9.4 The spleen channel sinews.

9.4 The Spleen Channel Sinews

Pathway: Beginning at the medial side of the large toe these sinews proceed to bind at the medial maleolus and ascend to the knee where they bind at the medial aspect of the tibia. Following up the yin side of the thigh these sinews bind at the inguinal region and gather at the genitals. They then ascend to the abdomen, bind at the navel and proceed to bind to the ribs and disperse in the chest. These sinews also attach internally to the side of the spine.

Main pathologic signs: Strain of the large toe (inability to stretch or support the toe); pain at the medial malleolus; cramp and pain in the gastrocnemius; pain in the medial aspect of the knee; pain in the inner thigh and inguinal region; cutting pain in the genitals (this pain may extend up to the navel and ribs or up into the chest or back to the spine).

Repletion: generalized aching and pain.

Vacuity: weakness at the limbs and joints.

9.5 The Great Connecting Vessel of the Spleen

Pathway: This connecting vessel issues from 3 inches below the axilla and spreads over the chest and lateral costal region.

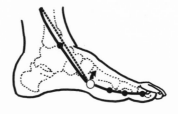

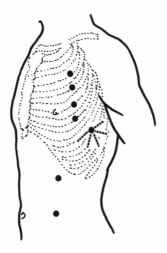

Figure 9.5 The great connecting vessel of the spleen.

147

SP-1
隱白
yǐn bái

"Hidden White"

Location: On the medial side of the big toe, about 0.1" proximal to the corner of the nail.

Classical Location: On the inner side of the big toe, the width of a Chinese leek leaf from the corner of the nail. *(The Great Compendium)*

Local Anatomy: The dorsal digital artery. On the anastomosis of the dorsal digital nerve derived from the superficial peroneal nerve and the plantar digital proprial nerve.

Functions: Regulates and manages the blood; supports and warms the spleen; clears the heart and stabilizes the spirit; warms yang and returns inversion.

Indications: Abdominal distention; metrorrhagia; mania and withdrawal; excessive dreaming; fright wind.

Supplementary Indications: Dyspnea; cold qi in the abdomen; intestinal heat with fulminant diarrhea; heat disease with persistent nosebleed; vexation; sighing; sorrowfulness; cold in the foot and lower leg; dreaming with pressure sensation as if being held down by a ghost; persistent menstruation; blood ejection; blood in stool and urine; infantile chronic fright wind.

Stimulation: 0.1" upward oblique insertion.
Moxa: 3-7 cones; pole 5-20 min.
Needle Sensation: Localized pain.

Point Categories & Associations: Well-jing (wood) point; first of the thirteen ghost points.

SP-2
大都
dà dū

"Great Metropolis"

Location: On the medial side of the big toe, distal and inferior to the 1st metatarsophalangeal joint, at the border of the red and white skin.

Classical Location: On the inner side of the big toe, in the depression formed by the cleft of the bone behind the base joint, on the border of the red and white flesh. *(The Great Compendium)*

Local Anatomy: Branches of the medial plantar artery and vein. The plantar digital proprial nerve derived from the medial plantar nerve.

Functions: Fortifies the spleen and harmonizes the stomach; returns yang and stems counterflow.

Indications: Abdominal distention; stomach pain; adiaphoretic heat diseases.

Supplementary Indications: Heat diseases with sweating and inversion; cold in the extremities; fulminant diarrhea; pain in the stomach and cardiac region; untransformed digestate; retching counterflow; evacuation difficulty; all forms of dysentery; lumbar pain.

Illustrative Point Combinations & Applications: KI-11 and SP-2 provide emergency treatment for qi-stagnation lumbar pain that prevents the patient from standing. *(Ode of Xi Hong)*

Stimulation: 0.3″ perpendicular insertion.
Moxa: 1-3 cones; pole 5-20 min.

Point Categories & Associations: Spring-ying (fire) point.

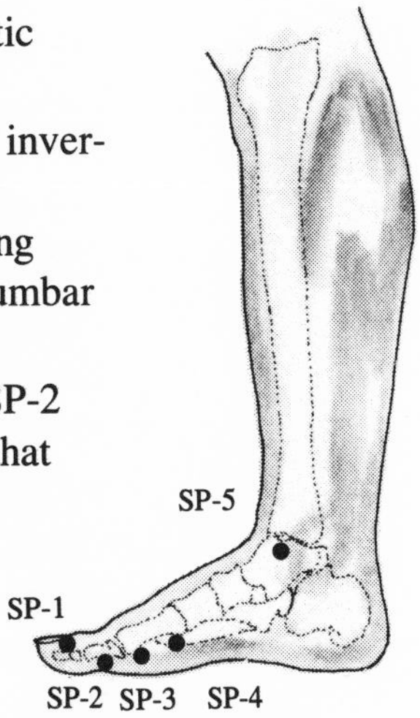

Figure 9.6

SP-3
太白
tài bái

"Supreme White"

Location: Proximal and inferior to the head of the 1st metatarsal bone, at the border of the red and white skin.

Classical Location: Back along the inside of the toe from SP-2, in the depression under the ball bone. *(The Golden Mirror)*

Local Anatomy: The dorsal venous network of the foot, the medial plantar artery and branches of the medial tarsal artery. Branches of the saphenous nerve and superficial peroneal nerve.

Functions: Supports spleen-earth; harmonizes the central burner; regulates qi dynamic; helps movement and transformation.

Indications: Stomach pain; abdominal distention; generalized heaviness; dysentery; constipation; vomiting and diarrhea; foot qi.

Supplementary Indications: Heat diseases starting with pain in the head and face; fullness and oppression preventing the patient from assuming a reclining posture; untransformed digestate; distention in the chest and lateral costal region; rumbling intestines and stabbing pain; pain in the stomach and cardiac region; retching and vomiting; cholera and counterflow frigidity; evacuative difficulty; diarrhea with pus and blood in the stool; hemorrhoids and fistulae; lumbar pain preventing movement; heaviness of the body and bone pain.

Stimulation: 0.3″ perpendicular insertion.
Moxa: 3 cones; pole 5-10 min.
Needle Sensation: Localized distention and pain.

Point Categories & Associations: Stream-shu (earth) and source-yuan point.

SP-4
公孫
gōng sūn
"Yellow Emperor"

Location: In the depression distal and inferior to the base of the 1st metatarsal bone, at the border of the red and white flesh.
Classical Location: One inch behind the base joint of the great toe. (The Systematized Canon)
Local Anatomy: The medial tarsal artery and the dorsal venous network of the foot. The saphenous nerve and the branch of the superficial peroneal nerve.

Functions: Supports the spleen and stomach; rectifies qi dynamic; regulates the sea of blood; harmonizes the penetrating vessel.
Indications: Stomach pain; vomiting; borborygmi; abdominal pain; diarrhea; dysentery.
Illustrative Point Combinations & Applications: SP-4 and PC-6 treat abdominal pain.
(Song of Point Applications for Miscellaneous Disease)

Stimulation: 0.5-1.0″ oblique or perpendicular insertion.
Moxa: 3 cones; pole 3-5 min.
Needle Sensation: Localized needle stimulus sensation and pain.

Point Categories & Associations: Connecting-luo point connecting to the stomach channel and a confluence-jiaohui point of the eight extraordinary channels (related to the penetrating vessel).

SP-5
商丘
shāng qiū
"Shang Hill"

Location: In the depression distal and inferior to the medial malleolus, midway between the tuberosity of the navicular bone and the tip of the medial malleolus.
Classical Location: In the slight depression under the inner ankle bone, between LV-4 in front and KI-6 behind.
(The Great Compendium)
Local Anatomy: The medial tarsal artery and the great saphenous vein. The medial crural cutaneous nerve and branch of the superficial peroneal nerve.

Functions: Fortifies the spleen and disinhibits damp.

Indications: Borborygmi; abdominal distention; pain and stiffness at the root of the tongue; constipation; diarrhea; ankle pain.

Supplementary Indications: Splenic vacuity; thin-stool diarrhea; heart sorrow; constipation; fever and chills and retching; pain in the venter; jaundice; untransformed digestate; gastric reflux; pain in the thighs; breast pain; hemorrhoids; shan causing lower abdominal pain; hypertonicity of the sinews; impaired bending and stretching of the knee with inability to walk; pain in the inner ankle; infertility; child fright wind (convulsions); throat bi; glomus; bone bi.

Illustrative Point Combinations & Applications: SP-5, ST-41 and GB-40 treat foot pain. *(Ode of the Jade Dragon)*

Stimulation: 0.3-1.0″ oblique or perpendicular insertion.
Moxa: 3 cones; pole 5-10 min.

Needle Sensation: Localized needle stimulus sensation and pain.

Point Categories & Associations: River-jing (metal) point.

Location: 3″ directly above the tip of the medial malleolus, on the posterior border of the tibia, on a line drawn from the medial malleolus to SP-9.

Classical Location: In the protuberance beneath the bone, three inches above the tip of the ankle. *(The Great Compendium)*

Local Anatomy: The great saphenous vein, the posterior tibial artery and vein. Superficially, the medial crural cutaneous nerve; deeper, in the posterior aspect, the tibial nerve.

SP-6
三陰交
sān yīn jiāo
"Three Yin Intersection"

Functions: Supplements spleen earth; helps movement and transformation; frees qi stagnation; courses the lower burner; regulates the blood chamber and the palace of essence; dispels wind-damp from the channels and connecting vessels.

Indications: Rumbling intestines; abdominal distention; thin stool with untransformed digestate; irregular menses; metrorrhagia; vaginal discharge; prolapse of the uterus; menstrual block; non-conception; difficult labor; seminal emission; genital pain; hernia; inhibited urination; enuresis; loss of locomotive ability of the lower extremities; insomnia.

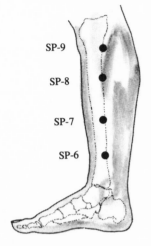

SP-9

SP-8

SP-7

SP-6

Figure 9.7

Functions: Warms and moves the central burner; regulates the spleen; transforms damp; regulates the waterways; dispels wind-cold.

Indications: Abdominal distention; water swelling; jaundice; diarrhea; inhibited urination or incontinence; genital pain; seminal emission; knee pain.

Supplementary Indications: Cold in the abdomen; qi distention in the abdomen; throughflux diarrhea with undigested food in the stool; no desire for food; inhibited urination or incontinence; genital pain; seminal emission; bi pain; pain in the lumbus, thigh and knee; foot qi with water swelling; shan conglomeration.

Illustrative Point Combinations & Applications: In urinary stoppage, draining SP-9 and ST-36 causes the urine to flow. *(Song of Point Applications for Miscellaneous Disease)*

Glomus and fullness in the chest and diaphragm is treated by first needling SP-9, then BL-57. This restores normal eating. *(Song of Point Applications for Miscellaneous Disease)*

SP-9 and CV-9 treat water swelling in the umbilical region. *(Ode of a Hundred Patterns)*

Stimulation: 0.5-1.0 ″ perpendicular insertion.
Moxa: 3 cones; pole 3-5 min.

Needle Sensation: Localized needle stimulus sensation and distention, sometimes spreading downward and outward.

Point Categories & Associations: Uniting-he (water) point.

SP-10
血海
xuè hǎi

"Sea of Blood"

Location: When the knee is flexed, the point is 2 ″ above the mediosuperior border of the patella, on the bulge of the medial portion of the quadriceps muscle of the thigh (m. vastus medialis). Another way to locate this point is to cup your right palm over the patient's left knee, with the thumb on its medial side and the four other fingers directed proximally. The point will be found where the tip of your thumb rests.

Classical Location: Two and a half inches above the knee cap, on the border of the white flesh on the inner side.
(The Great Compendium)

Local Anatomy: Muscular branches of the femoral artery and vein. The anterior femoral cutaneous nerve and the muscular branch of the femoral nerve.

Functions: Regulates and clears the blood; perfuses the lower burner.

Indications: Irregular menses; menstrual block; metrorrhagia; pain on the inside of the thigh; eczema.

Supplementary Indications: Malign blood discharge from the womb; painful, itching sores or red, swollen purulent sores on the inner side of the thigh; genital sores; the five stranguries.

Illustrative Point Combinations & Applications:

SP-8 and SP-10 regulate the menses. *(Ode of a Hundred Patterns)*

CV-6 and SP-10 treat the five stranguries. *(Ode of Spiritual Light)*

Stimulation: 0.5-1.2 ″ perpendicular insertion.
Moxa: 3-5 cones; pole 5-10 min.

Needle Sensation: Localized needle stimulus sensation and distention, sometimes spreading into the knee joint, or to the hip.

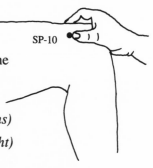

SP-10

Figure 9.8

Location: 6 ″ above SP-10, on the line drawn from SP-10 to SP-12.

Classical Location: Moving up from SP-10, on to the fish's belly and between the two sinews, a pulse can be felt at the point.

Local Anatomy: Superficially, the great saphenous vein; deeper, on the lateral side, the femoral artery and vein. The anterior femoral cutaneous nerve; deeper, the saphenous nerve.

Functions: Clears the head and disinhibits damp; promotes free flow through the waterways.

Indications: Urinary stoppage; enuresis; painful swelling of the groin.

Supplementary Indications: Dribbling urine with urinary inhibition; difficult urination.

Stimulation: 0.3-0.5 ″ perpendicular insertion.
Moxa: 3 cones; pole 3-10 min.

SP-11
箕門
jī mén
"Winnower Gate"

Location: Along the inguinal groove, on the lateral side of the femoral artery, at the level of the upper border of symphysis pubis, 3.5 ″ lateral to CV-2.

Classical Location: One inch below SP-13 at the pulsating vessel in the creases at the extremity of the pubic bone.

(The Great Compendium)

SP-12
衝門
chōng mén
"Surging Gate"

Functions: Clears heat and disinhibits damp; frees bowel qi.

Indications: Abdominal pain; untransformed digestate in the stool; constipation; dysentery.

Supplementary Indications: Abdominal cold pain; umbilical pain; dysentery with the pus and blood.

Stimulation: 0.5-1.0″ perpendicular insertion.
Moxa: 5 cones; pole 10-20 min.

Point Categories & Associations: Intersection-jiaohui point of the foot tai yin spleen channel and the yin linking vessel.

SP-17
食竇
shí dòu

"Food Hole"

Location: 6″ lateral to the midline, 2″ lateral to the mammillary line, in the 5th intercostal space.

Classical Location: One inch and six fen below SP-18, and six inches from the midline. *(The Great Compendium)*

Local Anatomy: The thoracoepigastric vein. The lateral cutaneous branch of the 5th intercostal nerve.

Functions: Rectifies qi and disinhibits water; courses the triple burner.

Indications: Pain and distention in the lateral costal region.

Supplementary Indications: Thunderous rumbling in the diaphragm region; major detriment to splenic qi; branching fullness in the chest and lateral costal region; postpartum abdominal distention and water swelling; urinary stoppage.

Stimulation: 0.3-0.5″ outward oblique insertion.
Moxa: 3-5 cones; pole 5-20 min.

SP-18
天溪 (天谿)
tiān xī

"Celestial Ravine"

Location: 2″ lateral to the nipple, in the 4th intercostal space.

Classical Location: One inch and six fen above SP-17, six inches from the midline. The point is located in supine posture. *(The Golden Mirror)*

Local Anatomy: Branches of the lateral thoracic artery and vein, the thoracoepigastric artery and vein, the 4th intercostal artery and vein. The lateral cutaneous branch of the 4th intercostal nerve.

Functions: Loosens the chest and rectifies qi; downbears counter-flow and suppresses cough.

Indications: Thoracic pain and distention; cough; mammary yong; scant breast milk.

Supplementary Indications: Cough counterflow qi ascent; throat rattle.

Stimulation: 0.4-0.5″ outward oblique insertion.
Moxa: 5 cones; pole 5-20 min.

Location: Above SP-18, in the 3rd intercostal space, 6″ lateral to the midline.

Classical Location: One inch and six fen above SP-18, six inches from the midline. The point is found in supine posture. *(The Golden Mirror)*

Local Anatomy: The lateral thoracic artery and vein, the 3rd intercostal artery and vein. The lateral cutaneous branch of the 3rd intercostal nerve.

Functions: Diffuses and downbears lung qi; suppresses cough and stabilizes dyspnea.

Indications: Pain and distention in the lateral costal region.

Supplementary Indications: Branching fullness in the chest and lateral costal region; pain referred from the chest to the back; inability to turn over; cough.

Stimulation: 0.4″ outward oblique insertion.
Moxa: 5 cones; pole 5-20 min.

SP-19
胸鄉
xiōng xiāng
"Chest Village"

Location: Above SP-19, below LU-1, in the 2nd intercostal space, 6″ lateral to the midline.

Classical Location: One inch and six fen above SP-19, six inches from the midline. The point is found in supine posture. *(The Golden Mirror)*

Local Anatomy: The lateral thoracic artery and vein, the 2nd intercostal artery and vein. The muscular branch of the anterior thoracic nerve, the lateral cutaneous branch of the 2nd intercostal nerve.

SP-20
周榮
zhōu róng
*"All-Round
Flourishing"*

159

Functions: Diffuses and downbears lung qi; suppresses cough and stabilizes dyspnea.

Indications: Distention and fullness in the chest and lateral costal region; cough.

Supplementary Indications: Spitting of foul pus; difficult ingestion.

Stimulation: 0.4-0.5″ outward oblique insertion.
Moxa: 5 cones; pole 5-20 min.

SP-21
大包

dà bāo

"Great
Embracement"

Location: On the mid-axillary line, 6″ below the axilla, midway between the axilla and the free end of the 11th rib.

Classical Location: Downward and outward from SP-20, crossing the shao yang gallbladder channel, three inches below GB-22, a little over six inches below the armpit. *(The Golden Mirror)*

Local Anatomy: The thoracodorsal artery and vein, the 7th intercostal artery and vein. The 7th intercostal nerve and the terminal branch of the long thoracic nerve.

Functions: Regulates qi and blood; leashes sinew and bone.

Indications: Pain in the chest and lateral costal region; asthma; generalized pain; limp, weak limbs.

Supplementary Indications: Connecting vessel repletion: generalized pain in the whole body; Connecting vessel vacuity: laxity of the hundred joints.

Stimulation: 0.3-0.5″ outward oblique insertion.
Moxa: 3 cones; pole 10-20 min.

Point Categories & Associations: Great connecting-luo point of the spleen. This channel presides over yin and yang, and via the spleen, irrigates the five viscera.

Foot Tai Yin Spleen Channel			
Point	**Location**	**Indications**	
		Primary	**Secondary**
*SP-1	Toe	Abdominal distention profuse menstruation	Mania and withdrawal
SP-2		Abdominal distention stomach pain	Heat disease
*SP-3	Foot	Abdominal distention diarrhea stomach pain	
SP-4		Stomach pain vomiting diarrhea, abdominal distention	Dysenteric disease
SP-5	Ankle	Abdominal distention diarrhea constipation foot and ankle pain	
*SP-6	Lower leg	Intestinal rumbling abdominal distention menstrual disorders seminal emission inhibited urination enuresis	Insomnia
SP-7		Abdominal distention intestinal rumbling paralysis of the lower limbs	
*SP-8		Abdominal pain, dysentery inhibited urination menstrual disorders painful menstruation seminal emission	
*SP-9		Abdominal distention diarrhea inhibited urination knee pain	Edema

Point	Location	Indications	
		Primary	**Secondary**
*SP-10	Upper leg	Menstrual disorders	Dormant papules eczema
SP-11		Inhibited urination enuresis	
Lower limb: Primarily disorders of the stomach and spleen; secondarily menstrual and genitourinary disorders			
SP-12	Abdomen	Abdominal pain	Hernia
SP-13		Abdominal pain	Hernia
SP-14		Abdominal pain	Hernia
*SP-15		Constipation diarrhea abdominal pain	
SP-16		Abdominal pain indigestion constipation dysenteric disease	
Abdomen: Gastric and intestinal disorders			
SP-17	Chest	Pain and distention of the chest and lateral costal region	
SP-18		Cough chest pain mammary yong	
SP-19		Pain and distention of the chest and lateral costal region	
SP-20		Cough fullness and distention of the chest and lateral costal region	
*SP-21		Dyspnea pain in the chest and lateral costal region	
Chest: Disorders of the chest and lung			

Table title: **Foot Tai Yin Spleen Channel** (continued)

10. The Heart Channel System (Hand Shao Yin) 手少陰心經

10.1 The Primary Heart Channel

Pathway: The hand shao yin heart channel starts in the heart, emerging through the blood vessels surrounding this organ. Traveling downward, it passes through the diaphragm to connect to the small intestine.

Another branch separates from the heart, traveling upward along the side of the esophagus to meet the tissues behind the eye and connect with the brain.

A further channel separates from the heart and travels directly up into the lung, and then veers downwards to emerge below the axilla. It travels down the medial aspect of the upper arm, medial to the hand tai yin lung and hand jue yin pericardium channels, and passes over the antecubital fossa. It continues down the anteromedial margin of the forearm to the capitate bone on the wrist, and then travels along the radial side of the fifth metacarpal bone to terminate at the tip of the little finger.

Main pathologic signs associated with the external course of the channel: general fever; headache; pain in the eyes; pain in the chest and back muscles; dry throat; thirst with the urge to drink; hot or painful palms; ~~inversion~~ frigidity of the limbs; pain in the scapular region and/or the medial aspect of the forearm.

Main pathologic signs associated with the organ: cardialgia; fullness and pain in the chest and lateral costal region; pain in the hypochondriac region; vexation; rapid breathing; discomfort when recumbent; dizziness with fainting spells; essence-spirit disorders.

10.2 The Connecting Vessel of the Heart

Pathway: The vessel separates from the primary channel at HT-5. It connects to the hand tai yang small intestine channel. It moves upward along the primary channel and enters into the heart and rises up to connect to the root of the tongue and the region behind the eye.

Main pathologic signs:

Repletion: distention and fullness in the region of the diaphragm and chest.

Vacuity: inability to speak.

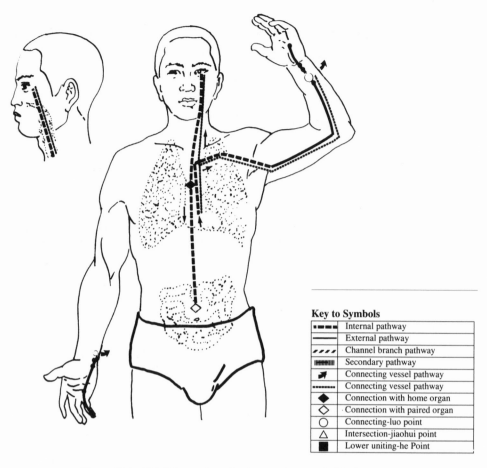

Key to Symbols

▪▬▬▪	Internal pathway
——	External pathway
⁄⁄⁄⁄	Channel branch pathway
▦▦▦	Secondary pathway
➚	Connecting vessel pathway
▪▪▪▪▪	Connecting vessel pathway
◆	Connection with home organ
◇	Connection with paired organ
○	Connecting-luo point
△	Intersection-jiaohui point
■	Lower uniting-he Point

Figure 10.1 - 10.2 Primary channel and connecting vessel of the heart.

10.3 The Heart Channel Divergence

Pathway: This divergence leaves the primary channel at the axillary fossa (at GB-22) and enters the chest and homes to the heart. It then runs up the throat emerging at the face and uniting with the hand tai yang small intestine channel at the inner canthus.

10.4 The Heart Channel Sinews

Pathway: The sinews originate at the medial aspect of the little finger and bind at the wrist (pisiform) bone; they then ascend the arm and bind at the medial aspect of the elbow. Proceeding upward the sinews enter the chest below the axilla, intersect the hand tai yin channel sinews at the breast and bind in the chest. They finally follow the diaphragm downward and connect to the umbilicus.

Main pathologic signs: Internal tension or cramping; infracardiac deep-lying beam; pain and cramping as strain along the course of the sinews.

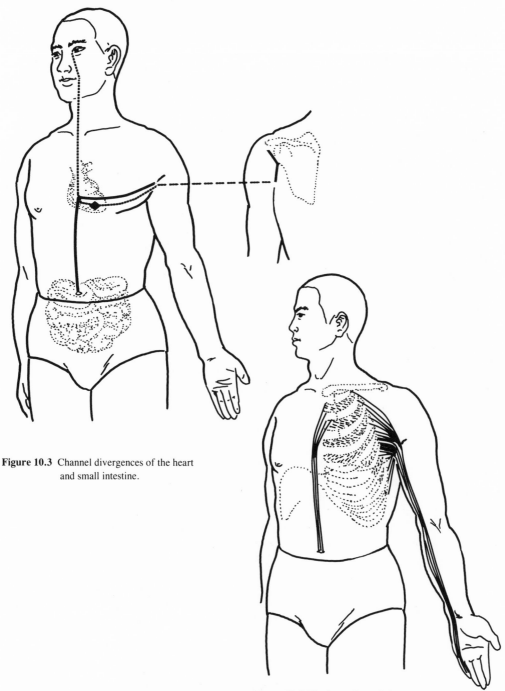

Figure 10.3 Channel divergences of the heart and small intestine.

Figure 10.4 The heart channel sinews.

165

HT-1
極泉
jí quán

"Highest Spring"

Location: In the center of the axilla, on the medial side of the axillary artery.

Classical Location: In the armpit, on the inner side of the arm, where the pulsating vessel enters the chest.
(The Great Compendium)

Local Anatomy: Laterally, the axillary artery. The ulnar nerve, median nerve and medial brachial cutaneous nerve.

Functions: Rectifies qi and loosens the chest; frees the channels and quickens the connecting vessel.

Indications: Pain in the ribs and the region of the heart; scrofula; cold and pain in the elbow and arm.

Supplementary Indications: Cardiac bi; dry retching; cardiac pain; thirst with desire to drink; fullness and pain in the lateral costal region; inversion cold in the arm and elbow.

Stimulation: 0.5″ perpendicular insertion.
Moxa: 1-3 cones; pole 5-10 min.

HT-2
青靈
qīng líng

"Cyan Spirit"

Location: When the elbow is flexed, the point is 3″ above the medial end of the transverse cubital crease (HT-3), in the groove medial to the biceps brachii muscle.

Classical Location: Three inches above the elbow, as located when the arm is raised and the elbow stretched out.
(The Great Compendium)

Local Anatomy: The basilic vein, the superior ulnar collateral artery. The medial antebrachial cutaneous nerve, the medial brachial cutaneous nerve and the ulnar nerve.

Functions: Frees the channels and quickens the connecting vessel; regulates qi and blood.

Indications: Yellowing of the sclera; lateral costal pain; shoulder and arm pain.

Supplementary Indications: Inability to lift the arm; headache and quivering with cold.

Stimulation: 0.3-0.5″ perpendicular insertion.
Moxa: 3-7 cones; pole 5-10 min.

Location: When the elbow is flexed, the point is at the medial end of the transverse cubital crease, in the depression anterior to the medial epicondyle of the humerus.

Classical Location: On the inner side of the elbow, behind the joint, off the big bone, five fen from the tip of the elbow when the arm is flexed toward the head. *(The Great Compendium)*

Local Anatomy: The basilic vein, the inferior ulnar collateral artery, the ulnar recurrent artery and vein. The medial antebrachial cutaneous nerve.

Functions: Courses heart qi; clears the pericardium; stabilizes the spirit-disposition; transforms phlegm-drool.

Indications: Pain in the region of the heart; numbness of the arm; trembling hands; hypertonicity of the elbow; pain in the axillary and lateral costal region; scrofula.

Supplementary Indications: Toothache; headache and dizziness; vomiting of foamy drool; trembling hands and hypertonicity of the elbow; axillary pain; poor memory; mania; qi counterflow; numbness in both arms; cardiac pain.

Illustrative Point Combinations & Applications: For numbness in both arms use HT-3 with LI-10. *(Ode of a Hundred Patterns)*

Stimulation: 0.3-0.8″ perpendicular insertion.
Moxa: 3-5 cones; pole 5-15 min.

Point Categories & Associations: Uniting-he (water) point

HT-3
少海
shào hǎi

"Lesser Sea"

Location: 1.5″ proximal to the transverse wrist crease on the palmar aspect of the forearm. On the radial side of the tendon of the ulnar flexor muscle of the wrist (m. flexor carpi ulnaris).

Classical Location: One inch and five fen behind the hand. *(The Great Compendium)*

Local Anatomy: The ulnar artery. The medial antebrachial cutaneous nerve; on the ulnar side, the ulnar nerve.

Functions: Nourishes the heart and quiets the spirit; soothes the sinews and quickens the connecting vessel.

Indications: Pain in the region of the heart; sudden loss of voice; hypertonicity of the elbow and arm; convulsive spasm.

HT-4
靈道
líng dào

"Spirit Pathway"

167

Supplementary Indications: Visceral agitation; clonic spasm; sorrow and fear.

Stimulation: 0.3-0.5 ″ perpendicular insertion.
Moxa: 1-3 cones; pole 10-20 min.

Point Categories & Associations: River-jing (metal) point

HT-5
通里
tōng lǐ

"Connecting Li"

Location: 1 ″ proximal to the transverse wrist crease. On the radial side of the tendon of the ulnar flexor muscle of the wrist (m. flexor carpi ulnaris).
Classical Location: In the depression one inch behind the hand. *(The Great Compendium)*
Local Anatomy: See HT-4.

Functions: Quiets the spirit and regulates heart qi.
Indications: Palpitations and racing of the heart; dizziness; sore, swollen throat; sudden loss of voice; stiff tongue preventing speech; pain in the wrist and arm.
Supplementary Indications: Throat bi; profuse menstruation; visceral agitation.
Illustrative Point Combinations & Applications: For lazy speech and prostrate exhaustion, use HT-5 and KI-4.
(Ode of a Hundred Patterns)

Stimulation: 0.3-0.5 ″ perpendicular insertion.
Moxa: 1-3 cones; pole 10-20 min.
Needle Sensation: Localized distention and needle stimulus sensation dispersing up and down the arm.

Point Categories & Associations: Connecting-luo point of the heart channel connecting to the small intestine channel.

HT-6
陰郄
yīn xī

"Yin Cleft"

Location: 0.5 ″ proximal to the transverse wrist crease. On the radial side of the tendon of the ulnar flexor muscle of the wrist (m. flexor carpi ulnaris).
Classical Location: In the vessel behind the hand, five fen from the wrist. *(The Great Compendium)*
Local Anatomy: See HT-4.

Functions: Clears heart fire; subdues vacuous yang; quiets the spirit-disposition; secures the exterior.

Indications: Cardiac pain; fright palpitations; night sweating.

Supplementary Indications: Dizziness; fright palpitations; nosebleed; throat bi; infantile steaming bone fever; loss of voice; fullness in the chest; fright inversion.

Illustrative Point Combinations & Applications: Profuse night sweats can be treated with SI-3 and HT-6.
(Ode of a Hundred Patterns)

Stimulation: 0.3-0.5″ perpendicular insertion.
Moxa: 3 cones; pole 10-20 min.

Point Categories & Associations: Cleft-xi point of the heart channel.

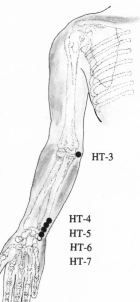

HT-7
神門
shén mén
"Spirit Gate"

Location: On the transverse crease on the palmar side of the wrist, in the articular region between the pisiform bone and the ulna, in the depression on the radial side of the tendon of the ulnar flexor muscle of the wrist (m. flexor carpi ulnaris).

Classical Location: Behind the hand, in the depression at the end of the extremity of the ulna. *(The Great Compendium)*

Local Anatomy: See HT-4.

Functions: Quiets the heart and spirit; clears fire and cools construction; clears heart heat; regulates qi counterflow.

Indications: Cardiac pain; vexation; mania and withdrawal; poor memory; racing of the heart; fright palpitations; insomnia; yellowing of the eyes; pain in the lateral costal region; heat in the palms.

Supplementary Indications: Dizziness; feeblemindedness; epilepsy; retching or spitting of blood; visceral agitation; throat bi; dryness of the throat with no desire to eat; dyspnea counterflow qi ascent; red facial complexion and tendency to laugh.

Illustrative Point Combinations & Applications: SI-3, CV-15 and HT-7 treat the five epilepsies. *(Song More Precious than Jade)*

Stimulation: 0.3-0.5″ perpendicular insertion.
Moxa: 1-3 cones; pole 10-20 min.

Point Categories & Associations: Stream-shu (earth) and source-yuan point.

HT-3

HT-4
HT-5
HT-6
HT-7

Figure 10.5

169

HT-8
少府
shào fǔ

"Lesser Mansion"

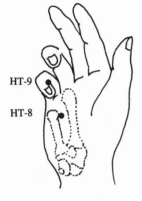

HT-9

HT-8

Figure 10.6

Location: On the palmar surface, between the 4th and 5th meta-carpal bones, proximal to the metacarpal joint. When a fist is made, the point will be found where the tip of the little finger rests.

Classical Location: Behind the base joint of the little finger, the gap between the bones, level with PC-8.
(The Great Compendium)

Local Anatomy: The common palmar digital artery and vein. The 4th common palmar digital nerve derived from the ulnar nerve.

Functions: Quiets the heart and regulates the spirit.

Indications: Palpitations; chest pain; hypertonicity of the fingers; heat in the palm; itchy skin; inhibited urination; enuresis.

Supplementary Indications: Genital itch; vexation, fullness, and diminished qi; sorrow, fear, and fearfulness of people.

Stimulation: 0.3-0.5 ″ perpendicular insertion.
Moxa: 3 cones; pole 5-10 min.

Point Categories & Associations: Spring-ying (fire) point.

Location: On the radial side of the little finger, about 0.1″ proximal to the corner of the nail.

Classical Location: On the inner side of the little finger, the width of a Chinese leek leaf away from the corner of the nail.
(The Great Compendium)

Local Anatomy: The arterial and venous network formed by the palmar digital proprial artery and vein. The palmar digital proprial nerve derived from the ulnar nerve.

Functions: Opens the cardiac portals; clears the spirit-disposition; resuscitates; discharges pathogenic heat.

Indications: Palpitations; cardiac pain; pain in the chest and lateral costal region; mania and withdrawal; heat diseases; clouding inversion.

Supplementary Indications: Jaundice; throat bi; heat diseases with vexation and agitation; emergency treatment of wind strike; pain in the root of the tongue.

Illustrative Point Combinations & Applications: For animal smell of the genitals, first drain LV-13, and then HT-9.
(The Great Compendium)

Stimulation: 0.1″ upward oblique insertion.
Moxa: 1 cone; pole 10 min.

Point Categories & Associations: Well-jing (wood) point.

HT-9
少衝
shào chōng
"Lesser Surge"

Point	Location	Indications Primary	Secondary
*HT-1	Armpit	Cardiac pain pain and aching in the lateral costal region	Scrofula
HT-2	Upper arm	Lateral costal pain upper arm and shoulder pain	
*HT-3	Elbow	Cardiac pain pain and hypertonicity of the elbow and upper arm	Scrofula
HT-4		Cardiac pain pain and hypertonicity of the elbow and upper arm	Clonic spasm
*HT-5	Forearm	Palpitations racing of the heart	Stiff tongue with inability to speak sudden loss of voice
HT-6		Cardiac pain fright palpitations	Night sweating
*HT-7	Wrist joint	Cardiac pain vexation racing of the heart impaired memory insomnia mania, withdrawal, and epilepsy pain in the chest and lateral costal region	
HT-8	Palm	Palpitations chest pain	Inhibited urination pain and itching of the genitals
*HT-9	Finger	Palpitations cardiac pain pain in the chest and lateral costal region mania and withdrawal	Stupor heat disease

Hand Shao Yin Heart Channel

Upper limb: Disorders of the heart and chest; mental disorders

11. The Small Intestine Channel System (Hand Tai Yang) 手太陽小腸經

11.1 The Primary Small Intestine Channel

Pathway: The hand tai yang small intestine channel starts on the outside edge of the little finger tip and travels along the ulnar side of the hand to the wrist, emerging at the ulnar styloid process. Continuing up the posterior aspect of the ulna, it passes between the olecranon of the ulna and the medial epicondyle of the humerus on the medial side of the elbow. It then runs up the posteromedial side of the upper arm, emerging behind the shoulder joint and circling around the superior and inferior fossae of the scapula. At the top of the shoulder it intersects the foot tai yang bladder channel at BL-41 and BL-11, connecting with the governing vessel at GV-14 before turning downward into the supraclavicular fossa. Here it submerges, connects with the heart, and follows the esophagus down through the diaphragm to the stomach. It then intersects with the conception vessel internally at CV-13 and CV-12 before homing to the small intestine.

A branch separates from the channel at the supraclavicular fossa and runs up the neck to the cheek. It then travels to the outer canthus of the eye where it meets the foot shao yang gallbladder channel at GB-1, and then turns back across the temple to enter the ear at SI-19.

Another branch breaks off at the mandible, rises to the infraorbital region, and continues to the inner canthus where it meets the foot tai yang bladder channel at BL-1. It then crosses horizontally to the zygomatic region.

The *Spiritual Axis* claims that another branch descends internally from the small intestine to emerge at ST-39, the lower uniting-he point of the small intestine.

Main pathologic signs associated with the external course of the channel: erosion of the glossal and oral mucosa; pain in the cheeks; sore pharynx; lachrymation; [*tearing of eyes*] stiffness of the neck; pain on the lateral aspect of the shoulder and upper arm.

Main pathologic signs associated with the internal organ: Lower abdominal pain and distention with the pain stretching around to the lumbar region; lower abdominal pain radiating into the testicles; diarrhea; pain in the stomach with dry feces and constipation. [*b/c SI pathology tends to be hot*]

11.2 The Connecting Vessel of the Small Intestine Channel

Pathway: This vessel separates from the primary channel and SI-7 and connects to the hand shao yin heart channel. A branch also proceeds up the arm past the elbow and connects to the top of the shoulder (near LI-15).

Main pathologic signs of repletion: looseness of the joints; atony of the sinews in the elbow region.

Main pathologic sign of vacuity: small wart-like excresences.

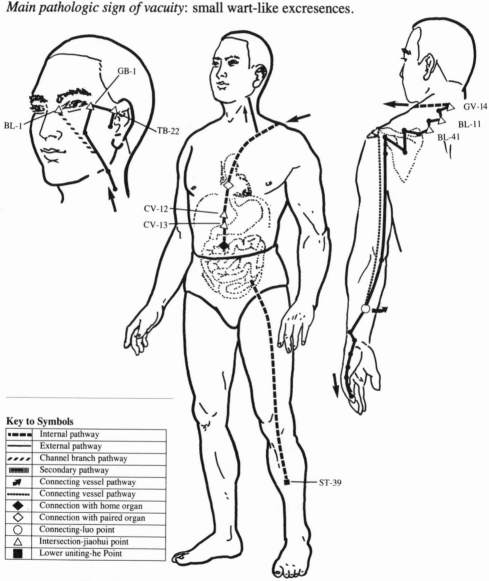

Key to Symbols

■━■━	Internal pathway
────	External pathway
⁄⁄⁄⁄	Channel branch pathway
▥▥▥▥	Secondary pathway
◢	Connecting vessel pathway
▪▪▪▪▪	Connecting vessel pathway
◆	Connection with home organ
◇	Connection with paired organ
○	Connecting-luo point
△	Intersection-jiaohui point
■	Lower uniting-he Point

Figure 11.1 - 11.2 Primary channel and connecting vessel of small intestine.

11.3 The Small Intestine Channel Divergence

Pathway: The divergence separates from the primary channel at the shoulder, enters at the axilla, goes to the heart and proceeds downward to connect to the small intestine.

11.4 The Small Intestine Channel Sinews

Pathway: These sinews originate at the dorsal aspect of the little finger and bind at the wrist. They then ascend along the arm, binding at the elbow (the medial condyle of the humerus) and again below the axilla.

A branch travels from the posterior aspect of the axilla to wrap the scapula. Proceeding up the neck following anterior to the foot tai yang bladder channel sinews, it binds to the bone behind the ear. From here, a branch enters into the ear, then issues at the top of the ear and descends to bind at the submandibular region. This branch then rises to home to the outer canthus. Another branch forks out from the mandible, curves upward past the teeth and rises in front of the ear, homing to the outer canthus and binding to the corner of the forehead.

Main pathologic signs: Strain and inability to support the little finger; pain at the medial aspect of the elbow, the yin aspect of the upper arm and the axilla. Axilla pain that extends back over the scapula and neck; pain (and tinnitus) in the ear that may extend to the submandibular region; the need to close the eyes for a while to get them to focus. Spasms or tension of the neck sinews resulting in sinew atony or swelling at the neck.

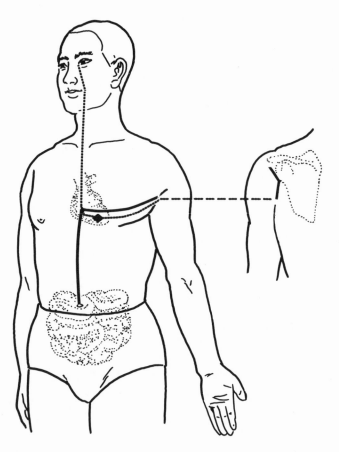

Figure 11.3 Channel divergences of the small intestine and heart channels.

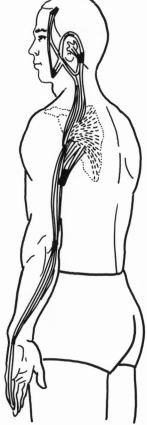

Figure 11.4 The small intestine channel sinews.

Location: On the ulnar side of the little finger, about 0.1″ proximal to the corner of the nail. *(The Great Compendium)*

Classical Location: On the outer side of the little finger, in the depression one fen from the corner of the nail. *(The Great Compendium)*

Local Anatomy: The arterial and venous network formed by the palmar digital proprial artery and vein and the dorsal digital artery and vein.

Functions: Clears heart fire; dissipates depressed heat; frees the channels and quickens the connecting vessels; opens the portals; disinhibits breast milk.

Indications: Heat disease; clouding inversion; scant breast milk; sore, swollen throat; eye screens.

Supplementary Indications: Fever and chills without sweating; headache; quivering from cold; throat bi; curled tongue; heat in the mouth and vexation; shortness of breath; jaundice; nosebleed; swelling of the breasts; postpartum absence of milk; wind strike; loss of the use of the little finger; dry pharynx.

Illustrative Point Combinations & Applications: Swelling of the breast in women can be treated with SI-1 and M-HN-9. *(Ode of the Jade Dragon)*

Stimulation: 0.1″ slightly upward oblique insertion.
Moxa: 1-3 cones; pole 5-10 min.

Needle Sensation: Localized needle stimulus sensation and pain.

Point Categories & Associations: Well-jing (metal) point.

SI-1
少澤
shào zé
"Lesser Marsh"

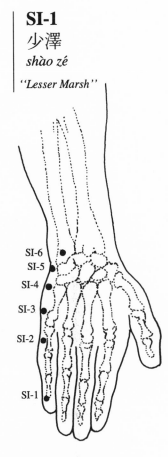

Figure 11.5

Location: When a loose fist is made, the point is distal to the metacarpophalangeal joint, at the border of the red and white skin.

Classical Location: On the outer side of the little finger, in the depression in front of the base joint. *(The Great Compendium)*

Local Anatomy: The dorsal digital artery and vein arising from the ulnar artery and vein. The dorsal digital nerve and palmar digital proprial nerve derived from the ulnar nerve.

SI-2
前谷
qián gǔ
"Front Valley"

Functions: Courses wind and resolves heat; disperses swelling.
Indications: Numbness of the fingers; heat diseases.
Supplementary Indications: Cough and thoracic fullness; headache; swelling and stiffness of the neck; swollen pharynx; postpartum absence of milk; tinnitus; nosebleed; nasal congestion with yellow snivel.

Stimulation: 0.1-0.3″ perpendicular insertion.
Moxa: 1-3 cones; pole 5-10 min.

Point Categories & Associations: Spring-ying (water) point.

SI-3
後溪
hòu xī

"Back Ravine"

Location: When a loose fist is made, the point is proximal to the head of the 5th metacarpal bone on the ulnar side, in the depression at the border of the red and white skin.

Classical Location: On the outer side of the little finger, in the depression behind the base joint, located by making a fist.
(The Great Compendium)

Local Anatomy: The dorsal digital artery and vein, the dorsal venous network of the hand. The dorsal branch derived from the ulnar nerve.

Functions: Clears the spirit-disposition; dispels interior heat; frees the governing vessel; secures the exterior.
Indications: Headache; stiff neck; reddening of the eyes; deafness; hypertonicity of the elbow, arm, and fingers; heat diseases; epilepsy; malarial disease; night sweating.
Supplementary Indications: Cardiac pain; dark-colored urine; mania and withdrawal; headache and neck pain; gastric reflux.
Illustrative Point Combinations & Applications: HT-6 and SI-3 treat profuse night sweating.

Needling SI-3 and GB-30 relieves pain in the thigh.
(Ode of a Hundred Patterns)

SI-3, CV-15 and HT-7 bring immediate improvement for the five epilepsies. *(Song More Precious than Jade)*

Stimulation: 0.3-0.7″ perpendicular insertion.
Moxa: 1-3 cones; pole 5-15 min.

Needle Sensation: Distention and numbness, sometimes spreading down the little finger.

Point Categories & Associations: Stream-shu (wood) point; confluence-jiaohui point of the eight extraordinary vessels; related to the governing vessel.

Location: On the ulnar side of the palm, in the depression between the base of the 5th metacarpal bone and the triquetral bone.

Classical Location: On the outer side of the hand, in the depression by the protruding bone in front of the wrist.
(The Great Compendium)

Local Anatomy: The posterior carpal artery (the branch of the ulnar artery), the dorsal venous network of the hand. The dorsal branch of the ulnar nerve.

Functions: Courses tai yang channel pathogens; clears small intestinal damp-heat.

Indications: Headache; stiff neck; eye screens; pain in the lateral costal region; jaundice; heat diseases.

Supplementary Indications: Absence of sweating in heat diseases; throat bi; nasal congestion; clear, runny snivel; nosebleed; wasting thirst; hypertonicity of the finger; pain in the forearm; weak, aching wrist.

Illustrative Point Combinations & Applications: For splenic vacuity jaundice, use SI-4 and CV-12. *(Ode of the Jade Dragon)*

Stimulation: 0.2-0.5″ perpendicular insertion.
Moxa: 3 cones; pole 5-20 min.

Point Categories & Associations: Source-yuan point.

SI-4
腕骨
wàn gŭ
"Wrist Bone"

Location: On the ulnar side of the wrist, in the depression between the styloid process of the ulna and the triquetral bone.
Classical Location: At the wrist, in the depression at extremity of the ulna. *(The Great Compendium)*
Local Anatomy: The posterior carpal artery. The dorsal branch of the ulnar nerve.

SI-5
陽谷
yáng gŭ
"Yang Valley"

Functions: Resolves heat and disperses swelling; quiets the spirit and settles tetany.

Indications: Swelling of the neck and submandibular region; pain along the lateral aspect of the arm; pain in the wrist; heat diseases.

Supplementary Indications: Heat disease without sweating; pain in the lateral costal region; deafness and tinnitus; visual dizziness and eye pain; infantile clonic spasm; madness; throat bi; sensation of obstruction of the pharynx; stiffness of the tongue in infants that prevents suckling; toothache among the upper and lower teeth; painful hemorrhoids.

Stimulation: 0.2-0.4″ perpendicular insertion.
Moxa: 3 cones; pole 5-20 min.

Point Categories & Associations: River-jing (fire) point.

SI-6
養老
yăng lăo

"Nursing the Aged"

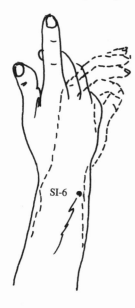

SI-6

Figure 11.6
A depression appears
at SI-6 when the wrist
is rotated.

Location: On the dorsal aspect of the head of the ulna. When the palm faces the chest, the point is in the bony cleft on the radial side of the styloid process of the ulna.

Classical Location: Moving up from the wrist bone, one inch behind SI-4. *(The Great Compendium)*

Local Anatomy: The terminal branches of the posterior interosseous artery and vein, the dorsal venous network of the wrist. The anastomotic branches of the posterior antebrachial cutaneous and dorsal branch of the ulnar nerve.

Functions: Frees the channels and quickens the connecting vessels; brightens the eyes.

Indications: Blurred vision; pain in the shoulder, arm, and elbow.

Supplementary Indications: Lumbar pain preventing turning over; hypertonicity of the sinews and bi of the foot; redness and swelling of the outer face of the elbow.

Stimulation: 0.3-0.5″ perpendicular insertion.
Moxa: 3 cones; pole 5-20 min.

Point Categories & Associations: Cleft-xi point of the small intestine channel.

Location: 5″ proximal to the wrist, on the line joining SI-5 and SI-8. On the medial edge of the ulna.

Classical Location: Five inches behind the wrist.
(The Great Compendium)

Local Anatomy: The terminal branches of the posterior interosseous artery and vein. Superficially, the branch of the medial antebrachial cutaneous nerve; deeper, on the radial side, the posterior interosseous nerve.

Functions: Clears the spirit-disposition; resolves exterior heat; courses channel pathogens.

Indications: Stiff neck; hypertonicity of the elbow; pain in the fingers; heat diseases; mania and withdrawal.

Supplementary Indications: Quivering from cold; fever and chills; headache; loss of grasping ability of the fingers; heat diseases with sweating; madness; fright, fear, sorrow and anxiety; lumbar pain.

Illustrative Point Combinations & Applications: For visual dizziness, use SI-7 and BL-58. *(Ode of a Hundred Patterns)*

Stimulation: 0.3-0.5″ perpendicular insertion.
Moxa: 3-5 cones; pole 5-20 min.

Point Categories & Associations: Connecting-luo point of the small intestine channel connecting to the heart channel.

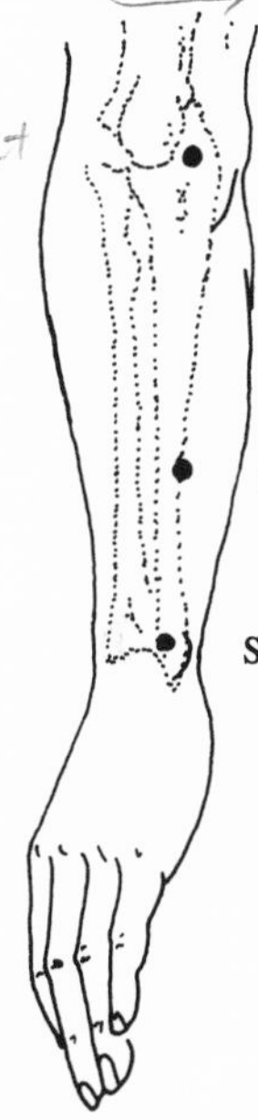

SI-7
支正
zhī zhèng

"Branch to the Correct"

Figure 11.7

Location: In the shallow depression on the flat area between the olecranon of the ulna and the medial epicondyle of the humerus, when the elbow is flexed.

Classical Location: On the outer side of the outside major bone of the elbow, in the depression five fen from the tip of the elbow. The point is found by flexing the arm toward the head.
(The Great Compendium)

Local Anatomy: The superior and inferior ulnar collateral arteries and veins, the ulnar recurrent artery and vein. The branches of the medial antebrachial cutaneous nerve, the ulnar nerve.

SI-8
小海
xiǎo hǎi

"Small Sea"

181

Cramp
constipation

Functions: Dissipates tai yang channel pathogens; frees small intestinal heat bind; dispels wind qi; clears the spirit-disposition.

Indications: Swelling of the cheek; pain in the nape and lateroposterior aspect of the shoulder and arm; epilepsy.

Supplementary Indications: Madness; heat diseases without sweating; aversion to cold; tooth decay; dizziness; neck pain; lower abdominal pain; vexation in the heart.

Stimulation: 0.3-0.8″ oblique insertion.
Moxa: 5-7 cones; pole 5-20 min.

Point Categories & Associations: Uniting-he (earth) point.

SI-9
肩貞
jiān zhēn

"*True Shoulder*"

Location: On the back, inferior to the shoulder joint. 1″ above the posterior end of the axillary fold when the arm is adducted.

Classical Location: Between the two bones below the scapula, in the depression behind LI-15. *(The Great Compendium)*

Local Anatomy: The circumflex scapular artery and vein. Branch of the axillary nerve; deeper in the superior aspect, the radial nerve.

Functions: Courses wind and quickens the connecting vessels; dissipates binds and relieves pain.

Indications: Pain in the shoulder blade; pain and inhibited movement of the hand and arm.

Supplementary Indications: Cold damage fever and chills; swelling of the submandibular region; tinnitus and deafness; pain in the supraclavicular fossa; toothache.

Stimulation: 0.5-1.0″ perpendicular insertion.
Moxa: 3 cones; pole 5-20 min.

SI-10
臑俞
nào shū

"*Upper Arm Shu*"

Location: With the arm adducted, the point is directly above SI-9, in the depression inferior to the scapular spine. On the medial aspect of the acromial angle.

Classical Location: Behind TB-14, below the large bone, in the depression above the shoulder blade. The point is found with the arm raised. *(The Great Compendium)*

Local Anatomy: The posterior circumflex humeral artery and vein; deeper, the suprascapular artery and vein. The posterior cutaneous nerve of the arm, the axillary nerve; deeper, the suprascapular nerve.

Functions: Quickens the blood and frees the connecting vessels; soothes the sinews and dissipates binds.

Indications: Pain and lack of strength in the shoulder and arm.

Supplementary Indications: Fever and chills; inability to move the shoulder and arm; shoulder pain that extends to the scapula.

Stimulation: 0.5-1.0″ perpendicular insertion.
Moxa: 3 cones; pole 5-20 min.

Point Categories & Associations: Intersection-jiaohui point of the hand tai yang small intestine channel and the yang linking and yang motility vessels.

SI-11
天宗
tiān zōng
"Celestial Gathering"

Location: In the infrascapular fossa, midway between the medial and lateral borders and one third of the distance between the lower border of the scapular spine and the inferior angle of the scapula.

Classical Location: Behind SI-12, in the depression of the shoulder blade. *(The Great Compendium)*

Local Anatomy: The muscular branches of the circumflex scapular artery and vein. The suprascapular nerve.

Functions: Resolves tai yang channel pathogens; diffuses qi stagnation in the chest and lateral costal region.

Indications: Pain in the shoulder blade and the lateroposterior aspect of the arm and elbow.

Supplementary Indications: Branching fullness in the chest and lateral costal region; cough counterflow; swelling of the lateral cheek and submandibular region.

Stimulation: 0.5-1.0″ oblique or perpendicular insertion.
Moxa: 3 cones; pole 5-20 min.

Needle Sensation: Distention and numbness, sometimes spreading over the shoulder.

SI-15
肩中俞
jiān zhōng shū

"Central Shoulder Shu"

Location: 2″ lateral to the lower border of the spinous process of the 7th cervical vertebra (GV-14).
Classical Location: On the inner side of the shoulder blade, two inches from the spinal column. *(The Great Compendium)*
Local Anatomy: See SI-14.

Functions: Diffuses the lung and clears heat; transforms phlegm and brightens the eyes.
Indications: Cough, asthma; shoulder and back pain.
Supplementary Indications: Fever and chills; unclear vision; spitting of blood.

Stimulation: 0.3-0.6″ perpendicular insertion.
Moxa: 5-10 cones; pole 5-20 min.

SI-16
天窗
tiān chuāng

"Celestial Window"

Location: On the lateral aspect of the neck, on the posterior border of the sternocleidomastoid muscle (m. sternocleidomastoideus), posterosuperior to LI-18.
Classical Location: In the cleft in the major sinew of the neck, below the corner of the jaw, and behind LI-18, in the depression where a pulsating vessel can be felt. (dà chéng)
Local Anatomy: The ascending cervical artery. The cutaneous cervical nerve, the emerging portion of the great auricular nerve.

Functions: Dispels wind and quickens the connecting vessels; quiets the spirit and nourishes the heart.
Indications: Deafness and tinnitus; sore, swollen throat; pain and rigidity of the neck.
Supplementary Indications: Painful swelling of the cheek; wind strike with loss of voice; throat bi; mania.

Stimulation: 0.3-0.8″ perpendicular insertion.
Moxa: 3 cones; pole 5-10 min.

Location: Immediately posterior to the angle of the mandible, in the depression on the anterior border of the sternocleidomastoid muscle (m. sternocleidomastoideus).

Classical Location: Below the ear, behind the corner of the jaw. *(The Great Compendium)*

Local Anatomy: Anteriorly, the external jugular vein; deeper, the internal carotid artery and internal jugular vein. Superficially, the anterior branch of the great auricular nerve, the cervical branch of the facial nerve; deeper, the superior cervical ganglion of the sympathetic trunk.

Functions: Soothes the sinews and quickens connecting vessels; clears heat and disperses swelling.

Indications: Deafness and tinnitus; sore, swollen throat; sensation of throat being obstructed; swelling of the cheek.

Supplementary Indications: Thoracic fullness hampering respiration; retching counterflow and ejection of foam; clenched teeth.

Stimulation: 0.3-0.8″ perpendicular insertion toward the root of the tongue.
Moxa: 3 cones; pole 5-10 min.

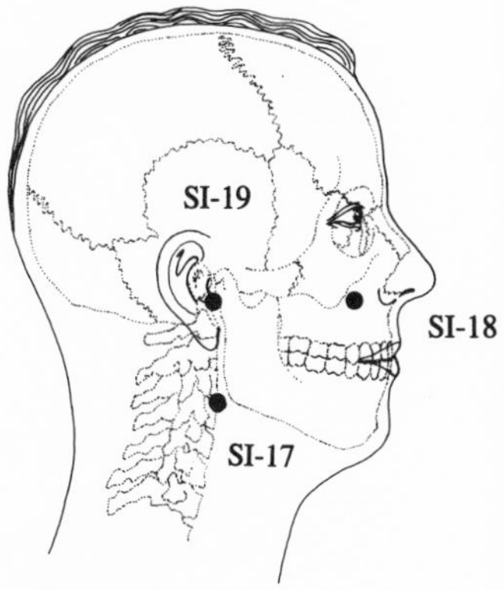

SI-17
天容
tiān róng

"Celestial
    Countenance"

Figure 11.9

Location: Directly below the outer canthus, in the depression beneath the lower border of the zygoma.

Classical Location: In the depression below the protuberance of the cheek bone. *(The Great Compendium)*

Local Anatomy: Branches of the transverse facial artery and vein. The facial and infraorbital nerves.

Functions: Relieves pain and tetany.

Indications: Wryness of the mouth and eyes; twitching of the eyelids; toothache; yellowing of the eyes.

Supplementary Indications: Pain and swelling of the cheek.

Stimulation: 0.2-0.3″ oblique or perpendicular insertion.

Contraindications: Contraindicated for moxibustion.

SI-18
顴髎
quán liáo

"Cheek Bone-Hole"

SI-19

聽宮

tīng gōng

"Auditory Palace"

Location: Between the tragus of the ear and the mandibular joint, where a depression is formed when the mouth is open wide.

Classical Location: At the pearl in the ear (which is the size of an adzuki bean). *(The Great Compendium)*

Local Anatomy: The auricular branches of the superficial temporal artery and vein. Branch of the facial nerve, the auriculotemporal nerve.

Functions: Frees the channel and connecting vessels; opens the ear portals; relieves pain; boosts visual and hearing acuity.

Indications: Deafness; tinnitus; purulent ear discharge.

Supplementary Indications: Arm pain; toothache; cardioabdominal pain; madness.

Illustrative Point Combinations & Applications: SI-19 and BL-20 eliminate sorrow and sadness below the heart.
(Ode of a Hundred Patterns)

Stimulation: 0.2-1.0 " perpendicular insertion.
Moxa: 3-5 cones; pole 5 min.

Needle Sensation: Distention, sometimes spreading into the ear.

Hand Tai Yang Small Intestine Channel			
Point	**Location**	**Indications**	
		Primary	**Secondary**
*SI-1	Finger	Headache eye screen pain and swelling of the throat	Shortage of breast milk heat disease
SI-2		Headache numbness of the fingers pain and swelling of the throat	Heat disease
*SI-3	Side of palm	Pain and stiffness of the head and neck red eyes deafness	Mania, withdrawal, and epilepsy
*SI-4	Anterior to wrist	Pain and stiffness of the head and neck eye screen hypertonicity of the fingers wrist pain	Jaundice heat disease
SI-5	Wrist	Visual dizziness tinnitus deafness wrist pain	Madness swelling of the neck
*SI-6	Forearm	Dim vision	Lumbar pain
*SI-7		Stiff neck hypertonicity of the elbow	Madness heat disease
SI-8		Arm and elbow pain	Mania and withdrawal
Hand to elbow: Disorders of the head, neck, ears, eyes and throat; heat disease; mental disorders			

Point	Location	Indications	
		Primary	**Secondary**
SI-9		Pain and aching of the shoulder and arm	
SI-10		Shoulder and upper arm pain	
*SI-11	Shoulder	Shoulder and upper arm pain	Mammary yong
SI-12		Shoulder and upper arm pain	
SI-13		Shoulder and upper arm pain	
SI-14		Pain and aching of the shoulder and back rigidity of the neck	
SI-15	Back	Shoulder and back pain	
Shoulder: Disorders of the scapular region			
SI-16	Neck	Tinnitus deafness pain and swelling of the throat	
SI-17		Tinnitus deafness pain and swelling of the throat	Swelling of the cheek
Neck: Disorders of the throat and ears			
*SI-18	Face	Wry mouth and eyes eyelid spasm toothache	
*SI-19	Ear	Tinnitus deafness	
Face: Disorders of the mouth, teeth, and ears			

Hand Tai Yang Small Intestine Channel (continued)

12. The Bladder Channel System
(Foot Tai Yang) 足太陽膀胱經

12.1 The Primary Bladder Channel

UB1 (handwritten)

Pathway: The foot tai yang bladder channel starts at the inner canthus of the eye, travels upwards over the forehead, intersecting the governing vessel at GV-24 and the foot shao yin gallbladder channel at GB-15. It travels on up to the vertex and again meets the governing vessel at GV-20.

A branch separates at the vertex and goes down to the area just above the ear, meeting the foot shao yang gallbladder channel at GB-7, GB-8, GB-10, GB-11, and GB-12.

A vertical branch enters the brain from the vertex to meet the governing vessel at GV-17, and reemerges to run down the nape of the neck and the muscles of the medial aspect of the scapula, meeting the governing vessel again at GV-14 and GV-13. It continues downward, parallel to the spine, to the lumbar region. Here the channel submerges, follows the paravertebral muscles, and connects with the kidney before homing to the bladder.

A branch separates in the lumbar region and runs down the buttocks and the posterior midline of the thighs to the popliteal fossa behind the knee.

A further branch separates from the main channel at the nape of the neck, descending lateral to the paravertebral branch mentioned above along the medial border of the scapula and down to the gluteal region, where it crosses the buttocks and intersects the gallbladder channel at GB-30. It then passes down the posterolateral aspect of the thigh to meet the other branch of the same channel in the popliteal fossa. The channel continues downward through the gastrocnemius muscle, (calf) emerges posterior to the lateral malleolus, and then runs along the lateral margin of the fifth metatarsal bone, crossing its tuberosity, to the lateral tip of the little toe at BL-67.

Main pathologic signs associated with the exterior course of the channel: chills and fever; headache; stiff neck; pain in the lumbar region and along the spine; nasal congestion; ocular pain and lachrymation; pain in the posterior thigh, popliteal region, gastrocnemius, and foot. *calf* (handwritten)

Main pathologic signs associated with the internal organ: pain and distention in the lower abdomen; inhibited micturition; urinary block and enuresis; mental disorders; opisthotonos. *(bladder there)* (handwritten)

urination (handwritten)

arching of neck + back contraction (handwritten)
head (handwritten)
heels (handwritten)

191

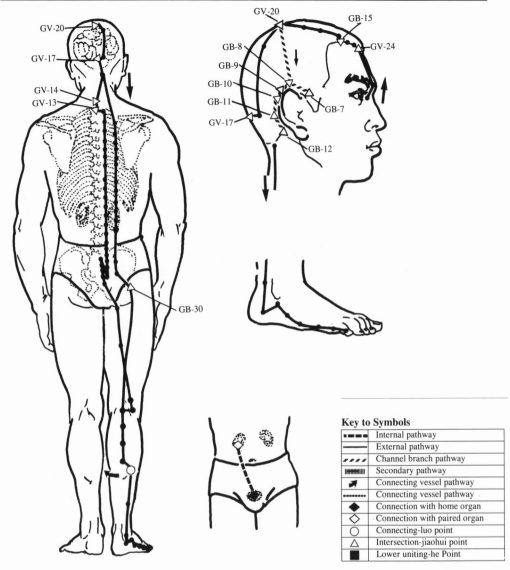

Figure 12.1 - 12.2 Primary channel and connecting vessel of the bladder.

12.2 The Connecting Vessel of the Bladder Channel

Pathway: This vessel breaks from the primary channel at BL-58 and connects to the foot shao yin kidney channel.

Main pathologic signs:

Repletion: nasal congestion with clear nasal discharge; headache; back pain.

Vacuity: clear nasal discharge; nosebleed.

12.3 The Bladder Channel Divergence

Pathway: This divergence leaves the primary channel at the popliteal fossa and ascends to a point 5 body inches below the coccyx where it enters the anal region, homes to the bladder, disperses over that organ and then follows the spine upward to the neck where it homes to the primary channel.

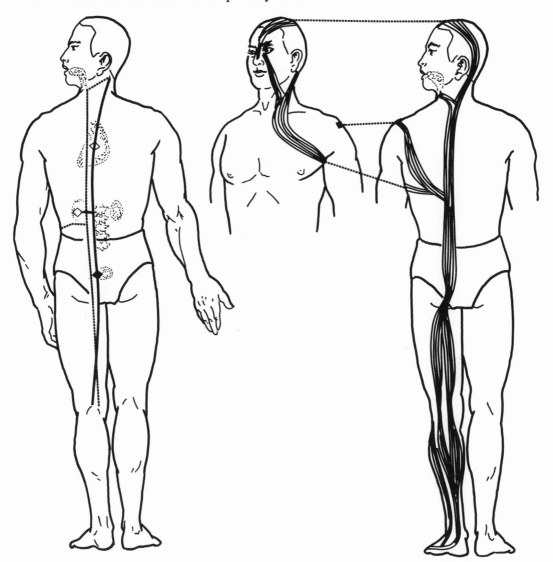

Figure 12.3 Channel divergences of the bladder and kidney.

Figure 12.4 The bladder channel sinews.

12.4 The Bladder Channel Sinews

Pathway: These sinews originate at the little toe, bind at the lateral malleolus and then slant upward to bind at the knee. Another branch follows below the first. It travels under the lateral malleolus, binds at the heel and rises to bind again at the popliteal fossa. Another branch breaks off at the mid-calf and proceeds upward to bind at the medial aspect of the popliteal fossa.

The two branches proceed from the popliteal fossa up the posterior of the thigh and together bind in the gluteal region. As one sinew group they rise along the side of the spine to the nape of the neck. A branch enters to bind at the root of the tongue. Another branch binds to the occipital bone and rises over the head to bind to the nose. A branch goes to the area above the eye (ie: the sinews that control opening and closing of the eye) and then binds at the side of the nose.

From the posterolateral aspect of the axilla a branch binds to the top of the shoulder. Another branch enters below the axilla and rises to issue at the supraclavicular fossa where it rises to bind to the bone behind the ear. A final branch slants up from its issuance at the supraclavicular fossa to the side of the nose.

Main pathologic signs:

Strain or inability to support the little toe; pain and swelling of the heel; spasm or tension in the popliteal region; opisthotonos; spasm or tension in the neck sinews; inability to raise the arm; muscular discomfort in the axilla; strained muscles in the supraclavicular fossa.

Location: 0.1″ superior to the inner canthus. To locate the point, have the patient close her eyes.

Classical Location: In the depression one fen outward from the inner canthus. *(The Golden Mirror)*

Local Anatomy: The angular artery and vein; deeper, superiorly, the ophthalmic artery and vein. Superficially, the supratrochlear and infratrochlear nerves; deeper, branches of the oculomotor nerve, the opthalmic nerve.

Functions: Courses wind and discharges heat; nourishes water and brightens the eyes.

Indications: Pain and swelling of the eyes; tearing on exposure to wind; itching of the canthus; night blindness; color blindness.

Supplementary Indications: Abhorrence of cold with headache; visual dizziness; nearsightedness.

Illustrative Point Combinations & Applications: Unsufferable reddening and swelling of the eyes and aversion to light is treated by needling BL-1 and M-HN-7, and letting blood from M-HN-9. *(Song of the Jade Dragon)*

Stimulation: 0.3″ perpendicular insertion along the orbital wall.

Point Categories & Associations: Intersection-jiaohui point of the hand tai yang small intestine, foot tai yang bladder, and foot yang ming stomach channels and the yin motility and yang motility vessels.

BL-1
睛明
jīng míng
"Bright Eyes"

Location: At the medial end of the eyebrow, in the supraorbital notch.

Classical Location: In the depression on the eyebrow above BL-1. *(The Golden Mirror)*

Local Anatomy: The frontal artery and vein. The medial branch of the frontal nerve.

Functions: Dispels wind qi; brightens the eyes.

BL-2
攢竹
zǎn zhú
"Bamboo Gathering"

195

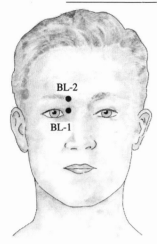

Indications: Headache; visual dizziness; pain in the superciliary ridge; blurring of vision; tearing on exposure to wind; redness, pain and swelling of the eye; twitching of the eyelids.

Supplementary Indications: Wind dizziness; painful hemorrhoids; infantile epilepsy with the eyes looking upwards; aversion to wind and cold; stiff neck.

Illustrative Point Combinations & Applications: BL-2 and ST-8 treat eye pain and headache. *(Ode of the Jade Dragon)*

Stimulation: 0.3-0.5″ transverse insertion in inferior lateral direction; bleed with three-edged needle. Moxa: pole 1-3 min.

Figure 12.5

BL-3
眉衝
méi chōng

"Eyebrow Ascension"

Location: Above BL-2. 0.5″ within the anterior hairline, between GV-24 and BL-4.

Classical Location: Above the (inner) border of the eyebrow, between GV-24 and BL-4. *(The Great Compendium)*

Local Anatomy: See BL-2.

Functions: Dispels wind and clears heat; brightens the eyes.

Indications: Headache; dizziness; epilepsy.

Supplementary Indications: Nasal congestion; the five epilepsies.

Stimulation: 0.3-0.5″ upward transverse insertion. Moxa: pole 5-10 min.

BL-4
曲差
qū chāi

"Deviating Turn"

Location: 1.5″ lateral to the midline, 0.5″ within the anterior hairline, one-third of the distance from GV-24 to ST-8.

Classical Location: Lateral to BL-3 within the hairline, one inch and five fen either side of GV-24. *(The Golden Mirror)*

Local Anatomy: The frontal artery and vein. The lateral branch of the frontal nerve.

Functions: Discharges heat and opens the portals; clears the head and brightens the eyes.

Indications: Frontal vertical headache; visual dizziness; eye pain; nasal congestion; nosebleed.

Supplementary Indications: Headache; body fever; vexation and fullness in the heart; absence of sweating; blurred vision; nose sores; clear, runny snivel with nosebleed.

Stimulation: 0.3-0.5″ upward transverse insertion. Moxa: 3-5 cones; pole 5-15 min.

Location: Posterior to BL-4, 1″ inside the anterior hairline.
Classical Location: Five fen back from BL-4, one inch and five fen each side of GV-23. *(The Golden Mirror)*
Local Anatomy: See BL-4.

Functions: Diffuses and discharges wind-heat; clears the head and brightens the eyes.
Indications: Headache; visual dizziness; epilepsy.
Supplementary Indications: Heaviness of the head; clonic spasm; opisthotonos; wind bi.

Stimulation: 0.3-0.5″ backward transverse insertion.
Moxa: 3 cones; pole 5-15 min.

BL-5
五處
wǔ chù

"Fifth Place"

Location: 1.5″ posterior to BL-5, 1.5″ lateral to the governing vessel.
Classical Location: One inch and five fen behind BL-5. *(The Great Compendium)*
Local Anatomy: The anastomotic network of the frontal artery and vein, the superficial temporal artery and vein and the occipital artery and vein. The anastomotic branch of the frontal nerve and the great occipital nerve.

Functions: Clears heat and eliminates vexation; brightens the eyes and opens the portals.
Indications: Headache; visual dizziness; nasal congestion.
Supplementary Indications: Absence of sweating in heat diseases; vomiting; vexation; loss of smell; nasal congestion with copious snivel; eye screens; wind dizziness; wryness of the mouth.

Stimulation: 0.3-0.5″ backward transverse insertion.
Moxa: pole 2-5 min.

BL-6
承光
chéng guāng

"Light Guard"

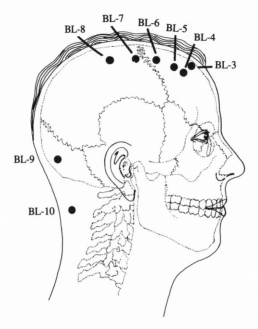

Figure 12.6

BL-7
通天

tōng tiān

"Celestial Connection"

Location: 1.5 ″ posterior to BL-6, 1.5 ″ lateral to the governing vessel.

Classical Location: One inch and five fen behind BL-6, one inch and five fen each side of GV-20. *(The Golden Mirror)*

Local Anatomy: The anastomotic network of the superficial temporal artery and vein and the occipital artery and vein. The branch of the great occipital nerve.

Functions: Dispels wind and resolves the exterior; frees and disinhibits the nose.

Indications: Headache; dizziness; nasal congestion; nosebleed; deep-source nasal congestion.

Supplementary Indications: Nose sores; nasal polyps; hemilateral wind; wryness of the mouth; stiff neck; dyspnea.

Stimulation: 0.2-0.3 ″ transverse insertion.
Moxa: 3 cones; pole 5-15 min.

Location: 1.5″ posterior to BL-7, 1.5″ lateral to the governing vessel.

Classical Location: One inch and five fen behind BL-7. *(The Great Compendium)*

Local Anatomy: Branches of the occipital artery and vein. Branch of the great occipital nerve.

Functions: Dissipates wind and clears heat; clears the head and brightens the eyes.

Indications: Dizziness; tinnitus; mania and withdrawal.

Supplementary Indications: Nasal congestion; clonic spasm; manic movement; retching and vomiting.

Stimulation: 0.3-0.5″ transverse insertion.
Moxa: 3 cones; pole 5-10 min.

BL-8
絡却
luò què
"Declining Connection"

Location: 1.3″ lateral to GV-17, on the lateral side of the superior border of the external occipital protuberance.

Classical Location: One inch and five fen behind BL-8, one inch and three fen to each side of GV-17. *(The Great Compendium)*

Local Anatomy: The occipital artery and vein.

Functions: Dispels wind and quickens the connecting vessels; frees the portals and brightens the eyes.

Indications: Headache; eye pain; nasal congestion.

Supplementary Indications: Insufferable wind headache; dizzy or heavy head; upturned eyes; blurred vision; pain and reddening of the eyes; nasal congestion and sore pharynx; stiff neck; aversion to cold; absence of sweating in heat diseases.

Stimulation: 0.3-0.5″ downward transverse insertion.
Moxa: pole 5-15 min.

BL-9
玉枕
yù zhěn
"Jade Pillow"

Location: 1.3″ lateral to GV-15, 0.5″ within the posterior hairline, on the lateral side of the trapezius muscle (m. trapezius).

Classical Location: At the hairline on either side of the nape, in the depression on the outer face of the major sinew. *(The Great Compendium)*

BL-10
天柱
tiān zhù
"Celestial Pillar"

Local Anatomy: The occipital artery and vein.

Functions: Dispels wind and dissipates cold; soothes the sinews and quickens the connecting vessels; clears the head and brightens the eyes; relieves pain.

Indications: Headache; stiff neck; nasal congestion; shoulder and back pain.

Supplementary Indications: Dizzy or heavy head; nearsightedness; blurry vision with red painful eyes; tearing; eyes fit to burst from their sockets; pain in the vertex as if the top of the head were being pried off; nasal congestion and pharyngeal swelling; stiff neck; aversion to cold; absence of sweating in heat diseases; child fright epilepsy; other forms of epilepsy.

Illustrative Point Combinations & Applications: For blurry vision, needle SI-6 and BL-10. *(Ode of a Hundred Patterns)*

Stimulation: 0.5″ perpendicular insertion. Moxa: pole 5-15 min.

BL-11
大杼

dà zhù

"Great Shuttle"

Location: 1.5″ lateral to the lower border of the spinous process of the 1st thoracic vertebra, about 2 finger breadths from the governing vessel.

Classical Location: On the nape of the neck, one inch and five fen either side of the spine, below the first vertebra. The point is found in sitting posture. *(The Golden Mirror)*

Local Anatomy: The medial cutaneous branches of the posterior branches of the intercostal artery and vein. The medial cutaneous branches of the posterior rami of the 1st and 2nd thoracic nerves; deeper, their lateral cutaneous branches.

Functions: Dispels the wind pathogen; resolves exterior heat; soothes the sinews and vessels; regulates the bones and joints.

Indications: Cough; fever; headache; pain in the shoulder blade; rigidity of the neck.

Supplementary Indications: Headache and quivering from cold; lumbar and back pain; throat bi; thoracic fullness and dyspnea; malarial disease; absence of sweating in cold damage; body fever; painful knee that cannot bend or stretch; vexation and fullness with abdominal urgency.

Illustrative Point Combinations & Applications: Wind bi with atony and inversion cold in the limbs is miraculously treated by needling BL-11 and LV-8. *(Song to Keep Up Your Sleeve)*

Stimulation: 0.5″ downward oblique insertion.
Moxa: 3-7 cones; pole 10-20 min.
Needle Sensation: Distention and numbness, sometimes spreading
over the back of the shoulder.

Point Categories & Associations: Meeting-hui point of the bones;
intersection-jiaohui point of the foot tai yang bladder, hand tai
yang small intestine, foot shao yang gallbladder and hand shao
yang triple burner channels.

Location: 1.5″ lateral to the lower border of the spinous process
of the 2nd thoracic vertebra.
Classical Location: One inch and five fen either side of the spine,
below the second vertebra. The point is found in sitting posture.
(The Great Compendium)
Local Anatomy: The medial cutaneous branches of the posterior
branches of the intercostal artery and vein. Superficially, the
medial cutaneous branches of the posterior rami of the 2nd and 3rd
thoracic nerves; deeper, their lateral cutaneous branches.

BL-12
風門
fēng mén
"Wind Gate"

Functions: Dispels wind and diffuses the lung; courses the channels and resolves the exterior.
Indications: Wind damage; cough; fever; headache; stiff neck;
pain in the back and lumbus.
Supplementary Indications: Wind dizziness and headache; nasal
congestion and runny nose; heavy eyes; sneezing; counterflow qi
ascent retching; pain in the back and chest; heat in the chest; yong
or ju on the back; jaundice.
Illustrative Point Combinations & Applications: BL-13 and BL-12
address productive cough. *(Song of Needle Practice)*

Stimulation: 0.5″ downward oblique insertion.
Moxa: 3 cones; pole 10-20 min.

Point Categories & Associations: Intersection-jiaohui point of the
governing vessel and the foot tai yang bladder channel.

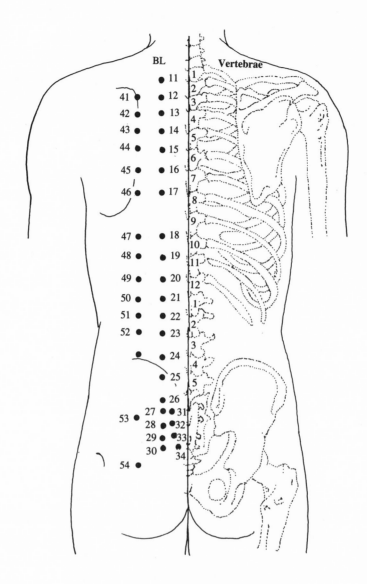

Figure 12.7

BL-13
肺俞
fei shū

"*Lung Shu*"

Location: 1.5″ lateral to the lower border of the spinous process of the 3rd thoracic vertebra.

Classical Location: One inch and five fen either side of the spine, below the third vertebra. *(The Great Compendium)*

The Golden Mirror points out that if you hang your hand contralaterally over your back, the end of your middle finger touches the point.

Local Anatomy: The medial cutaneous branches of the posterior branches of the intercostal artery and vein. The medial cutaneous branches of the posterior rami of the 3rd and 4th thoracic nerves; deeper, their lateral branches.

Functions: Regulates lung qi; supplements taxation and detriment; clears vacuity heat; harmonizes construction and blood.

Indications: Cough; asthma; blood ejection; steaming bone tidal fever; night sweating.

Supplementary Indications: Pulmonary atony; consumption; thoracic fullness and qi ascent; cough and dyspnea; tension and stiffness in the back; branching fullness in the chest and lateral costal region; no pleasure in eating; absence of sweating; throat bi; persistent cough in children.

Illustrative Point Combinations & Applications: For wind damage with constant coughing that eventually develops into consumption, needle BL-13 to treat the cough and ST-40 to eliminate copious phlegm. *(Song of the Jade Dragon)*

Stimulation: 0.5 ″ downward oblique insertion.
Moxa: 5-10 cones; pole 10-15 min.

Needle Sensation: Distention and numbness spreading downward and outward.

Point Categories & Associations: Associated-shu point of the lung.

BL-14
厥陰俞
jué yīn shū
"*Jue Yin Shu*"

Location: 1.5 ″ lateral to the lower border of the spinous process of the 4th thoracic vertebra.

Classical Location: One inch and five fen either side of the spine, below the fourth vertebra. The point is found in sitting posture. *(The Great Compendium)*

Local Anatomy: The medial cutaneous branches of the posterior branches of the intercostal artery and vein. The medial cutaneous branches of the posterior rami of the 4th and 5th thoracic nerves; deeper, their lateral branches.

Functions: Frees the channels and quickens the connecting vessels; soothes the liver and rectifies qi.

Indications: Cough; cardiac pain; thoracic oppression; vomiting.

Supplementary Indications: Qi accumulation pain in the chest and diaphragm; toothache.

Stimulation: 0.5 " downward oblique insertion.
Moxa: 5-7 cones; pole 10-20 min.

Point Categories & Associations: Associated-shu point of the
pericardium (jue yin).

BL-15
心俞
xīn shū

"Heart Shu"

Location: 1.5 " lateral to the lower border of the spinous process
of the 5th thoracic vertebra.
Classical Location: One inch and five fen either side of the spine,
below the fifth vertebra. The point is found in sitting posture.
(The Great Compendium)

Local Anatomy: The medial cutaneous branches of the posterior
branches of the intercostal artery and vein. Medial cutaneous
branches of the posterior rami of the 5th and 6th thoracic nerves;
deeper, their lateral branches.

Functions: Nourishes the heart and quiets the spirit; clears heat
and stabilizes the disposition; loosens the chest and regulates qi.
Indications: Epilepsy; fright palpitations; poor memory; vexation;
cough; blood ejection.

Supplementary Indications: Fever and chills; cardiac pain; vexation and oppression in the heart and chest; coughing of malign
blood; retching, vomiting and difficult ingestion; mania, withdrawal and epilepsy; heat in the palms and soles; seminal emission
and white turbid urethral discharge; poor memory; shortness of
breath; clear, runny snivel; eye pain and tearing; not speaking for
years.
Illustrative Point Combinations & Applications: BL-15 and BL-23
treat kidney vacuity dream emission with lumbar weakness.
(Ode of the Jade Dragon)

Gallbladder cold characterized by susceptibility to fright, as well
as seminal emission and white turbid urethral discharge or dreaming of sexual intercourse with ghosts, are treated by needling BL-
15 and BL-30. *(Song of the Jade Dragon)*

Stimulation: 0.3-0.5 " downward oblique insertion.
Moxa: 3-7 cones; pole 3 min.
Needle Sensation: Distention and numbness spreading forward to
the region of the heart.

Functions: Associated-shu point of the heart.

BL-16

督俞

dū shū

"Governing Shu"

Location: 1.5″ lateral to the lower border of the spinous process of the 6th thoracic vertebra.

Classical Location: One inch and five fen either side of the spine, below the sixth vertebra. The point is found in sitting posture. *(The Great Compendium)*

Local Anatomy: Medial branches of the posterior branches of the intercostal artery and vein, the descending branch of the transverse cervical artery. The dorsal scapular nerve, the medial cutaneous branches of the posterior rami of the 6th and 7th thoracic nerves; deeper, their lateral branches.

Functions: Loosens the chest and rectifies qi; promotes regulated flow through the triple burner.

Indications: Cardiac pain; abdominal pain.

Supplementary Indications: Thunderous rumbling of the intestines; counterflow qi.

Stimulation: 0.3-0.5″ downward oblique insertion. Moxa: 3-5 cones; pole 5-10 min.

BL-17

膈俞

gě shū

"Diaphragm Shu"

Location: 1.5″ lateral to the lower border of the spinous process of the 7th thoracic vertebra.

Classical Location: One inch and five fen either side of the spine, below the seventh vertebra. The point is found in sitting posture. *(The Great Compendium)*

Local Anatomy: Medial branches of the posterior branches of the intercostal artery and vein. Medial branches of the posterior rami of the 7th and 8th thoracic nerves; deeper, their lateral branches.

Functions: Clears blood heat; rectifies vacuity and detriment; harmonizes stomach qi; loosens the chest and diaphragm.

Indications: Vomiting; hiccough; difficult ingestion; asthma; cough; blood ejection; tidal fever; night sweating.

Supplementary Indications: Back pain and stiffness of the spine; vomiting of food eaten the previous day; abdominal pain or distention; steaming bone night sweats; tidal fever; fever without sweating; generalized bi; all blood patterns; evacuation difficulty; mania and withdrawal.

Stimulation: 0.3-0.5″ downward oblique insertion.
Moxa: 5-7 cones; pole 20-30 min.

Point Categories & Associations: Meeting-hui point of the blood.

BL-18
肝俞
gān shū

"Liver Shu"

Location: 1.5″ lateral to the lower border of the spinous process
of the 9th thoracic vertebra.
Classical Location: One inch and five fen either side of the spine,
below the ninth vertebra. The point is found in sitting posture.
(The Great Compendium)
Local Anatomy: Medial branches of the posterior branches of the
intercostal artery and vein. Medial cutaneous branches of the posterior rami of the 9th and 10th thoracic nerves; deeper, their
lateral branches.

Functions: Supplements construction-blood; disperses stasis;
dispels hepatocystic damp-heat; stabilizes the spirit and brightens
the eyes.
Indications: Jaundice; pain in the lateral costal region; blood ejection; nosebleed; reddening of the eyes; visual dizziness; night
blindness; pain in the spine and back; mania and withdrawal;
epilepsy.
Supplementary Indications: Painful accumulations, gatherings and
glomi; cough causing acute pain in the chest and lateral costal
region; nosebleed; lower abdominal pain; shortness of breath.
Illustrative Point Combinations & Applications: Sufferers of liver
disorders with diminished blood and clouded, flowery vision
should be supplemented at BL-18 and drained at ST-36.
(Song of the Jade Dragon)

Stimulation: 0.5″ downward oblique insertion.
Moxa: 3-7 cones; pole 20-30 min.
Needle Sensation: Distention and numbness spreading downward
or forward along the ribs.

Point Categories & Associations: Associated-shu point of the
liver.

Location: 1.5″ lateral to the lower border of the spinous process of the 10th thoracic vertebra.

Classical Location: One inch and five fen either side of the spine, below the tenth vertebra. The point is found in sitting posture. *(The Great Compendium)*

Local Anatomy: Medial branches of the posterior branches of the intercostal artery and vein. Medial cutaneous branches of the posterior rami of the 10th and 11th thoracic nerves; deeper, their lateral branches.

Functions: Clears gallbladder fire; dispels damp-heat; harmonizes the stomach; loosens the diaphragm; brightens the eyes.

Indications: Jaundice; bitter taste in the mouth; pain in the lateral costal region; pulmonary tuberculosis; tidal fever.

Supplementary Indications: Dry retching; pain in the throat; difficult ingestion; irascibility; headache and quivering from cold; yellowing of the eyes; steaming bone taxation fever; vacuity taxation; semen in the urine; axillary swelling; branching fullness in the chest and lateral costal region that prevents turning over; shortness of breath.

Stimulation: 0.3-0.5″ downward oblique insertion.
Moxa: 3-7 cones; pole 10-20 min.

Point Categories & Associations: Associated-shu point of the gallbladder.

BL-19

膽俞

dǎn shū

"Gallbladder Shu"

Location: 1.5″ lateral to the lower border of the spinous process of the 11th thoracic vertebra.

Classical Location: One inch and five fen either side of the spine, below the eleventh vertebra. *(The Systematized Canon)*

Local Anatomy: Medial branches of the posterior branches of the intercostal artery and vein. Medial cutaneous branches of the posterior rami of the 11th and 12th thoracic nerves; deeper, their lateral branches.

BL-20

脾俞

pí shū

"Spleen Shu"

Functions: Supports earth to dispel water-damp; rectifies the spleen to improve movement and transformation.

Indications: Abdominal distention; jaundice; vomiting; diarrhea; dysentery; untransformed digestate; water swelling; back pain.

Supplementary Indications: Pain and distention in the lateral costal region and abdomen; fulminant pain in the chest and lateral costal region; cough and vomiting; accumulations, gatherings and lump glomi; lassitude and prostrate exhaustion; thinness despite large food intake, or no pleasure in eating; drum distention; chronic infantile fright wind; phlegm patterns; clonic spasm; fever and chills.

Illustrative Point Combinations & Applications: SI-19 and BL-20 treat sorrow below the heart. Also, splenic vacuity with untransformed digestate is treated through BL-20 and BL-28. *(Ode of a Hundred Patterns)*

Stimulation: 0.5″ downward oblique insertion.
Moxa: 3-7 cones; pole 20-30 min.

Needle Sensation: Distention and numbness spreading downwards or forward along the ribs.

Point Categories & Associations: Associated-shu point of the spleen.

BL-21

胃俞

wèi shū

"Stomach Shu"

Location: 1.5″ lateral to the lower border of the spinous process of the 12th thoracic vertebra.

Classical Location: One inch and five fen either side of the spine, below the twelfth vertebra. The point is found in sitting posture. *(The Great Compendium)*

Local Anatomy: Medial branches of the posterior branches of the subcostal artery and vein. Medial cutaneous branch of the posterior ramus of the 12th thoracic nerve; deeper its lateral branch.

Functions: Regulates the center and harmonizes the stomach; transforms damp and disperses stagnation; supports center qi to eliminate vacuity.

Indications: Pain in the chest and lateral costal region; pain in the venter; abdominal distention; gastric reflux; vomiting; rumbling intestines; untransformed digestate.

Supplementary Indications: Stomach cold; abdominal distention and rumbling intestines; diarrhea; water swelling and drum distention; marked emaciation; tension and pain in the back; hypertonic sinews; difficult ingestion; prolapse of the rectum; accumulation lumps persisting for many years; no pleasure in eating; jaundice.

Illustrative Point Combinations & Applications: Untransformed digestate due to stomach cold is treated through BL-47 and BL-21. *(Ode of a Hundred Patterns)*

Stimulation: 0.5″ downward oblique insertion.
Moxa: 3-7 cones; pole 20-30 min.
Needle Sensation: Distention and numbness often spreading forward along the ribs.

Point Categories & Associations: Associated-shu point of the stomach.

Location: 1.5″ lateral to the lower border of the spinous process of the 1st lumbar vertebra.
Classical Location: One inch and five fen either side of the spine, below the thirteenth vertebra. The point is found in sitting posture. *(The Great Compendium)*
Local Anatomy: The posterior rami of the 1st lumbar artery and vein. The lateral cutaneous branch of the posterior ramus of the 10th thoracic nerve; deeper, the lateral branch of the posterior ramus of the 1st lumbar nerve.

BL-22
三焦俞
sān jiāo shū
"*Triple Burner Shu*"

Functions: Regulates qi and disinhibits water.
Indications: Abdominal distention; rumbling intestines; untransformed digestate; vomiting; diarrhea and dysentery; water swelling; pain and stiffness of the lumbus.
Supplementary Indications: Visual dizziness; headache; body fever; jaundice; difficult ingestion; alternating fever and chills; large accumulations and gatherings in the lower abdomen.

Stimulation: 0.5″ downward oblique insertion.
Moxa: 3-7 cones; pole 20-30 min.
Needle Sensation: Distention and numbness, often spreading downwards and outwards.

Point Categories & Associations: Associated-shu point of the triple burner.

BL-23
腎俞

shèn shū

"Kidney Shu"

Location: 1.5″ lateral to the lower border of the spinous process of the 2nd lumbar vertebra.

Classical Location: One inch and five fen either side of the spine, below the fourteenth vertebra, at the level of the navel. The point is found in sitting posture. *(The Great Compendium)*

Local Anatomy: The posterior ramus of the 2nd lumbar artery and vein. Branch of the posterior ramus of the 1st lumbar nerve.

Functions: Supplements the kidney; strengthens transformative action of qi; dispels water-damp; strengthens the lumbar and spine; boosts water and invigorates fire; brightens the eyes and sharpens the hearing.

Indications: Seminal emission; impotence; enuresis; irregular menses; vaginal discharge; backache and weakness of the knee; clouded vision; tinnitus; deafness; edema.

Supplementary Indications: Vacuity taxation and emaciation; bloody urine; turbid urine containing semen; aching lumbus and frigid knees; fullness in the lateral costal region; acute pain in the lower abdomen; wasting thirst; cough, dyspnea and diminished qi; headache; genital pain; throughflux diarrhea and untransformed digestate; wind-strike deafness and paralysis of the limbs; rumbling intestines; accumulation of frigid qi giving rise to taxation in females; emaciation in females due to intercourse during menstruation; alternating fever and chills.

Illustrative Point Combinations & Applications: BL-15 and BL-23 treat kidney vacuity dream emission with lumbar weakness. *(Ode of the Jade Dragon)*

Stimulation: 0.5-1.0″ perpendicular insertion.
Moxa: 3-7 cones; pole 10-20 min.

Needle Sensation: Distention and numbness, often spreading downwards and outwards and sometimes spreading over the buttocks and down the legs.

Point Categories & Associations: Associated-shu point of the kidney.

Location: 1.5″ lateral to the lower border of the spinous process of the 3rd lumbar vertebra.

Classical Location: One inch and five fen either side of the spine, below the fifteenth vertebra. The point is found in sitting posture. *(The Great Compendium)*

Local Anatomy: The posterior rami of the 3rd lumbar artery and vein. The lateral cutaneous branch of the posterior ramus of the 2nd lumbar nerve.

Functions: Regulates and supplements qi and blood; strengthens the lumbus and knees.

Indications: Lumbar pain.

Supplementary Indications: Hemorrhoids and fistulae.

Stimulation: 0.5-1.0″ perpendicular insertion.
Moxa: 3-7 cones; pole 10-20 min.

BL-24
氣海俞
qì hǎi shū
"Sea-of-Qi Shu"

Location: 1.5″ lateral to the lower border of the spinous process of the 4th lumbar vertebra, approximately at the level of the upper border of the iliac crest.

Classical Location: One inch and five fen either side of the spine, below the sixteenth vertebra. The point is found in prostrate posture. *(The Great Compendium)*

Local Anatomy: The posterior rami of the 4th lumbar artery and vein. The posterior ramus of the 3rd lumbar nerve.

Functions: Courses and regulates the large and small intestine; rectifies qi and transforms stagnation.

Indications: Abdominal pain and distention; rumbling intestines; diarrhea; constipation; lumbar pain.

Supplementary Indications: Intestinal pi diarrhea; difficult ingestion; cutting pain in the umbilical region; emaciation despite large food intake; inhibited urination and defecation; gripping pain in the lower abdomen.

Stimulation: 0.5-1.0″ perpendicular insertion.
Moxa: 5-10 cones; pole 20-30 min.

BL-25
大腸俞
dà cháng shū
"Large Intestine Shu"

Needle Sensation: needle stimulus sensation and distention, often spreading downward.

Point Categories & Associations: Associated-shu point of the large intestine.

BL-26
關元俞

guān yuán shū

"Origin Pass Shu"

Location: 1.5″ lateral to the lower border of the spinous process of the 5th lumbar vertebra.

Classical Location: One inch and five fen either side of the spine, below the 17th vertebra. The point is found in prostrate posture. *(The Great Compendium)*

Local Anatomy: Posterior branches of the lowest lumbar artery and vein. The posterior ramus of the 5th lumbar nerve.

Functions: Frees the channels and quickens the connecting vessels; courses wind and dissipates cold; regulates the lower burner.

Indications: Abdominal distention; diarrhea; lumbar pain.

Supplementary Indications: Wasting thirst; frequent or difficult urination; concretions and conglomerations; vacuity distention; enuresis; wind taxation.

Illustrative Point Combinations & Applications: BL-26 combined with BL-28 treats wind taxation lumbar pain (wind lumbar pain that lingers and becomes taxation). *(Life-Promoting Canon)*

Stimulation: 0.7-1.0″ perpendicular insertion.
Moxa: 3-7 cones; pole 5-10 min.

BL-27
小腸俞

xiǎo cháng shū

"Small Intestine Shu"

Location: At the level of the 1st sacral foramen, 1.5″ lateral to the governing vessel.

Classical Location: One inch and five fen either side of the spine, below the eighteenth vertebra. The point is found in prostrate posture. *(The Great Compendium)*

Local Anatomy: The posterior branches of the lateral sacral artery and vein. The lateral branch of the posterior ramus of the 1st sacral nerve.

Functions: Rectifies the small intestine; transforms stagnation and accumulation; promotes the separation of the clear and turbid; regulates the bladder.

Indications: Seminal emission; hematuria; enuresis; lower abdominal pain and distention; dysentery.

Supplementary Indications: Hemorrhoids; shan qi; dark-colored urine; dry mouth; vaginal discharge; swelling of the feet; vexation.

Stimulation: 0.5-1.0″ perpendicular insertion.
Moxa: 3-7 cones; pole 20-30 min.

Needle Sensation: Distention and numbness often spreading downward and outward.

Point Categories & Associations: Associated-shu point of the small intestine.

Location: At the level of the 2nd sacral foramen, 1.5″ lateral to the governing vessel, in the depression between the medial border of the posterior superior iliac spine and the sacrum.

Classical Location: One inch and five fen either side of the spine, below the nineteenth vertebra. The point is found in prostrate posture. *(The Great Compendium)*

Local Anatomy: Posterior branches of the lateral sacral artery and vein. Lateral branches of the posterior rami of the 1st and 2nd sacral nerves.

Functions: Regulates the bladder; perfuses the lower burner; disinhibits the lumbus; dispels wind-damp; supplements the lower origin.

Indications: Urinary stoppage; enuresis; diarrhea; constipation; pain and stiffness of the lumbus.

Supplementary Indications: Wind patterns; vacuity taxation; spermaturia; hard binds, accumulations, and gatherings; genital sores or swelling; turbid strangury; rough micturition with dark-colored urine; cold and weakness in the knee and lower leg; abdominal fullness; evacuation difficulty; cold and hypertonicity of the lower leg preventing bending and stretching; diminished qi; female conglomerations and gatherings; untransformed digestate due to splenic vacuity.

Illustrative Point Combinations & Applications: Splenic vacuity untransformed digestate is treated by needling BL-28 and BL-20. *(Ode of a Hundred Patterns)*

BL-28
膀胱俞
páng guāng shū
"Bladder Shu"

Stimulation: 0.5-1.0″ perpendicular insertion.
Moxa: 3-7 cones; pole 20-30 min.
Needle Sensation: Distention and numbness, sometimes spreading over the buttocks.

Point Categories & Associations: Associated-shu point of the bladder.

BL-29
中膂俞
zhōng lǚ shū

"Central Backbone Shu"

Location: At the level of the 3rd sacral foramen, 1.5″ lateral to the governing vessel.
Classical Location: One inch and five fen either side of the spine, below the twentieth vertebra. The point is found in prostrate posture. *(The Great Compendium)*
Local Anatomy: Posterior branches of the lateral sacral artery and vein, branches of the inferior gluteal artery and vein. The lateral branches of the posterior rami of the 3rd and 4th sacral nerves.

Functions: Strengthens the lumbar spine; warms yang and dissipates cold.
Indications: Dysentery; hernia; pain and stiffness of the lumbus.
Supplementary Indications: Intestinal frigidity; kidney vacuity wasting thirst; absence of sweating; lateral costal pain; abdominal distention.

Stimulation: 0.7-1.0″ perpendicular insertion.
Moxa: 3-7 cones; pole 20-30 min.

BL-30
白環俞
bái huán shū

"White Ring Shu"

Location: At the level of the 4th sacral foramen, 1.5″ lateral to the governing vessel.
Classical Location: One inch and five fen either side of the spine, below the twenty-first vertebra. The point is found in prostrate posture. *(The Great Compendium)*
Local Anatomy: The inferior gluteal artery and vein; deeper, the internal pudendal artery and vein. Lateral branches of the posterior rami of the 3rd and 4th sacral nerves, the inferior gluteal nerve.

Functions: Warms yang and regulates the menses; courses the channels and rectifies the lower burner.

Indications: Seminal emission; irregular menses; vaginal discharge; hernia; pain in the lower back and hip joint.

Supplementary Indications: Inhibited urination and defecation; vacuity heat block.

Illustrative Point Combinations & Applications: For pain in the back and lumbus, needle BL-30 and BL-40.
(Ode of a Hundred Patterns)

Stimulation: 0.7-1.0″ perpendicular insertion.
Moxa: pole 5-10 min.

Location: In the 1st sacral foramen, about midway between the posterior superior iliac spine and the governing vessel.

Classical Location: In the first opening one inch below the lumbar bone, in the depression either side of the spine.
(The Systematized Canon)

Local Anatomy: Posterior branches of the lateral sacral artery and vein. The site where the posterior ramus of the 1st sacral nerve passes.

BL-31
上髎
shàng liáo
"Upper Bone-Hole"

Functions: Frees the channels and quickens the connecting vessels; supplements the lower burner; strengthens the lumbus.

Indications: Lumbar pain; irregular menses; vaginal protrusion; vaginal discharge; inhibited defecation and urination.

Supplementary Indications: Genital itch; red and white vaginal discharge; turbid strangury; counterflow retching; nosebleed; infertility; malarial fever and chills.

Stimulation: 0.7-1.0″ perpendicular insertion.
Moxa: 3-7 cones; pole 20-30 min.

Needle Sensation: Distention and numbness spreading down towards the legs.

Location: In the 2nd sacral foramen, about midway between the lower border of the posterior superior iliac spine and the governing vessel.

Classical Location: In the second opening, in the depression either side of the spine. *(The Great Compendium)*

BL-32
次髎
cì liáo
"Second Bone-Hole"

Local Anatomy: Posterior branches of the lateral sacral artery and vein. The course of the posterior ramus of the 2nd sacral nerve.

Functions: Frees the channels and rectifies qi; quickens the blood and relieves pain; regulates the menses and treats vaginal discharge.

Indications: Lumbar pain; irregular menses; vaginal discharge; hernia; loss of locomotive ability of the lower limbs.

Supplementary Indications: Turbid strangury; insensitivity from the lumbar down to the feet; rumbling intestines and outpour diarrhea; hardness and distention below the heart.

Stimulation: 0.7-1.0″ perpendicular insertion.
Moxa: 3-7 cones; pole 10-20 min.
Needle Sensation: Distention and numbness spreading down towards the legs.

BL-33
中髎
zhōng liáo
"Central Bone-Hole"

Location: In the 3rd sacral foramen, between BL-29 and the governing vessel.
Classical Location: In the third opening, in the depression on either side of the spine. *(The Great Compendium)*
Local Anatomy: Posterior branches of the lateral sacral artery and vein. The course of the posterior ramus of the 3rd sacral nerve.

Functions: Frees the channels and quickens the blood; dissipates cold and relieves pain; regulates the menses and treats vaginal discharge.

Indications: Irregular menses; vaginal discharge; lumbar pain; inhibited urination; constipation.

Supplementary Indications: Red and white vaginal discharge; turbid strangury; abdominal distention and diarrhea; swill diarrhea; the five taxations and the seven affect damages.

Stimulation: 0.7-1.0″ perpendicular insertion.
Moxa: 3-7 cones; pole 20-30 min.

BL-34
下髎
xià liáo
"Lower
   Bone-Hole"

Location: In the 4th sacral foramen, between BL-30 and the governing vessel.
Classical Location: In the fourth opening, in the depression on either side of the spine. *(The Great Compendium)*
Local Anatomy: Branches of the inferior gluteal artery and vein. The course of the posterior ramus of the 4th sacral nerve.

Functions: Disinhibits the stools and urine; frees the channels and relieves pain.

Indications: Lower abdominal pain; constipation; inhibited urination; lumbar pain.

Supplementary Indications: Rumbling intestines; diarrhea; evacuation of blood with the stool; vaginal discharge; cold shan; pain and itching in the genitals.

Stimulation: 0.5-1.0″ perpendicular insertion.
Moxa: 5-7 cones; pole 20-30 min.

Location: On either side of the tip of the coccyx, 0.5″ lateral to the governing vessel.

Classical Location: On either side of the tail bone.
(The Systematized Canon)

Local Anatomy: Branches of the inferior gluteal artery and vein. The coccygeal nerve.

BL-35
會陽
huì yáng
"Meeting of Yang"

Functions: Clears and discharges lower burner damp-heat.

Indications: Vaginal discharge; impotence; dysentery; hemafecia; hemorrhoids; diarrhea.

Supplementary Indications: Menstrual lumbar pain; painful frigidity in the abdomen; intestinal pi; genital sweating; leg pain.

Stimulation: 0.5-0.8″ perpendicular insertion.
Moxa: 3-7 cones; pole 10-20 min.

Location: In the middle of the transverse gluteal fold. Locate the point in prone position.

Classical Location: In the crease below the buttock and above the inner face of the thigh. *(The Great Compendium)*

Local Anatomy: The artery and vein running alongside the sciatic nerve. Superficially, the posterior femoral cutaneous nerve; deeper, the sciatic nerve.

BL-36
承扶
chéng fú
"Support"

Functions: Soothes the sinews and quickens the connecting vessels.

Indications: Hemorrhoids; pain in lumbar, sacral, gluteal and femoral regions.

Supplementary Indications: Enduring hemorrhoids with swelling of the buttocks; inhibited urination; genital pain; evacuation difficulty.

Stimulation: 0.7-1.5 ″ perpendicular insertion.
Moxa: 3 cones; pole 5-10 min.
Needle Sensation: Distention and numbness, spreading towards the knees or feet.

BL-37
股門

yīn mén

"Gate of
Abundance"

Location: 6″ below BL-36, on the line joining BL-36 and BL-40.
Classical Location: Six inches below BL-36.
(The Great Compendium)
Local Anatomy: Laterally, the 3rd perforating branches of the deep femoral artery and vein. The posterior femoral cutaneous nerve.

Functions: Strengthens the lumbar spine; soothes the sinews and quickens the connecting vessels; relieves pain.
Indications: Pain in the lumbus and thigh; loss of locomotive ability of the lower limbs.
Supplementary Indications: Outpour diarrhea with malign blood in the stool; swelling of the outer thigh.

Stimulation: 0.7-1.5 ″ perpendicular insertion.
Moxa: 3-5 cones; pole 5-10 min.

BL-38
浮郄

fú xī

"Superficial Cleft"

Location: 1 ″ above BL-39, on the medial side of the tendon of the biceps muscle of the thigh (m. biceps femoris). The point is located with the knee slightly flexed.
Classical Location: One inch above BL-39. The point is found with the knee flexed. *(The Great Compendium)*
Local Anatomy: The superolateral genicular artery and vein. The posterior femoral cutaneous nerve and the common peroneal nerve.

Functions: Soothes the sinews and quickens the connecting vessels; quickens the blood and relieves pain; clears and disinhibits the lower burner.
Indications: Numbness of the gluteal region; hypertonicity of the popliteal sinews.
Supplementary Indications: Small intestinal heat; large intestinal bind; tension in the outer thigh.

Stimulation: 0.5-1.0 ″ perpendicular insertion.
Moxa: 3-7 cones; pole 5-10 min.

Location: On the popliteal crease lateral to BL-40, on the medial border of the biceps femoris tendon of the biceps muscle of the thigh (m. biceps femoris).

Classical Location: One cubit and six inches below BL-36. The point is in front of the foot tai yang and behind the shao yang, between the two sinews on the outer face of the popliteal fossa. *(The Great Compendium)*

Local Anatomy: See BL-38.

Functions: Disinhibits the triple burner and courses the waterways; frees the channels, quickens the connecting vessels and relieves pain.

Indications: Stiffness and pain of the lumbus; lower intestinal distention and fullness; inhibited urination; pain and hypertonicity of the leg and foot.

Supplementary Indications: Axillary swelling; hemorrhoids; hypertonicity of the knee.

Illustrative Point Combinations & Applications: BL-39 combined with PC-1 quickly disperses axillary swelling. *(Ode of a Hundred Patterns)*

Stimulation: 0.5-1.0″ perpendicular insertion. Moxa: 3-7 cones; pole 3-5 min.

Point Categories & Associations: Lower uniting-he point of the triple burner channel.

BL-39

委陽

wěi yáng

"Bend Yang"

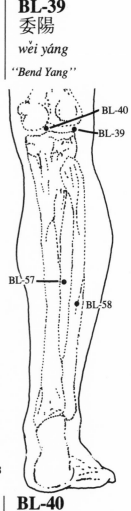

Figure 12.8

Location: At the midpoint of the transverse crease of the popliteal fossa, between the tendons of biceps muscle of the thigh (m. biceps femoris) and semitendinosus muscle (m. semitendinosus). This point is located with the patient in a prone posture or with flexed knee.

Classical Location: At the pulsating vessel in the center of the popliteal crease. *(The Systematized Canon)*

BL-40

委中

wěi zhōng

"Bend Middle"

Local Anatomy: Superficially, the femoropopliteal vein; deeper and medially, the popliteal vein; at the deepest level, the popliteal artery. The posterior femoral cutaneous nerve, the tibial nerve.

Functions: Clears the blood and discharges heat; soothes the sinews and frees the connecting vessels; dispels wind-damp; disinhibits the lumbus and knees.

relieving stagnation

Indications: Lumbar pain; inhibited movement of the hip joint; hypertonicity of the popliteal sinews; loss of locomotive ability of the lower limbs; hemiplegia; abdominal pain; vomiting and diarrhea.

Supplementary Indications: Absence of sweating in heat disease; persistent nosebleed; vacuity and night sweating; wind-damp loss of locomotive ability; cholera with gripping cardioabdominal pain; clove sores; aching among the lower teeth; throat disorders.

Stimulation: 0.5-1.5″ perpendicular insertion; bleed with three-edged needle (avoid deep lancing). Moxa: 3-5 cones; pole 5 min.

Needle Sensation: Distention and numbness, sometimes spreading to the soles of the feet.

Illustrative Point Combinations & Applications: For back and lumbar pain, needle BL-30 and BL-40. *(Ode of a Hundred Patterns)*

CV-4, CV-6 and BL-40 address vacuity.
(Song of Needle Practice)

Point Categories & Associations: Uniting-he (earth) point; command point of the back.

BL-41
附分

fū fēn

"Attached Branch"

Location: 3″ lateral to the lower border of the spinous process of the 2nd thoracic vertebra, just medial to the vertebral border of the scapula.

Classical Location: Below the second vertebra, on the inner border of the shoulder blade, three inches either side of the spine. *(The Systematized Canon)*

Local Anatomy: The descending branch of the transverse cervical artery, lateral branches of the posterior branches of the intercostal artery and vein. Lateral cutaneous branches of the posterior rami of the 1st and 2nd thoracic nerves; deeper, the dorsal scapular nerve.

Functions: Courses wind and dissipates cold; soothes the sinews and quickens the connecting vessels.

Indications: Hypertonicity of the shoulder and back; stiffness and pain in the neck; numbness of the elbow and arm.

Supplementary Indications: Insensitivity of the elbow and arm; wind taxation.

Stimulation: 0.3-0.5″ oblique insertion.
Moxa: 3-7 cones; pole 10-20 min.

Point Categories & Associations: Intersection-jiaohui point of the foot tai yang bladder and hand tai yang small intestine channels.

Location: 3″ lateral to the lower border of the spinous process of the 3rd thoracic vertebra.

BL-42
魄戶
pò hù
"Po Door"

Classical Location: Below BL-41, three inches either side of the spine, below the third vertebra. The point is found in sitting posture. *(The Great Compendium)*

Local Anatomy: The posterior branch of the intercostal artery, the descending branch of the transverse cervical artery. Medial cutaneous branches of the posterior rami of the 2rd and 3rd thoracic nerve; deeper, their lateral branches and the dorsal scapular nerve.

Functions: Diffuses lung qi; calms dyspnea and suppresses cough.

Indications: Pulmonary tuberculosis; cough; asthma; stiffness of the neck; pain in the shoulder and back.

Supplementary Indications: Retching and vomiting with vexation and fullness; vacuity taxation; pulmonary atony; steaming bone tidal fever.

Illustrative Point Combinations & Applications: BL-42 and BL-43 provide the way to treat consumption.
(Ode of a Hundred Patterns)

Stimulation: 0.3-0.5″ downward oblique insertion.
Moxa: 3-7 cones; pole 20-30 min.

BL-43
膏肓俞

gāo huāng shū

"Gao Huang
Shu"

Location: 3″ lateral to the lower border of the spinous process of the 4th thoracic vertebra.

Classical Location: Three inches either side of the spine, below the fourth vertebra and just above the fifth.
(The Glorious Anthology of Acupuncture)

Local Anatomy: The posterior branch of the intercostal artery and the descending branch of the transverse cervical artery. Medial cutaneous branches of the posterior rami of the 2nd and 3rd thoracic nerves; deeper, their lateral branches and the dorsoscapular nerve.

Functions: Supplements the lung and fortifies the spleen; treats taxation and detriment; stabilizes the heart and banks up the kidney; supports the origin.

Indications: Pulmonary tuberculosis; cough; asthma; blood ejection; night sweating; poor memory; seminal emission; untransformed digestate.

Supplementary Indications: Esophageal constriction; gastrosplenic vacuity; dream emission; back pain; wind taxation; vacuity detriment and the five taxations; affect damage.

Illustrative Point Combinations & Applications: ST-36 treats emaciation related to the five taxations. Hua Tuo adds BL-43.
(Wo Yan's Efficacious Point Applications)

Stimulation: 0.3-0.5″ downward oblique insertion.
Moxa: 7-15 cones; pole 20-50 min.

Note: Most older texts mention that BL-43 is only suitable for moxibustion and further that moxibustion at that point should be followed by needling points in the lower body such as CV-4 and ST-36 to prevent vacuity fire from upflaming.

Needle Sensation: Distention spreading downward and outward.

BL-44
神堂

shén táng

"Spirit Hall"

Location: 3″ lateral to the lower border of the spinous process of the 5th thoracic vertebra.

Classical Location: In the depression three inches either side of the spine, below the fifth vertebra. The point is found in sitting posture. *(The Great Compendium)*

Local Anatomy: Posterior branches of the intercostal artery and vein, the descending branch of the transverse cervical artery. Medial cutaneous branches of the posterior rami of the 4th and 5th thoracic nerves; deeper, their lateral branches and the dorsal scapular nerve.

Functions: Loosens the chest and rectifies qi; suppresses cough and stabilizes dyspnea; soothes the sinews and quickens the connecting vessels.

Indications: Asthma; cough; pain and stiffness of the back.

Supplementary Indications: Fullness in the chest and abdomen.

Stimulation: 0.5 ″ oblique insertion toward corner of the shoulder blade. Moxa: 7-15 cones; pole 5-10 min.

Location: 3 ″ lateral to the lower border of the spinous process of the 6th thoracic vertebra.

Classical Location: Three inches either side of the spine, below the sixth vertebra. When firm pressure is applied, the patient cries ''ee shee'' (thus the point name), indicating that the point has been found. *(The Golden Mirror)*

Local Anatomy: Posterior branches of the intercostal artery and vein. Medial cutaneous branches of the posterior rami of the 5th and 6th thoracic nerves; deeper, their lateral branches.

Functions: Resolves the exterior and clears heat; diffuses the lung and rectifies qi; frees the channels and quickens the connecting vessels.

Indications: Cough; asthma; shoulder and back pain.

Supplementary Indications: Lower rib pain associated with lower abdominal pain and distention; visual dizziness; chest pain associated with pain on the inner side of the shoulder and arm; malaria, heat disease.

Stimulation: 0.5 ″ downward oblique insertion.
Moxa: 3-7 cones; pole 10-30 min.

BL-45
譩譆
yì xī
"Yi Xi"

Location: 3 ″ lateral to the lower border of the spinous process of the 7th thoracic vertebra, approximately level with the inferior angle of the scapula.

Classical Location: In the depression three inches either side of the spine, below the seventh vertebra. The point is found in sitting posture. *(The Great Compendium)*

Local Anatomy: Posterior branches of the intercostal artery and vein. Medial cutaneous branches of the posterior rami of the 6th and 7th thoracic nerves; deeper, their lateral branches.

BL-46
膈關
gé guān
"Diaphragm Pass"

Functions: Fortifies the spleen and disinhibits damp; harmonizes the stomach and abducts stagnation; soothes the sinews and quickens the connecting vessels.

Indications: Difficult ingestion; vomiting; eructation; pain and stiffness of the back.

Supplementary Indications: Blood disorders; yellow urine; body pain.

Stimulation: 0.5″ downward oblique insertion.
Moxa: 3-7 cones; pole 5-20 min.

BL-47
魂門
hún mén
"Hun Gate"

Location: 3″ lateral to the lower border of the spinous process of the 9th thoracic vertebra.

Classical Location: In the depression three inches either side of the spine, below the ninth vertebra. The point is found in sitting posture. *(The Great Compendium)*

Local Anatomy: Posterior branches of the intercostal artery and vein. Lateral branches of the posterior rami of the 7th and 8th thoracic nerves.

Functions: Courses the liver and rectifies qi; fortifies the spleen and harmonizes the stomach; frees and regulates bowel qi.

Indications: Pain in the chest and lateral costal region; backache; vomiting; diarrhea.

Supplementary Indications: Difficult ingestion; rumbling intestines and diarrhea; dark-colored urine; irregular defecation; hypertonicity of the sinews and bone pain.

Illustrative Point Combinations & Applications: Stomach frigidity hampering the transformation of ingested food is treated through BL-47 and BL-21. *(Ode of a Hundred Patterns)*

Stimulation: 0.5″ downward oblique insertion.
Moxa: 3-7 cones; pole 5-20 min.

BL-48
陽綱
yáng gāng
"Yang Headrope"

Location: 3″ lateral to the lower border of the spinous process of the 10th thoracic vertebra.

Classical Location: In the depression three inches either side of the spine, below the tenth vertebra. The point is found in sitting posture. *(The Great Compendium)*

Local Anatomy: Posterior branches of the intercostal artery and vein. Lateral branches of the posterior rami of the 8th and 9th thoracic nerves.

Functions: Clears the gallbladder and stomach; transforms damp-heat.

Indications: Borborygmi; abdominal pain; diarrhea; jaundice.

Supplementary Indications: Difficult ingestion; abdominal fullness and vacuity distention; irregular defecation.

Illustrative Point Combinations & Applications: Yellowing of the eyes is treated through BL-48 and BL-19.
(Ode of a Hundred Patterns)

Stimulation: 0.5ʺ downward oblique insertion.
Moxa: 3-7 cones; pole 5-10 min.

Location: 3ʺ lateral to the lower border of the spinous process of the 11th thoracic vertebra.

Classical Location: Three inches either side of the spine, below the eleventh vertebra. The point is found in sitting posture.
(The Great Compendium)

Local Anatomy: Posterior branches of the intercostal artery and vein. Lateral branches of the posterior rami of the 10th and 11th thoracic nerves.

BL-49
意舍
yì shè

"Reflection Abode"

Functions: Courses and discharges damp-heat; fortifies splenic yang.

Indications: Abdominal distention; borborygmi; diarrhea; vomiting; difficult ingestion.

Supplementary Indications: Back pain; aversion to wind and cold; abdominal fullness and vacuity distention; efflux diarrhea; wasting thirst; jaundice and yellowing of the eyes; dark-colored urine.

Illustrative Point Combinations & Applications: Thoracic fullness with esophageal constriction is relieved by needling LU-1 and BL-49. *(Ode of a Hundred Patterns)*

Stimulation: 0.5ʺ downward oblique insertion.
Moxa: 3-7 cones; pole 5-30 min.

BL-50

胃倉

wèi cāng

"Stomach Granary"

Location: 3ʺ lateral to the lower border of the process of the 12th thoracic vertebra.

Classical Location: Three inches either side of the spine, below the twelfth vertebra. The point is found in sitting posture. *(The Great Compendium)*

Local Anatomy: Posterior branches of the subcostal artery and vein. The lateral branch of the posterior ramus of the 11th thoracic nerve.

Functions: Harmonizes the stomach and transforms damp; rectifies qi and disinhibits the center.

Indications: Abdominal distention; pain in the venter; back pain.

Supplementary Indications: Water swelling; infantile digestate accumulation.

Stimulation: 0.5ʺ downward oblique insertion.
Moxa: 3-7 cones; pole 10-30 min.

BL-51

肓門

huāng mén

"Huang Gate"

Location: 3ʺ lateral to the lower border of the spinous process of the 1st lumbar vertebra.

Classical Location: In the depression either side of the spine, below the thirteenth vertebra. The point is located in sitting posture. *(The Great Compendium)*

Local Anatomy: Posterior branches of the 1st lumbar artery and vein. The lateral branch of the 12th thoracic nerve.

Functions: Disperses digestate and abducts stagnation; softens hardness.

Indications: Epigastric pain; lump glomus; constipation.

Supplementary Indications: Mammary diseases; major hardness below the heart.

Stimulation: 0.5-1.0ʺ perpendicular insertion.
Moxa: 3-7 cones; pole 10-30 min.

Location: 3″ lateral to the lower border of the spinous process of the 2nd lumbar vertebra.

Classical Location: In the depression three inches either side of the spine, below the fourteenth vertebra. The point is found in sitting posture. *(The Great Compendium)*

Local Anatomy: The lateral branch of the posterior ramus of the 12th thoracic nerve and the lateral branch of the 1st lumbar nerve.

Functions: Supplements the kidney and boosts essence; disinhibits urine and abducts damp.

Indications: Seminal emission; impotence; inhibited urination; edema; pain and stiffness of the back.

Supplementary Indications: Abdominal distention; lateral costal fullness; pain and swelling of the genitals; dribbling urination; counterflow vomiting; untransformed digestate; cholera.

Stimulation: 0.7-1.0″ perpendicular insertion.
Moxa: 7-15 cones; pole 10-30 min.

Needle Sensation: Distention and numbness, spreading either downward or downward and outward.

BL-52
志室
zhì shì
"Will Chamber"

Location: 3″ lateral to the lower border of the spinous process of the 2nd sacral vertebra, level with BL-32.

Classical Location: In the depression three inches either side of the spine, below the nineteenth vertebra. The point is located in prostrate posture. *(The Great Compendium)*

Local Anatomy: The superior gluteal artery and vein. Superior cluneal nerves; deeper, the superior gluteal nerve.

Functions: Strengthens the lumbar spine; frees bowel qi; disinhibits the lower burner.

Indications: Borborygmus; abdominal distention; back pain.

Supplementary Indications: Urinary stoppage; abdominal pain.

Stimulation: 0.7-1.3″ perpendicular insertion.
Moxa: 7-15 cones; pole 10-30 min.

BL-53
胞肓
bāo huāng
"Bladder Huang"

BL-54
秩邊
zhì biān

"Sequential Limit"

Location: Directly below BL-53, 3" lateral to the governing vessel, about 4 finger breadths lateral to the sacral hiatus.

Classical Location: In the depression three inches either side of the spine, below the twentieth vertebra. The point is found in prostrate posture. *(The Great Compendium)*

Local Anatomy: The inferior gluteal artery and vein. The inferior gluteal nerve, the posterior femoral cutaneous nerve and sciatic nerve.

Functions: Courses the channels and connecting vessels; strengthens the knee and lumbus.

Indications: Lumbosacral pain; hemorrhoids; loss of locomotive ability of the lower limbs.

Supplementary Indications: Inhibited urination; genital pain.

Stimulation: 1.0-1.5" perpendicular insertion.
Moxa: 3-7 cones; pole 20-50 min.

Needle Sensation: Distention and numbness, spreading down the legs.

BL-55
合陽
hé yáng

"Yang Union"

Location: 2" directly below BL-40, between the medial and lateral heads of the gastrocnemius muscle (m. gastrocnemius), on the line joining BL-40 and BL-57.

Classical Location: Three inches below the crease of the knee. *(The Great Compendium)*

Local Anatomy: The small saphenous vein; deeper, the popliteal artery and vein. The medial sural cutaneous nerve; deeper, the tibial nerve.

Functions: Strengthens the lumbus and boosts the kidney; soothes the sinews and quickens the connecting vessels; regulates the penetrating and conception vessels.

Indications: Back pain; pain and paralysis of the lower limbs.

Supplementary Indications: Heat in the inner thigh; uterine bleeding and vaginal discharge; shan pain; fulminant genital pain; abdominal pain.

Stimulation: 0.7-1.0" perpendicular insertion.
Moxa: 3-5 cones; pole 5-10 min.

Location: Midway between BL-55 and BL-57, in the center of the belly of gastrocnemius muscle (m. gastrocnemius), between the two heads.

Classical Location: In the depression at the center of the calf, between BL-55 and BL-57. *(The Great Compendium)*

Local Anatomy: The small saphenous vein; deeper, the posterior tibial artery and vein. The medial sural cutaneous nerve; deeper, the tibial nerve.

Functions: Soothes the sinews and quickens the connecting vessels.

Indications: Pain in the lower leg; hemorrhoids; hypertonicity of the lumbar region and back.

Supplementary Indications: Cholera with cramps; axillary swelling; lower leg bi; dizziness and headache.

Stimulation: 0.5″ perpendicular insertion (see contraindication). Moxa: 3 cones; pole 5-20 min.

Contraindications: Some texts consider this point contraindicated for needling.

BL-56
承筋
chéng jīn
"Sinew Support"

Location: Directly below the body of the gastrocnemius muscle (m. gastrocnemius), on the line joining BL-40 and the Achilles tendon (t. calcaneus), about 8″ below BL-40.

Classical Location: Below BL-56, in the parting of the flesh at the lower tip of the belly of the calf. *(The Golden Mirror)*

Local Anatomy: See BL-56.

Functions: Soothes the sinews and cools the blood; harmonizes the intestines and eliminates hemorrhoids.

Indications: Lumbar pain; pain and cramp in the legs; hemorrhoids; constipation.

Supplementary Indications: Pain in the heel; no pleasure in eating; painful glomus in the chest and diaphragm; foot qi.

Stimulation: 0.5-0.8″ perpendicular insertion. Moxa: 3-7 cones; pole 5-15 min.

BL-57
承山
chéng shān
"Mountain Support"

Needle Sensation: Distention and numbness.

Illustrative Point Combinations & Applications: SP-9 treats fullness in the heart and chest, and the addition of BL-57 stirs the desire for food and drink. *(Ode of Xi Hong)*

BL-58
飛揚
fei yáng

"Taking Flight"

Location: 7″ above BL-60, on the posterior border of the fibula, on the lateral anterior border of the gastrocnemius muscle, about 1″ inferior and lateral to BL-57.

Classical Location: Moving obliquely [outward and downward] from BL-57, in the depression seven inches above the outer ankle bone. *(The Golden Mirror)*

Local Anatomy: The lateral sural cutaneous nerve.

Functions: Dispels tai yang channel pathogens; dissipates wind-damp in the channels and connecting vessels.

Indications: Headache; visual dizziness; nasal congestion; nosebleed; lumbar pain; weakness of the legs.

Supplementary Indications: Hemorrhoids; swelling and pain in the lower limbs.

Illustrative Point Combinations & Applications: Diminished qi with scant uterine bleeding in women is treated by needling KI-8 and BL-58. *(Ode of a Hundred Patterns)*

Stimulation: 0.7-1.0″ perpendicular insertion.
Moxa: 3-7 cones; pole 5-20 min.

Point Categories & Associations: Connecting-luo point of the bladder channel connecting to the kidney channel.

BL-59
跗陽
fū yáng

"Instep Yang"

Location: 3″ directly above BL-60, on the line connecting BL-58, BL-60.

Classical Location: Between the sinew and bone, three inches above the outer ankle bone. *(The Golden Mirror)*

Local Anatomy: The small saphenous vein; deeper, the terminal branch of the peroneal artery. The sural nerve.

Functions: Dispels tai yang channel pathogens; dissipates wind-damp in the channels and connecting vessels.

Indications: Heavy-headedness; headache; lumbosacral pain; redness and swelling of the external malleolus; paralysis.

Supplementary Indications: Dizziness; nasal congestion with clear runny snivel; pain and swelling of the lower limbs.

Stimulation: 0.5-1.0″ perpendicular insertion.
Moxa: 3-7 cones; pole 5-20 min.

Point Categories & Associations: Cleft-xi point of the yang motility vessel; intersection-jiaohui point of the foot tai yang bladder channel and the yang motility vessel.

Location: In the depression midway between the external malleolus and the Achilles tendon (t. calcaneus), level with the high point of the bone.
Classical Location: Five fen behind the outer ankle bone, in the depression above the heel bone where a fine pulsating vessel can be felt. *(The Golden Mirror)*
Local Anatomy: The small saphenous vein, the posteroexternal malleolar artery and vein. The sural nerve.

BL-60
崑崙
kūn lún

"Kunlun Mountains"

Functions: Dispels tai yang channel pathogens; rectifies uterine blood stagnation; soothes the sinews and transforms damp; strengthens the lumbar and kidney.
Indications: Headache; stiff neck; visual dizziness; nosebleed; hypertonicity of the shoulder and arm; lumbar pain; pain in the heel; infantile epilepsy; difficult delivery.
Supplementary Indications: Malarial disease; diseases of the head; aching among the upper teeth; thoracic fullness and fulminant dyspnea; abdominal pain and throughflux diarrhea; retention of afterbirth; hemilateral wind; infantile fright epilepsy.
Illustrative Point Combinations & Applications: Straw shoe wind (redness and swelling of the legs and feet starting in the upper thigh and spreading downward) must be attacked at BL-60; subsequent needling of BL-62 and KI-3 will bring relief to even enduring cases. *(Song of the Jade Dragon)*

Stimulation: 0.5″ perpendicular insertion.
Moxa: 3-7 cones; pole 5-20 min.

Point Categories & Associations: River-jing (fire) point.

BL-61
僕參
pū cān

*"Subservient
Visitor"*

Location: Below BL-60, in the depression of the calcaneum at the border of the red and white flesh.
Classical Location: In the depression below the heel bone. The point is found with the legs bent. *(The Great Compendium)*
Local Anatomy: The external calcaneal branches of the peroneal artery and vein. The external calcaneal branch of the sural nerve.

Functions: Frees the channels and quickens the connecting vessels; disperses swelling and relieves pain.
Indications: Atony of the lower limbs; pain in the heel.
Supplementary Indications: Lumbar pain; deathlike inversion; mania, withdrawal and epilepsy; turbid strangury; foot qi and swelling of the knees; choleraic cramp.

Stimulation: 0.3-0.5 ″ perpendicular insertion.
Moxa: 3-5 cones; pole 20-30 min.

BL-62
申脈
shēn mài

"Extending Vessel"

Figure 12.9

Location: In the depression directly below the external malleolus.
Classical Location: In the depression five fen below the outer ankle bone, between the two sinews below the ankle bone. *(The Great Compendium)*
Local Anatomy: The external malleolar arterial network. The sural nerve.

Functions: Courses exterior pathogens; treats wind diseases; stabilizes the spirit-disposition; soothes the sinews and vessels.
Indications: Epilepsy; mania and withdrawal; headache; dizziness; insomnia; pain in the lumbus and leg.
Supplementary Indications: Fever and chills; swelling of the neck and armpit; unilateral and ambilateral headache; heart fright; ringing in the ears; nosebleed; foot qi; wind strike with hemiplegia and loss of speech; wryness of the eyes and mouth; female blood and qi pain; difficulty in bending and stretching the knee and foot.
Illustrative Point Combinations & Applications: For head wind and headache needle BL-62 and BL-63.
(Ode to Elucidate Mysteries)

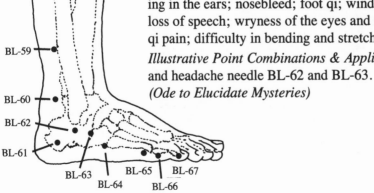

BL-59
BL-60
BL-62
BL-61
BL-63
BL-64
BL-65
BL-66
BL-67

Stimulation: 0.3″ perpendicular insertion.
Moxa: 2-3 cones; pole 3-5 min.

Point Categories & Associations: Confluence-jiaohui point of the
eight extraordinary vessels (related to the yang motility vessel);
intersection-jiaohui point of the foot tai yang bladder channel and
the yang motility vessel; fifth of the thirteen ghost points.

Location: Anterior and inferior to BL-62, in the depression inferior to the cuboid bone.
Classical Location: Slightly behind the outer ankle bone, behind
GB-40, in front of BL-62. *(The Great Compendium)*
Local Anatomy: The lateral plantar artery and vein. The lateral
dorsal cutaneous nerve of the foot; deeper, the lateral plantar
nerve.

Functions: Soothes the sinews and quickens the connecting
vessels; opens the portals and quiets the spirit.
Indications: Epilepsy; infantile fright wind (convulsions); lumbar
pain; pain in the external malleolus; bi pain in the lower limbs.
Supplementary Indications: Choleraic cramp; deathlike inversion;
lower abdominal pain; fulminant shan.
Illustrative Point Combinations & Applications: When cold damage alone sets both ears to ring, with BL-63 and GB-2 it will be
gone with the wind. *(Ode of Xi Hong)*

Stimulation: 0.5″ perpendicular insertion.
Moxa: 3 cones; pole 5-20 min.

Point Categories & Associations: Cleft-xi point of the bladder
channel; intersection-jiaohui point of the foot tai yang bladder
channel and the yang linking vessel.

BL-63
金門
jīn mén
"Metal Gate"

Location: On the lateral side of the dorsum of the foot, proximal
to the tuberosity of the 5th metatarsal bone, at the border of the
red and white skin.
Classical Location: On the outer side of the foot, below the large
bone, in the depression at the border of the red and white flesh.
(The Systematized Canon)

BL-64
京骨
jīng gŭ
"Capital Bone"

233

Local Anatomy: See BL-63.

Functions: Frees the channels and quickens the connecting vessels; quiets the heart and spirit; dissipates wind and clears heat.

Indications: Epilepsy; headache; stiff neck; pain in the lumbus and leg.

Supplementary Indications: Clear, runny snivel and nosebleed; eye screens; diarrhea; abdominal fullness; mania and withdrawal; fever and chills; malarial disease; palpitations; splitting headache.

Illustrative Point Combinations & Applications: Insufferable headache can be treated by needling the source points of the foot jue yin and tai yang channels (i.e., LV-3 and BL-64).
(Life-Preserving Collection)

Stimulation: 0.3-0.5″ perpendicular insertion.
Moxa: 3-7 cones; pole 5-20 min.

Point Categories & Associations: Source-yuan point of the bladder channel.

BL-65
束骨
shù gǔ

"Bundle Bone"

Location: On the lateral side of the dorsum of the foot, proximal to the head of the 5th metatarsal bone, at the border of the red and white flesh.

Classical Location: On the outer side of the small toe, in the depression behind the base joint.
(The Systematized Canon)

Local Anatomy: The 4th common plantar digital artery and vein. The 4th common plantar digital nerve and the lateral dorsal cutaneous nerve of the foot.

Functions: Courses wind and dispels pathogens; clears heat and resolves toxin; soothes the sinews and quickens the connecting vessels.

Indications: Mania and withdrawal; headache; stiff neck; visual dizziness; pain in the back, lumbus and posterior aspect of the lower limbs.

Supplementary Indications: Fever and chills; tinnitus; painful reddening of the eyes; yong, ju and dorsal effusions; clove sores; intestinal pi diarrhea; hemorrhoids; aversion to wind and cold in heat diseases; stiffness of the neck preventing movement.

Illustrative Point Combinations & Applications: Stiff neck and aversion to wind; needle BL-65 combined with BL-10. *(Ode of a Hundred Patterns)*

Dorsal yong should be treated by choosing points on the tai yang channel; choose from among BL-67, BL-66, BL-65, BL-60, and BL-40. *(Song of Point Applications for Miscellaneous Disease)*

Stimulation: 0.3" perpendicular insertion.
Moxa: 3-7 cones; pole 3-5 min.

Point Categories & Associations: Stream-shu (wood) point.

Location: In the depression distal and slightly inferior to the 5th metatarsophalangeal joint.
Classical Location: On the outer side of the small toe, in the depression in front of the base joint. *(The Great Compendium)*
Local Anatomy: The plantar digital artery and vein. The plantar digital proprial nerve and the lateral dorsal cutaneous nerve of the foot.

BL-66
足通谷
tōng gǔ
"Valley Passage"

Functions: Dissipates wind and clears heat; settles fright and quiets the spirit.
Indications: Headache; stiff neck; visual dizziness; nosebleed.
Supplementary Indications: Thoracic fullness; cough and dyspnea; untransformed digestate; susceptibility to fright; mania and withdrawal.

Stimulation: 0.2" perpendicular insertion.
Moxa: 3-7 cones; pole 5-20 min.

Point Categories & Associations: Spring-ying (water) point.

BL-67

至陰

zhì yīn

"Reaching Yin"

Location: On the lateral side of the small toe, about 0.1 " proximal to the corner of the nail.

Classical Location: On the outer side of the small toe, the width of a Chinese leek leaf away from the corner of the nail.
(The Great Compendium)

Local Anatomy: The network formed by the dorsal digital artery and plantar digital proprial artery. The plantar digital proprial nerve and the lateral dorsal cutaneous nerve of the foot.

Functions: Courses wind in the vertex; rectifies qi and quickens the blood; clears the brain and brightens the eyes.

Indications: Headache; nasal congestion; nosebleed; eye pain; heat in the soles of the feet; difficult delivery; malposition of the fetus.

Supplementary Indications: Nosebleed with clear snivel; eye screens; seminal emission; inhibited urination; generalized itching; pain and weakness of the limbs; retention of afterbirth; paralysis; vexation.

Illustrative Point Combinations & Applications: BL-67 combined with M-HN-9 and LU-7 treats unilateral headache; combined with GB-20, BL-10 and M-HN-9, it treats vertex headache.

Moxibustion at BL-67 can correct the position of the fetus; this combined with needling ST-36 can hasten delivery.

BL-67 combined with BL-23, CV-4, and SP-6 treats seminal loss.

Stimulation: 0.1 " upward oblique insertion.
Moxa: 3-5 cones; pole 3-5 min.

Point Categories & Associations: Well-jing (metal) point.

Foot Tai Yang Bladder Channel			
Point	**Location**	**Indications**	
		Primary	**Secondary**
*BL-1	Inner Canthus	Eye disease	
*BL-2	Eyebrow	Headache red, swollen, painful eyes	
BL-3	Front of Head	Headache visual dizziness nasal congestion	Epilepsy
BL-4		Headache visual dizziness nasal congestion nosebleed	Epilepsy
BL-5		Headache; dizziness	Epilepsy
BL-6		Headache nasal congestion	
BL-7		Headache dizziness nasal congestion nosebleed	
BL-8	Back of head	Dizziness tinnitus	Mania and withdrawal
BL-9		Head and neck pain eye pain nasal congestion	
*BL-10	Neck	Headache stiff neck nasal congestion	
Head & Neck: Disorders of the head, neck, eyes, and nose; mental disorders			
BL-11	Back	Cough fever stiff neck shoulder & back pain	
*BL-12		Wind damage cough stiff neck chest and back pain	

Foot Tai Yang Bladder Channel (continued)			
Point	**Location**	**Indications**	
		Primary	**Secondary**
*BL-13	Back	Cough dyspnea blood ejection steaming bone tidal fever	
BL-14		Cough; cardiac pain	
*BL-15		Cough blood ejection cardiac pain	Fright palpitations impaired memory epilepsy
The medial branch along the 1st to 7th thoracic vertebrae; disorders of heart and lung			
*BL-18	Back	Lateral costal pain blood ejection visual dizziness	Jaundice epilepsy mania and withdrawal
*BL-19		Lateral costal pain	Jaundice
*BL-20		Abdominal distention diarrhea dysenteric disease	Edema back pain
*BL-21		Pain in the venter back pain intestinal rumbling	
The medial branch along the 9th thoracic vertebrae to the 1st lumbar vertebrae: Primarily gastric & intestinal disorders; secondarily disorders of the chest & lung			
BL-22	Lumbus	Intestinal rumbling abdominal distention vomiting pain and stiffness in the lumbus	
*BL-23		Enuresis seminal emission impotence menstrual disorders lumbar pain	Edema tinnitus deafness
BL-24		Lumbar pain	
*BL-25		Abdominal distention diarrhea constipation lumbar pain	

Point	Location	Indications Primary	Secondary
Foot Tai Yang Bladder Channel (continued)			
BL-26	Buttocks	Diarrhea; lumbar pain	
BL-27		Abdominal pain diarrhea enuresis	
*BL-28		Urinary incontinence pain and stiffness of the lumbar spine	
BL-29		Diarrhea pain and stiffness of the lumbar spine	
BL-30		Seminal emission menstrual disorders white vaginal discharge lumbosacral pain	
BL-31	Sacrum	Inhibited urination vaginal discharge prolapse of the uterus lumbar pain	
*BL-32		Menstrual disorders vaginal discharge inhibited urination seminal emission lumbar pain	
BL-33		Menstrual disorders vaginal discharge inhibited urination lumbar pain	
BL-34		Inhibited urination vaginal discharge constipation	
BL-35	Buttocks	Diarrhea hemorrhoids vaginal discharge	
The medial branch from the 2nd lumbar vertebrae to the sacral region: Intestinal, gynecologic, and genitourinary disorders			

239

	Foot Tai Yang Bladder Channel (continued)		
Point	Location	Indications	
		Primary	Secondary
BL-36	Upper leg	Lumbosacral & buttock pain	
BL-37		Lumbar pain paralysis of the lower limbs	
BL-38		Pain and numbness of the lower buttocks	
*BL-39	Knee crease	Abdominal fullness inhibited urination hypertonicity and pain of the legs and feet	
*BL-40		lumbar pain paralysis of the lower limbs	Abdominal pain vomiting and diarrhea
Upper leg: Localized and intestinal disorders			
BL-41	Back	Stiff neck hypertonicity of the shoulders and back	
BL-42		Cough pulmonary consumption stiff neck back and shoulder pain	
*BL-43		Cough dyspnea pulmonary consumption	Impaired memory seminal emission
BL-44		Cough dyspnea oppression in the chest	
BL-45		Cough shoulder and back pain	Malaria heat disease
BL-46		Eructation vomiting	
The lateral branch along the 1st to 7th thoracic vertebrae: Disorders of the chest and lung			
BL-47	Back	Pain in the chest & lateral costal region vomiting back pain	

Point	Location	Indications	
		Primary	**Secondary**
BL-48	Back	Intestinal rumbling abdominal pain diarrhea	Jaundice
BL-49		Abdominal distention vomiting diarrhea	
BL-50		Pain in the venter abdominal distention	
BL-51		Constipation	
The lateral branch along the 9th thoracic vertebrae to the 1st lumbar vertebrae: Gastric and intestinal disorders			
*BL-52	Lumbus	Seminal emission inhibited urination pain and stiffness of the lumbar spine	
BL-53	Buttocks	Urinary block pain and stiffness of the lumbar spine	
BL-54		Inhibited urination hemorrhoidal disease lumbosacral pain	
The lateral branch along the 2nd to 9th lumbar vertebrae: Intestinal, gynecologic and genitourinary disorders			
BL-55	Lower leg	Pain and stiffness of the lumbar spine	
BL-56		Hemorrhoidal disease pain and hypertonicity of the legs & lumbar region	
*BL-57		Constipation hemorrhoidal disease pain and hypertonicity of the legs & lumbar region	
*BL-58		Headache visual dizziness pain in the legs & lumbar region	

Table title: **Foot Tai Yang Bladder Channel** (continued)

241

Point	Location	Indications	
		Primary	**Secondary**
BL-59	Lower leg	Headache lumbosacral pain paralysis of the lower limbs	
*BL-60	Ankle joint	Headache stiff neck visual dizziness lumbar pain	Difficult labor epilepsy
BL-61		Heel pain	Epilepsy mania and withdrawal
*BL-62		Red eyes insomnia headache dizziness pain in the legs & lumbar region	Epilepsy mania and withdrawal
BL-63		Lumbar pain	
BL-64	Foot	Headache stiff neck pain in the legs & lumbar region	Epilepsy
*BL-65		Headache stiff neck visual dizziness pain in the legs & lumbar region	Mania and withdrawal
BL-66		Headache stiff neck visual dizziness nosebleed	Mania and withdrawal
*BL-67		Headache eye pain nasal congestion nosebleed	Difficult labor malpositioned fetus

Foot Tai Yang Bladder Channel (continued)

Lower leg and foot: Disorders of the head, neck, eyes, nose, back, and lumbar region; hemorrhoidal disease; mental disorders; disorders of the posterior aspect of the lower limbs

13. The Kidney Channel System (Foot Shao Yin) 足少陰腎經

13.1 The Primary Kidney Channel

Pathway: The foot shao yin kidney channel starts on the underside of the little toe, crosses the sole of the foot obliquely, and emerges out of the arch of the foot under the navicular tuberosity at KI-2. It then proceeds posterior to the medial malleolus and continues into the heel. From there it travels up the rear medial aspect of the lower leg to intersect with the foot tai yin spleen channel at SP-6. Traveling up through the gastrocnemius muscle, it ascends across the medial aspect of the popliteal fossa and the posteromedial where it meets the governing vessel at GV-1. It continues up to link with the spinal column and home to the kidney, after which it turns downwards to connect with the bladder and intersect with the conception vessel at CV-4 and CV-3.

A branch ascends from the kidney, goes directly to the liver, crosses the diaphragm, enters the lung, and follows the throat up to the root of the tongue.

A further branch separates in the lung, links through to the heart and disperses in the chest.

Main pathologic signs associated with the external course of the channel: low back pain; counterflow frigidity of the legs; atony of the legs; dry mouth; sore pharynx; pain in the lateral gluteal region and in the posterior aspect of the thigh; there may also be pain in the soles of the feet.

Main pathologic signs associated with the internal organ: dizziness; facial edema; bleary eyes; ashen complexion; shortness of breath; short rapid breathing; somnolence or restlessness; enduring diarrhea; thin stool, or dry stool evacuated with difficulty; abdominal distention; nausea and vomiting; impotence.

13.2 The Connecting Vessel of the Kidney Channel

Pathway: The vessel leaves the primary channel at KI-4, behind the medial malleolus and skirts the heel before connecting to the foot tai yang bladder channel. A branch follows the primary channel to the region below the pericardium and from there it proceeds down to connect to the lumbar vertebrae.

Main pathologic signs:

Qi counterflow; vexation oppression.

Repletion: Blockage of the two yin (stool and urine).

Vacuity: low back pain.

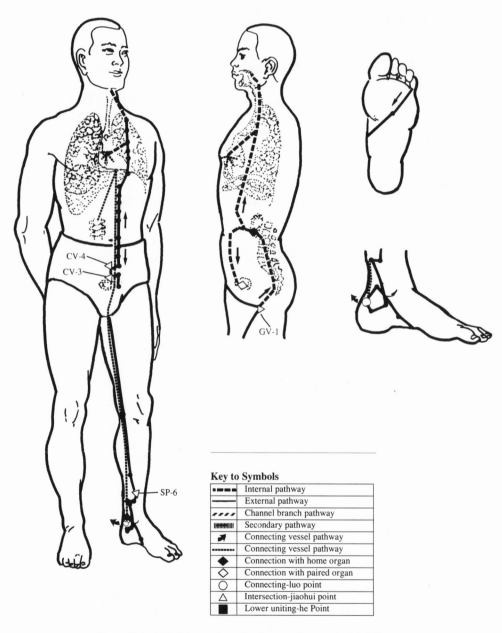

Key to Symbols

▄▄▄▄	Internal pathway
————	External pathway
⁄⁄⁄⁄	Channel branch pathway
▮▮▮▮▮▮	Secondary pathway
➚	Connecting vessel pathway
--------	Connecting vessel pathway
◆	Connection with home organ
◇	Connection with paired organ
○	Connecting-luo point
△	Intersection-jiaohui point
■	Lower uniting-he Point

Figure 13.1 - 13.2 Primary channel and connecting vessel of the kidney.

13.3 The Kidney Channel Divergence

Pathway: This divergence leaves the primary channel at the popliteal fossa and unites with the foot tai yang bladder channel divergence. It rises to the kidney and at the second lumbar vertebrae it homes to the girdling vessel. The divergence then rises to connect to the root of the tongue and moves out to the nape, where it unites with the foot tai yang bladder channel divergence.

13.4 The Kidney Channel Sinews

Pathway: This sinew originates beneath the little toe and enters the sole of the foot. It accompanies the foot tai yin spleen channel sinew by slanting below the medial malleolus and binding to the heel. Here it unites with the foot tai yang bladder channel sinew and rises to bind below the medial aspect of the knee. It joins the foot tai yin spleen channel sinew and rises up the medial side of the thigh to bind at the genitals. A branch ascends along the side of the spine to the nape where it binds to the occipital bone and unites with the foot tai yang bladder channel sinew.

Main pathologic signs: Cramping at the bottom of the foot; spasms, twisting or pain along the course of the sinews. The major symptoms associated with these sinews are the convulsions and spasms associated with epileptic diseases. If a disease attacks the back side the patient can not bend forward and if it affects the chest and abdomen the patient cannot lean backward. In yang diseases the upper body curves backward. In yin diseases the patient cannot lean backward.

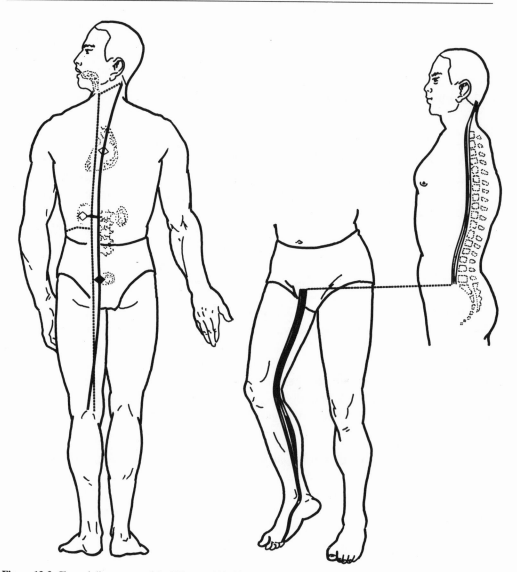

Figure 13.3 Channel divergences of the kidney and bladder.

Figure 13.4 The kidney channel sinews.

Location: In the depression appearing on the sole when the foot is in plantar flexion, one third of the distance from the base of the toes to the heel.

Classical Location: In the depression in the heart of the sole, as felt when the leg is stretched, the foot bent and the toes curled. *(The Great Compendium)*

Local Anatomy: At the deep level, the plantar arch. The 2nd common plantar digital nerve.

Functions: Clears kidney heat; downbears yin fire; stabilizes the spirit disposition; revives inversion patients.

Indications: Vertex headache; dizziness; flowery vision; sore throat; dry tongue; loss of voice; inhibited urination; difficult evacuation; infantile fright wind; heat in the soles of the feet; clouding inversion.

Supplementary Indications: Black complexion; susceptibility to fear; poor memory; irascibility; throat bi; swelling of the pharynx; dry tongue; nosebleed; cough and spitting of blood; water swelling; shan qi; impotence; running piglet; pain in the toes; lumbar pain; vexation; no pleasure in eating; cough and shortness of breath; cold stretching from the sole of the foot to the knee; backache; female infertility; madness; foot qi swelling; women's disorders; wind papules; child fright wind.

Illustrative Point Combinations & Applications: Pain in the lower abdomen and umbilical region is treated by first needling SP-9 and then KI-1. *(The Celestial Emperor's Secret)*

Stimulation: 0.3-0.5″ perpendicular insertion.
Moxa: 3 cones; pole 5-15 min.
Needle Sensation: Localized pain and distention.

Point Categories & Associations: Well-jing (wood) point; one of the nine needles for returning yang.

Location: In the depression inferior to the lower border of the tuberosity of the navicular bone.

Classical Location: In the depression below the large bone that lies in front of the inner ankle. *(The Great Compendium)*

KI-1
湧泉
yǒng quán
"Gushing Spring"

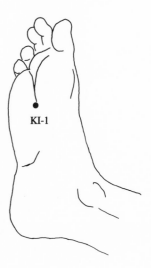

KI-1

Figure 13.5

KI-2
然谷
rán gǔ
"Blazing Valley"

Local Anatomy: Branches of the medial plantar and medial tarsal arteries. The terminal branch of the medial crural cutaneous nerve, the medial plantar nerve.

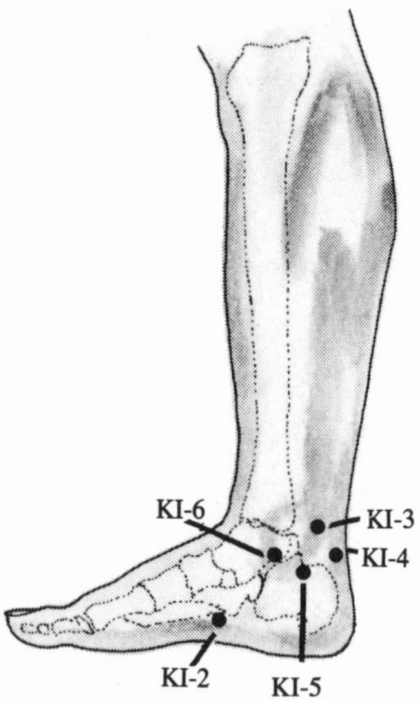

Functions: Abates kidney heat; courses inversion qi; rectifies the lower burner.

Indications: Genital itch; prolapse of the uterus; irregular menses; seminal emission; coughing of blood; diarrhea; painful swelling of the dorsum of the foot.

Supplementary Indications: Throat bi and swelling of the pharynx; spitting of blood; impotence; turbid white urethral discharge; thermic malaria; throughflux diarrhea; urinary stoppage; wasting thirst; jaundice; spontaneous and night sweating; swelling of the dorsum of the foot that prevents walking; cold shan with lower abdominal distention; infertility; pain in the lower leg that prevents standing for long periods; no pleasure in eating; vexation heat diseases; cold feet; heat in one foot and cold in the other; protracted tongue; vexation and fullness.

Illustrative Point Combinations & Applications: KI-2 drains kidney (heat), but should be combined with CV-7.
(Wo Yan's Efficacious Point Applications)

Stimulation: 0.3″ perpendicular insertion.
Moxa: 3 cones; pole 5-10 min.

Point Categories & Associations: Spring-ying (fire) point; also, a branch departs from the channel here and connects to SP-8.

Figure 13.6

KI-6   KI-3   KI-4   KI-2   KI-5

KI-3
太溪 (太谿)
tài xī

"Great Ravine"

Location: In the depression between the medial malleolus and the achilles tendon (t. calcaneus), level with the tip of the medial malleolus.

Classical Location: Five fen behind the inner ankle bone, in the depression above the heel bone where a pulsating vessel can be felt.

Figuring among the nine indicators of the three regions, KI-3 has diagnostic value: in severe diseases, the pulse at this point should be felt; if the pulse has expired, the patient cannot be saved.
(The Great Compendium)

Local Anatomy: Anteriorly, the posterior tibial artery and vein. The medial crural cutaneous nerve, on the course of the tibial nerve.

Functions: Enriches kidney yin; abates vacuity heat; invigorates original yang; and rectifies the womb.

Indications: Sore throat; toothache; deafness; coughing of blood; asthma; irregular menses; insomnia; seminal emission; impotence; urinary frequency; lumbar pain.

Supplementary Indications: Throat bi and swelling of the pharynx; toothache; kidney vacuity impotence and seminal emission; cold shan; difficult evacuation; mammary yong; cardiac pain; inversion cold in the extremities; damp itch and sores on the inside of the thigh; branching fullness in the chest and lateral costal region; kidney disease; heat disease with copious sweating; gluey sensation in the mouth; repletion dyspnea with fullness and phlegm tinnitus.

Illustrative Point Combinations & Applications: For lumbar pain, evacuation difficulty, cold hands and feet, needle KI-3, BL-40 and KI-4. *(The Shen Nong Canon)*

Stimulation: 0.3″ perpendicular insertion.
Moxa: 3 cones; pole 5-10 min.

Needle Sensation: Localized distention and numbness, the latter sometimes spreading over the soles of the feet.

Point Categories & Associations: Stream-shu (earth) and source-yuan point; one of the nine needles for returning yang.

KI-4
大鐘
dà zhōng
"Large Goblet"

Location: Posterior and inferior to KI-3, in the depression anterior to the angle formed by the achilles tendon (t. calcaneus) and the calcaneum.

Classical Location: At the back of the heel, between the two sinews above the large bone. *(The Great Compendium)*

Local Anatomy: The medial calcaneal branch of the posterior tibial artery. The medial crural cutaneous nerve, on the course of the medial calcaneal ramus derived from the tibial nerve.

Functions: Regulates the kidney and harmonizes the blood; supplements essence-spirit.

Indications: Coughing of blood; asthma; stiffness and pain in the lumbar region; inhibited urination; pain in the heel.

Supplementary Indications: Urinary block; constipation; lumbar pain; feeblemindedness; prostrate exhaustion; abdominal fullness; susceptibility to fright or anger; heat in the mouth; vexation and oppression; bleeding from the root of the tongue; insufficiency of spirit qi; sore pharynx; malarial disease.

Stimulation: 0.3″ oblique or perpendicular insertion.
Moxa: 3 cones; pole 5-20 min.

Point Categories & Associations: Connecting-luo point of the kidney channel connecting to the bladder channel.

KI-5
水泉
shuǐ quán

"Water Spring"

Location: 1″ directly below KI-3, in the depression anterior and superior to the medial side of the tuberosity of the calcaneum.
Classical Location: One inch below KI-3, below the inner ankle bone. *(The Great Compendium)*
Local Anatomy: See KI-4.

Functions: Regulates the menses; courses the lower burner.

Indications: Irregular menses; menstrual pain; prolapse of the uterus; inhibited urination; clouded or flowery vision.

Supplementary Indications: Absence of menstruation; oppression and pain below the heart; dribbling urination; nearsightedness; abdominal pain.

Illustrative Point Combinations & Applications: When the monthly tide fails to keep its times, needle KI-5 and ST-25.
(Ode of a Hundred Patterns)

Stimulation: 0.4″ oblique or perpendicular insertion.
Moxa: 5 cones; pole 5-10 min.

Point Categories & Associations: Cleft-xi point of the kidney channel.

KI-6
照海
zhào hǎi

"Shining Sea"

Location: 1″ below the medial malleolus.
Classical Location: Four fen below the inner ankle bone, in the depression bordered by sinews in front and behind, the ankle bone above, and the soft bone below. *(The Great Compendium)*
Local Anatomy: Posteroinferiorly, the posterior tibial artery and vein. The medial crural cutaneous nerve; deeper, the tibial nerve.

Functions: Frees the channels and harmonizes construction; drains fire and courses qi; clears the spirit-disposition; disinhibits the throat.

Indications: Irregular menses; prolapse of the uterus; genital itch; hernia; urinary frequency; epilepsy; dry, sore throat; insomnia.

Supplementary Indications: Vaginal discharge; abdominal pain; nocturnal epilepsy; sorrowfulness; no desire to eat; yellow urine; heat in the lower abdomen; pain and weakness of the limbs; thoracic oppression; phlegm-drool congestion; pharyngeal wind; running piglet; swelling and sagging of one testicle; difficult delivery; postpartum abdominal pain; persistent flow of lochia; female lassitude due to qi and blood vacuity; heat vexation in the five hearts; cramp in the hands and feet preventing movement; cholera with vomiting and diarrhea; cold-damp foot qi; fever; headache; swelling of the face and limbs; hemiplegia.

Illustrative Point Combinations & Applications: KI-6 and TB-6 free constipated bowels. *(Ode of the Jade Dragon)*

KI-6 is the choice of the skilled practitioner to clear a blocked throat. *(Ode to Elucidate Mysteries)*

Phlegm-drool congesting the throat, clenched jaws and throat wind can be treated by needling KI-6; bleeding this point with a three-edged needle brings immediate relief. *(Ode of the Dammed River)*

Stimulation: 0.3-0.5″ perpendicular insertion.
Moxa: 3 cones; pole 5-10 min.

Point Categories & Associations: A confluence-jiaohui point of the eight extraordinary vessels (related to the yin motility vessel); intersection-jiaohui point of the foot shao yin kidney channel and the yin motility vessel.

Location: 2″ above KI-3, on the anterior border of the achilles tendon (t. calcaneus).

Classical Location: In the depression two inches above the inner ankle bone. (The Systematized Canon)

Local Anatomy: At the deep level, anteriorly, the posterior tibial artery and vein. The medial sural and medial crural cutaneous nerves; deeper, the tibial nerve.

KI-7
復溜
fù liū
"Recover Flow"

Functions: Regulates the sweat pores; disinhibits the bladder; dispels dryness and disperses stagnation; enriches the kidney and moistens damp.

Indications: Diarrhea; rumbling intestines; edema; abdominal distention; swelling of the thighs; atony of the lower extremities; spontaneous or night sweating.

Supplementary Indications: The five stranguries; intestinal pi; abdominal pain; lumbar pain; cold in the lower leg; absence of sweating; abdominal distention; swelling of the limbs; bleeding hemorrhoids; heavy feeling in the rectum after diarrhea; pain in the nostrils; dry eructation; irascibility and talkativeness; curled tongue preventing speech; pus and blood in the stool; qi stagnation in the lumbus; pain on the dorsum of the foot.

Illustrative Point Combinations & Applications: Treat water swelling with CV-9 and KI-7.
(Song of Point Applications for Miscellaneous Disease)

Stimulation: 0.3-0.5 ″ perpendicular insertion.
Moxa: 5-7 cones; pole 5-8 min.

Needle Sensation: Localized numbness and distention sometimes spreading towards the feet.

Point Categories & Associations: River-jing (metal) point.

KI-8
交信

jiāo xìn

"Intersection Reach"

Location: 2 ″ above KI-3, 0.5 ″ anterior to KI-7, posterior to the medial border of the tibia.

Classical Location: Two inches above the inner ankle bone, between the bone and sinew.
(The Systematized Canon)

Local Anatomy: At the deep level, the posterior tibial artery and vein. The medial crural cutaneous nerve; deeper, the tibial nerve.

Functions: Supplements the kidney; regulates the penetrating and conception vessels; clears heat and eliminates damp.

Indications: Irregular menses; metrorrhagia; prolapse of the uterus; diarrhea; evacuative difficulty; pain and swelling of the testicles.

Supplementary Indications: Urinary block; shan.

Illustrative Point Combinations & Applications: KI-8 combined with BL-55 treats diminished qi scant uterine bleeding.
(Ode of a Hundred Patterns)

Stimulation: 0.4 ″ perpendicular insertion.
Moxa: 3 cones; pole 5-20 min.

Point Categories & Associations: Cleft-xi point of the yin motility vessel; intersection-jiaohui point of the foot shao yin kidney channel and the yin motility vessel.

Location: On the line drawn from KI-3 to KI-10, at the lower end of the body of the gastrocnemius muscle (m. gastrocnemius), on the anteromedial edge of the muscle, about 5″ above KI-3.

Classical Location: Five inches above the inner ankle, at the border of the calf. *(The Great Compendium)*

Local Anatomy: At the deep level, the posterior tibial artery and vein. The medial sural cutaneous nerve and medial crural cutaneous nerve; deeper, the tibial nerve.

Functions: Clears the heart and transforms phlegm; calms fright and quiets the spirit; resolves toxin and relieves pain.

Indications: Mania and withdrawal; pain on the medial aspect of the lower leg.

Supplementary Indications: Infantile womb-related shan; shan pain.

Stimulation: 0.5-0.8″ perpendicular insertion.
Moxa: 3 cones; pole 5-20 min.

Note: This point is mentioned in some texts as being effective for various types of food and drug toxicity. It is usually combined with the bleeding of BL-40.

Point Categories & Associations: Cleft-xi point of the yin linking vessel; intersection-jiaohui point of the foot shao yin kidney channel and the yin linking vessel.

KI-9
築賓
zhú bīn

"Guest House"

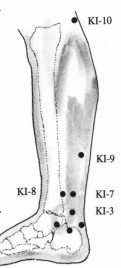

Figure 13.7

Location: On the medial side of the popliteal fossa, level with BL-40, between the tendons of the semitendinosus muscle (m. semitendinosus) and the semimembranosus muscle (m. semimembranosus) when the knee is flexed.

Classical Location: Below the knee, behind the inner leg bone, below the large sinew and above the small sinew.
(The Systematized Canon)

Local Anatomy: The medial superior genicular artery and vein. The medial femoral cutaneous nerve.

KI-10
陰谷
yīn gǔ

"Yin Valley"

253

Functions: Dispels damp and frees the urine; enriches the kidney and clears heat; courses inversion qi; disinhibits the lower burner.

Indications: Impotence; hernia; metrorrhagia; pain along the medial aspect of the knee and thigh.

Supplementary Indications: Difficult urination; urinary urgency; protracted tongue and drooling; shan pain; mania and withdrawal; abdominal distention.

Illustrative Point Combinations & Applications: To disinhibit urine and disperse water swelling, use KI-10, CV-9 and ST-36. *(Song of the Supreme Unity)*

Stimulation: 0.4-1.0″ perpendicular insertion.
Moxa: 3 cones; pole 3-5 min.

Point Categories & Associations: Uniting-he (water) point.

KI-11
橫骨
héng gǔ
"Pubic Bone"

Location: 5″ below the umbilicus, on the superior border of pubic symphysis, 0.5″ lateral to CV-2.

Classical Location: One inch below KI-12, on the pubic bone, one inch either side of the center line of the abdomen, in the depression shaped like an upturned moon. *(The Great Compendium)*

Local Anatomy: The inferior epigastric artery and external pudendal artery. The branch of the iliohypogastric nerve.

Functions: Boosts the stomach and disinhibits damp.

Indications: Pain in the genitals; seminal emission; impotence; urinary stoppage.

Supplementary Indications: Abdominal distention; lower abdominal pain; prolapse of the rectum persisting for years; painful protraction of the genitals; enuresis; the five stranguries; swelling of the lower extremities.

Illustrative Point Combinations & Applications: Qi stagnation lumbar pain making it difficult to stand can be treated through KI-11 and LV-1. *(Ode of Xi Hong)*

Stimulation: 0.3-0.8″ perpendicular insertion.
Moxa: 3-5 cones; pole 10-30 min.

Point Categories & Associations: Intersection-jiaohui point of the foot shao yin kidney channel and the penetrating vessel.

Location: 4″ below the umbilicus, 0.5″ lateral to CV-3.

Classical Location: One inch below KI-13 is the site of KI-12; five fen either side of the midline *(The Golden Mirror)*

Note: *The Great Compendium* places the points KI-12 through KI-17 1″ either side of the midline, while *The Golden Mirror* places them 5 fen from the midline.

Local Anatomy: The muscular branches of the inferior epigastric artery and vein. Branches of the subcostal nerve and iliohypogastric nerve.

Functions: Supplements kidney qi and regulates the penetrating and conception vessels.

Indications: Pain in the genitals; seminal emission; vaginal discharge.

Supplementary Indications: Genital retraction; pain in the penis.

Stimulation: 0.5-1.0″ perpendicular insertion.
Moxa: 3-5 cones; pole 10-30 min.

Point Categories & Associations: Intersection-jiaohui point of the foot shao yin kidney channel with the penetrating vessel.

KI-12

大赫

dà hè

"Great Manifestation"

Location: 3″ below the umbilicus, 0.5″ lateral to CV-4.

Classical Location: One inch above KI-12 is the site of KI-13, five fen from the midline. *(The Golden Mirror)*

Local Anatomy: See KI-12.

Functions: Supplements kidney qi; regulates the penetrating and conception vessels; rectifies the lower burner.

Indications: Irregular menses; diarrhea.

Supplementary Indications: Vaginal discharge; infertility; urinary stoppage; lumbar pain; running piglet.

Stimulation: 0.5-1.0″ perpendicular insertion.
Moxa: 3-5 cones; pole 10-30 min.

Point Categories & Associations: Intersection-jiaohui point of the foot shao yin kidney channel and the penetrating vessel.

KI-13

氣穴

qì xuè

"Qi Hole"

KI-14
四滿
sì mǎn

*"Fourfold
Fullness"*

Location: 2″ below the umbilicus, 0.5″ lateral to CV-5.

Classical Location: One inch above KI-14 is the site of KI-15, five fen either side of the midline. *(The Golden Mirror)*

Local Anatomy: See KI-12.

Functions: Supplements kidney qi; regulates the penetrating and conception vessels; promotes free flow through the waterways.

Indications: Metrorrhagia; irregular menses; postpartum abdominal pain; diarrhea.

Supplementary Indications: Acute pain due to malign blood; seminal emission; white turbid urethral discharge; cutting pain below the navel; running piglet; shan conglomeration.

Stimulation: 0.5-1.0″ perpendicular insertion.
Moxa: 3-5 cones; pole 10-30 min.

Point Categories & Associations: Intersection-jiaohui point of the foot shao yin kidney channel and the penetrating vessel.

KI-15
中注
zhōng zhù

"Central Flow"

Location: 1″ below the umbilicus, 0.5″ lateral to CV-7.

Classical Location: One inch above KI-14 is the site of KI-15, five fen from the midline. *(The Golden Mirror)*

Local Anatomy: The muscular branches of the inferior epigastric artery and vein. The 10th intercostal nerve.

Functions: Nourishes the kidney channel; regulates the penetrating and conception vessels; disinhibits the lower burner.

Indications: Irregular menses; lower abdominal pain; constipation; painful reddening of the eyes spreading from the inner canthus.

Supplementary Indications: Dry, hard stool; pain in the abdomen and lumbus; heat in the lower abdomen.

Stimulation: 0.5-1.0″ perpendicular insertion.
Moxa: 3-5 cones; pole 20-30 min.

Point Categories & Associations: Intersection-jiaohui point of the foot shao yin kidney channel and the penetrating vessel.

Location: 0.5″ lateral to the center of the umbilicus (CV-8).

Classical Location: One inch above KI-15 is the site of KI-16, five fen either side of the midline at the level of the navel. *(The Golden Mirror)*

Local Anatomy: The muscular branches of the inferior epigastric artery and vein. The 10th intercostal nerve.

Functions: Harmonizes the stomach and downbears counterflow; relieves pain.

Indications: Abdominal pain; vomiting; abdominal distention; constipation.

Supplementary Indications: Cold shan; dry stool.

Stimulation: 0.5-1.0″ perpendicular insertion.
Moxa: 5 cones; pole 20-30 min.

Point Categories & Associations: Intersection-jiaohui point of the foot shao yin kidney channel and the penetrating vessel.

KI-16
肓俞
huāng shū
''huang shu''

Location: 2″ above the umbilicus, 0.5″ lateral to CV-10.

Classical Location: Two inches above KI-16 is the site of KI-17, five fen either side of the midline. *(The Golden Mirror)*

Local Anatomy: Branches of the superior and inferior epigastric arteries and vein. The 9th intercostal nerve.

Functions: Fortifies the spleen and disinhibits damp; soothes the sinews and quickens the connecting vessel.

Indications: Abdominal fullness; diarrhea; constipation.

Supplementary Indications: Abdominal accumulations and gatherings with periodic cutting pain; pain in the intestines with no pleasure in eating; painful reddening of the eye spreading from the inner canthus.

Stimulation: 0.5-1.0″ perpendicular insertion.
Moxa: 5 cones; pole 20-30 min.

Point Categories & Associations: Intersection-jiaohui point of the foot shao yin kidney channel with the penetrating vessel.

KI-17
商曲
shāng qū
''Shang Bend''

KI-18
石關
shí guān

"Stone Pass"

Location: 3″ above the umbilicus, 0.5″ lateral to CV-11.

Classical Location: One inch above KI-17 is the site of KI-18, five fen from the midline. *(The Golden Mirror)*

Note: *The Great Compendium* places the point one inch and five fen from the midline.

Local Anatomy: Branches of the superior epigastric artery and vein. The 8th intercostal nerve.

Functions: Fortifies the center and harmonizes the stomach; frees the intestines and abducts stagnation.

Indications: Vomiting; pain in the venter; abdominal pain; constipation; postpartum abdominal pain.

Supplementary Indications: Infertility; copious spittle; malign blood surging upward in the abdomen; accumulations and gatherings; painful reddening of the eyes spreading from the inner canthus.

Illustrative Point Combinations & Applications: For non-conception, needle CV-7 and KI-18. *(Ode of a Hundred Patterns)*

Stimulation: 0.5-1.0″ perpendicular insertion.
Moxa: 5 cones; pole 20-30 min.

Point Categories & Associations: Intersection-jiaohui point of the foot shao yin kidney channel and the penetrating vessel.

KI-19
陰都
yīn dū

"Yin Metropolis"

Location: 4″ above the umbilicus, 0.5″ lateral to CV-12.

Classical Location: One inch above KI-18 is the site of KI-19, five fen from the midline. *(The Golden Mirror)*

Note: *The Great Compendium* places the point one inch and five fen from the midline.

Local Anatomy: See KI-18.

Functions: Fortifies the spleen and harmonizes the stomach; regulates qi dynamic and frees abdominal qi; regulates the penetrating and conception vessels.

Indications: Borborygmi; abdominal distention; abdominal pain.

Supplementary Indications: Counterflow qi with abdominal pain; heat and pain in the lateral costal region; difficult evacuation; infertility; vexation and fullness; painful reddening of the eyes spreading from the inner canthus.

Stimulation: 0.5-1.0″ perpendicular insertion.
Moxa: 3-5 cones; pole 20-30 min.

Point Categories & Associations: Intersection-jiaohui point of the foot shao yin kidney channel and penetrating vessel.

Location: 5″ above the umbilicus, 0.5″ lateral to CV-13.
Classical Location: The depression one inch above KI-19 is the site of KI-20, five fen either side of the midline.
(The Golden Mirror)

Note: *The Great Compendium* places the point one inch and five fen from the midline.

Local Anatomy: See KI-18.

Functions: Fortifies the spleen and harmonizes the stomach; loosens the chest and rectifies qi.

Indications: Abdominal pain; abdominal distention; vomiting; untransformed digestate.

Supplementary Indications: Accumulations and gatherings; bowstring and elusive masses; lodged rheum; pain in the chest and lateral costal region; retching; counterflow cough and dyspnea; epilepsy; sudden loss of voice; palpitations; abstraction.

Stimulation: 0.5-1.0″ perpendicular insertion.
Moxa: 5 cones; pole 20-30 min.

Point Categories & Associations: Intersection-jiaohui point of the foot shao yin kidney channel and the penetrating vessel.

KI-20
腹通谷
tōng gǔ
"Open Valley"

Location: 6″ above the umbilicus, 0.5″ lateral to CV-14.
Classical Location: The depression one inch above KI-20 is the site of KI-21, five fen from the midline. *(The Golden Mirror)*

Note: *The Great Compendium* places the point one inch and five fen from the midline.

Local Anatomy: Branches of the superior epigastric artery and vein. The 7th intercostal nerve.

KI-21
幽門
yōu mén
"Dark Gate"

259

Functions: Courses the liver and rectifies qi; fortifies the spleen and harmonizes the stomach; clears abdominal heat.

Indications: Abdominal pain; vomiting; diarrhea.

Supplementary Indications: Pain in the chest referring to the back and lumbus; glomus and distention below the heart; untransformed digestate; abdominal urgency; painful reddening of the eyes spreading from the inner canthus.

Stimulation: 0.5-1.0″ perpendicular insertion.
Moxa: 5 cones; pole 20-30 min.

Point Categories & Associations: Intersection-jiaohui point of the foot shao yin kidney channel and the penetrating vessel.

KI-22
步廊
bù láng
"Corridor Walk"

Location: In the 5th intercostal space, 2″ lateral to the conception vessel.

Classical Location: In the depression one inch and six fen above KI-21, two inches either side of the midline. The point is found in supine posture. *(The Golden Mirror)*

Local Anatomy: The 5th intercostal artery and vein. The anterior cutaneous branch of the 5th intercostal nerve; deeper, the 5th intercostal nerve.

Functions: Diffuses the lung and suppresses cough; downbears counterflow and stops vomiting.

Indications: Cough; asthma.

Supplementary Indications: Branching fullness in the chest and lateral costal region; nasal congestion; diminished qi; inability to move the arm.

Stimulation: 0.3-0.5″ oblique or perpendicular insertion.
Moxa: 5 cones; pole 5-10 min.

KI-23
神封
shén fēng
"Spirit Seal"

Location: In the 4th intercostal space, 2″ lateral to the conception vessel.

Classical Location: One inch and six fen above KI-22, two inches either side of the midline. The point is found in supine posture. *(The Golden Mirror)*

Local Anatomy: The 4th intercostal artery and vein. The anterior cutaneous branch of the 4th intercostal nerve; deeper, the 4th intercostal nerve.

Functions: Diffuses the lung and suppresses cough; harmonizes the stomach and downbears counterflow.

Indications: Cough; asthma; distention and fullness in the chest and lateral costal region; mammary yong.

Supplementary Indications: Branching fullness in the chest and lateral costal region; breathing difficulty; counterflow cough; shortness of breath; vomiting; no pleasure in eating.

Stimulation: 0.3-0.5″ oblique or perpendicular insertion.
Moxa: 5 cones; pole 5-20 min.

Location: In the 3rd intercostal space, 2″ lateral to the conception vessel.

Classical Location: One inch and six fen above KI-23, two inches either side of the midline. The point is found in supine posture. *(The Great Compendium)*

Local Anatomy: The 3rd intercostal artery and vein. The anterior cutaneous branch of the 3rd intercostal nerve; deeper, the 3rd intercostal nerve.

Functions: Opens the chest and downbears counterflow; clears heat and disperses swelling.

Indications: Cough; asthma; distention and fullness in the chest and lateral costal region; mammary yong.

Supplementary Indications: Branching fullness in the chest and lateral costal region; breathing difficulty; vomiting; no pleasure in eating; vexation and fullness.

Stimulation: 0.3-0.5″ oblique or perpendicular insertion.
Moxa: 5 cones; pole 5-20 min.

KI-24
靈墟
líng xū

"Spirit Ruins"

Location: In the 2nd intercostal space, 2″ lateral to the conception vessel.

Classical Location: One inch and six fen above KI-24, two inches either side of the midline. The point is found in supine posture. *(The Great Compendium)*

Local Anatomy: The 2nd intercostal artery and vein. The anterior cutaneous branch of the 2nd intercostal nerve; deeper, the 2nd intercostal nerve.

KI-25
神藏
shén cáng

"Spirit Storehouse"

261

Functions: Opens the chest; calms dyspnea and relieves cough; rectifies qi.

Indications: Cough; asthma; pain in the chest.

Supplementary Indications: Branching fullness in the chest and lateral costal region; vomiting; vexation and fullness; no pleasure in eating.

Illustrative Point Combinations & Applications: For thoracic fullness and stiffness in the neck, try needling KI-25 and CV-21. *(Ode of a Hundred Patterns)*

Stimulation: 0.3-0.5″ oblique or perpendicular insertion. Moxa: 5 cones; pole 5-20 min.

KI-26
彧中
yù zhōng

"Lively Center"

Location: In the 1st intercostal space, 2″ lateral to the conception vessel.

Classical Location: One inch and six fen above KI-25, in the depression two inches either side of the midline. The point is found in supine posture. *(The Golden Mirror)*

Local Anatomy: The 1st intercostal artery and vein. The anterior cutaneous branch of the 1st intercostal nerve, the medial supra-clavicular nerve; deeper, the 1st intercostal nerve.

Functions: Loosens the chest and promotes smooth flow of qi; calms dyspnea and relieves cough.

Indications: Cough; asthma; distention and fullness in the chest and lateral costal region.

Supplementary Indications: Branching fullness in the chest and lateral costal region; phlegm congestion; no pleasure in eating.

Stimulation: 0.3-0.5″ oblique or perpendicular insertion. Moxa: 3-5 cones; pole 5-20 min.

KI-27
俞府
shū fǔ

"Shu Mansion"

Location: In the depression on the lower border of the medial head of the clavicle, 2″ lateral to the conception vessel.

Classical Location: Below the clavicle, in the depression two inches from CV-21. *(The Systematized Canon)*

Local Anatomy: The anterior perforating branches of the internal mammary artery and vein. The medial supraclavicular nerve.

Functions: Diffuses the lung and downbears counterflow; calms dyspnea and suppresses cough; fortifies the spleen and harmonizes the stomach.

Indications: Cough; asthma; pain in the chest.

Supplementary Indications: Abdominal distention; vomiting; no pleasure in eating.

Illustrative Point Combinations & Applications: ST-18 and KI-27 treat qi cough (productive), and phlegm dyspnea.
(Ode of the Jade Dragon)

Stimulation: 0.3″ oblique or perpendicular insertion.
Moxa: 3-5 cones; pole 5-20 min.

| \multicolumn{4}{c}{**Foot Shao Yin Kidney Channel**} |

| Point | Location | Indications | |
		Primary	**Secondary**
*KI-1	Sole of foot	Pain and swelling of the throat inhibited urination constipation clouding inversion	Headache visual dizziness child fright wind mania and withdrawal
*KI-2		Menstrual disorders seminal emission coughing of blood	Wasting thirst
*KI-3		Pain and swelling of the throat coughing of blood menstrual disorders	Toothache insomnia tinnitus
*KI-4	Foot	Urinary blood constipation heel pain	Stupor
KI-5		Menstrual disorders menstrual pain inhibited urination	
*KI-6		Pain and dryness of the throat menstrual disorders constipation	Insomnia
Foot: Gynecologic, genitourinary, intestinal, lung, and throat disorders			

		Foot Shao Yin Kidney Channel (continued)	
Point	**Location**	**Indications**	
		Primary	**Secondary**
*KI-7	Lower leg	Abdominal distention diarrhea water swelling	Night sweating heat disease without sweat
KI-8		Menstrual disorders prolapse of the uterus	
KI-9		Hernia vomiting pain in the lower leg	Mania and withdrawal
KI-10	Knee crease	Impotence metrorrhagia inhibited urination	
Lower leg: gynecologic, genitourinary, and intestinal disorders			
KI-11	Lower abdomen	Seminal emission vaginal discharge	
KI-12		Seminal emission vaginal discharge	
KI-13		Menstrual disorders diarrhea	
KI-14	Lower abdomen	Menstrual disorders hernia diarrhea	
KI-15		Menstrual disorders constipation	
Lower abdomen: Gynecologic, genitourinary, and intestinal disorders			
KI-16	Upper abdomen	Abdominal pain constipation	
KI-17		Abdominal pain constipation diarrhea	
KI-18		Vomiting abdominal pain	
KI-19		Abdominal distention and pain	
KI-20		Vomiting abdominal pain	
KI-21		Abdominal pain vomiting diarrhea	
Upper abdomen: gastric and intestinal disorder			

Point	Location	Indications	
		Primary	**Secondary**
KI-22	Chest	Cough dyspnea distention and fullness of the chest and lateral costal region	
KI-23		Cough dyspnea distention and fullness of the chest and lateral costal region	
KI-24		Cough dyspnea distention and fullness of the chest and lateral costal region	
KI-25		Cough dyspnea chest pain	
KI-26		Cough dyspnea distention and fullness of the chest and lateral costal region	
*KI-27		Cough dyspnea chest pain	

Foot Shao Yin Kidney Channel (continued)

Chest: Disorders of the chest and lung

14. The Pericardium Channel System (Hand Jue Yin) 手厥陰心包經

14.1 The Primary Pericardium Channel

Pathway: The hand jue yin pericardium channel starts in the chest, where it homes to the pericardium. Descending through the diaphragm into the abdomen, it connects successively to the upper, middle, and lower burners.

A branch runs out horizontally from the center of the chest, emerges at the flank three body-inches below the anterior axillary fold, and then skirts around the axilla to the upper arm. It runs down the medial midline of the upper arm between the hand tai yin lung channel and the hand shao yin heart channel, crosses the center of the cubital fossa and then proceeds down the forearm between the tendons of the m. palmaris longus and m. flexor carpi radialis. It travels through the palm to the tip of the middle finger.

Another branch separates in the palm and proceeds along the lateral aspect of the fourth finger to its tip.

Main pathologic signs associated with the external course of the channel: stiffness of the neck; spasm in the limbs; red facial complexion; pain in the eyes; subaxillary swelling; hypertonicity of the elbow and arm inhibiting movement; hot palms.

Main pathologic signs associated with the internal organ: delirious speech; clouding inversion; vexation; fullness and oppression in the chest and lateral costal region; aphasia; palpitations; cardialgia; constant laughter and other essence-spirit disorders.

[handwritten margin note: unconsciousness]

14.2 The Connecting Vessel of the Pericardium Channel

Pathway: The pericardium connecting vessel separates from the primary channel at PC-6 and travels to the hand shao yang triple burner channel. It also follows the primary channel upward to the pericardium and then connects to the heart.

Main pathologic signs:

Repletion: heart pain.
Vacuity: vexation in the heart.

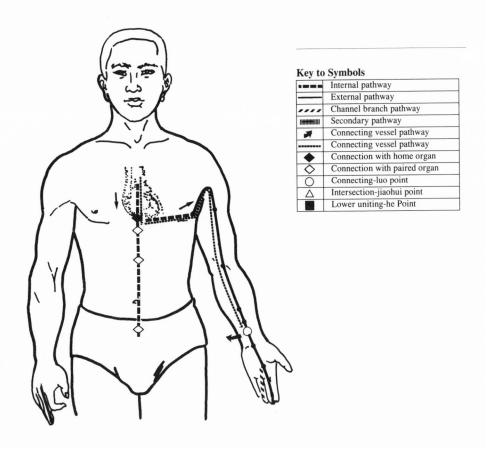

Figure 14.1 - 14.2 Primary channel and connecting vessel of the pericardium.

14.3 The Pericardium Channel Divergence

Pathway: This divergence leaves the primary channel three body inches below the axilla and extends in to the chest where it homes to each of the three burners. It then rises along the throat and issues behind the ear to unite with the hand shao yang triple burner channel (below the bone behind the ear).

14.4 The Pericardium Channel Sinews

Pathway: The channel sinews of the pericardium originate at the middle finger and accompany the hand tai yin lung channel sinews upward, binding at both the medial aspect of the elbow and below the axilla. From here the sinews disperse outward and downward over the ribcage. A branch also enters the chest at the axilla and disperses in the chest and binds to the diaphragm.

267

Main pathologic signs:

Spasms, stiffness, strain and pain along the course of the sinews; chest pain and a feeling of a palpable inverted cup below the lower right ribs.

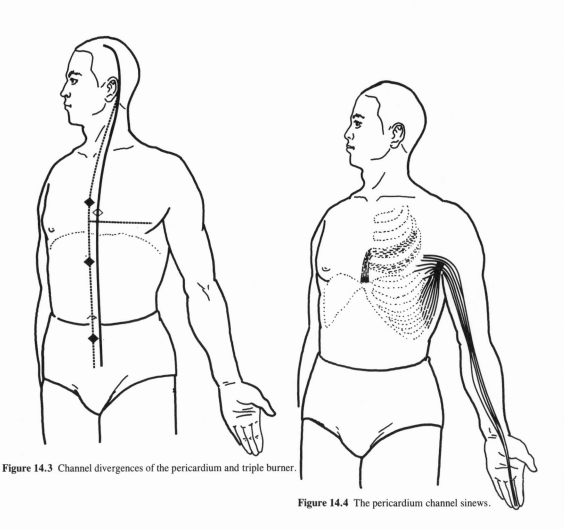

Figure 14.3 Channel divergences of the pericardium and triple burner.

Figure 14.4 The pericardium channel sinews.

Location: 1 " supralateral to the nipple, in the 4th intercostal space.

Classical Location: Three inches below the armpit, one or two inches behind the nipple, between the protuberances of the ribs. *(The Golden Mirror)*

Local Anatomy: The thoracoepigastric vein, branches of the lateral thoracic artery and vein. The muscular branch of the anterior thoracic nerve, the 4th intercostal nerve.

Functions: Opens the chest and rectifies qi; suppresses cough and calms dyspnea; diffuses the lung and clears heat.

Indications: Thoracic oppression; pain in the lateral costal region; pain and swelling of the axillary region.

Supplementary Indications: Cough with copious phlegm; dyspnea; saber and pearl-string lumps; malaria; headache; inability to move the limbs; throat rattle.

Illustrative Point Combinations & Applications: Needling BL-39 and PC-1 swiftly dissipates axillary swelling. *(Ode of a Hundred Patterns)*

Stimulation: 0.2 " outward oblique insertion; bleed with three-edged needle. Moxa: 1-5 cones; pole 5-19 min.

Point Categories & Associations: Intersection-jiaohui point of the hand jue yin pericardium, foot jue yin liver, and foot shao yang gallbladder channels.

PC-1

天池

tiān chí

"Celestial Pool"

Location: 2 " below the end of the anterior axillary fold, between the two heads of the biceps muscle of the arm (m. biceps brachii).

Classical Location: Two inches below the armpit fold. The point is located with the arm raised. *(The Great Compendium)*

Local Anatomy: The muscular branches of the brachial artery and vein. The medial brachial cutaneous nerve and musculocutaneous nerve.

Functions: Opens the chest and rectifies qi; nourishes the heart and calms the spirit; quickens the blood, transforms stasis, and relieves pain.

Indications: Cardiac pain; lateral costal distention; cough; pain in the anterior chest, back, shoulder blade, and medial aspect of the arm.

PC-2

天泉

tiān quán

"Celestial Spring"

Supplementary Indications: Palpitations; stone water swelling; blurred vision; aversion to wind and cold.

Stimulation: 0.3-0.7″ inward oblique or perpendicular insertion. Moxa: 5-8 cones; pole 5-10 min.

PC-3
曲澤

qū zé

"Marsh at the Bend"

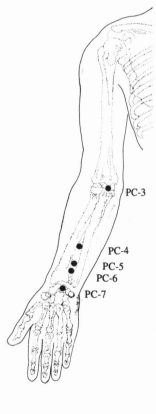

Figure 14.5

Location: At the elbow on the transverse cubital crease, on the ulnar side of the tendon of biceps muscle of the arm (m. biceps brachii).

Classical Location: On the inner side of the elbow, where a pulsating vessel can be felt on the inside of the large sinew on the transverse crease. *(The Great Compendium)*

Local Anatomy: The pathway of the brachial artery and vein. The median nerve. [in terms of heat Qi component of Blood]

Functions: Clears construction and cools the blood; downbears counterflow and stops vomiting; eliminates vexation and settles tetany. [spasmed muscle (opposite of atony)]

Indications: Stomach pain; vomiting; heat diseases; vexation and agitation; cardiac pain; palpitations; pain in the elbow and arm; trembling of the arm.

Supplementary Indications: Susceptibility to fright; body fever; vexation thirst and dry mouth; cold damage, seasonal thermic disease, scourges and pestilences; cholera; cramp; headache and visual dizziness; sha patterns; counterflow cough.

Illustrative Point Combinations & Applications: LU-11 and PC-3 are needled together for blood vacuity thirst.
(Ode of a Hundred Patterns)

Stimulation: 0.5-0.7″ perpendicular insertion; bleed for sha disorders. Moxa: 1-3 cones; pole 5-15 min.

Needle Sensation: Localized needle stimulus sensation, distention, and numbness. Sometimes the distention and numbness will spread down to the fingers.

Point Categories & Associations: Uniting-he (water) point.

Location: 5″ above the transverse crease of the wrist, on the line connecting PC-3 and PC-7, between the tendons of the long palmar muscle and the radial flexor muscle of the wrist (m. palmaris longus and m. flexor carpi radialis).

Classical Location: Below PC-3, five inches behind the wrist. *(The Golden Mirror)*

Local Anatomy: The median artery and vein; deeper, the anterior interosseous artery and vein. The medial antebrachial cutaneous nerve; deeper, the median nerve; deepest, the anterior interosseous nerve.

PC-4
郄門
xī mén
"Cleft Gate"

Functions: Quiets the heart and spirit; clears construction and cools the blood; loosens the chest and rectifies qi.

Indications: Cardiac pain; palpitations; retching of blood; nosebleed; clove sores.

Supplementary Indications: Vexation; pain in the chest; melancholy; insufficiency of spirit qi; fear and fright; fear of people.

Illustrative Point Combinations & Applications: PC-4 combined with LI-11 and TB-8 is especially effective in treating expectoration of blood. *(The Records of Dai Tian-Wen)*

Stimulation: 0.5-0.8″ perpendicular insertion.
Moxa: 5-7 cones; pole 5-20 min.

Needle Sensation: Distention and numbness, often spreading down to the fingers.

Point Categories & Associations: Cleft-xi point of the pericardium channel.

Location: 3″ above the transverse crease of the wrist, between the tendons of the long palmar muscle and the radial flexor muscle of the wrist (m. palmaris longus and m. flexor carpi radialis).

Classical Location: In the depression between the two sinews, three inches from the wrist. *(The Golden Mirror)*

Note: Before needling, apply forceful pressure with a fingernail to make a clear impression on the skin in order to prevent damage to the sinews.

PC-5
間使
jiān shǐ
"Intermediary Courier"

Local Anatomy: The median artery and vein; deeper, the anterior interosseous artery and vein. The medial and lateral antebrachial cutaneous nerves, the palmar cutaneous branch of the median nerve; at the deepest level, the anterior interosseous nerve.

Functions: Nourishes the heart and quiets the spirit; loosens the chest, transforms phlegm, and harmonizes the stomach; soothes the sinews and quickens the connecting vessels.

Indications: Cardiac pain; palpitations; stomach pain; vomiting; heat disease; vexation and agitation; malarial disease; mania and withdrawal; epilepsy; axillary swelling; hypertonicity of the elbow; pain in the arm.

Supplementary Indications: Cold damage chest bind; critical wind strike conditions of qi blockage, rising drool, and clouding; loss of voice; enduring malaria; menstrual irregularity and clotted discharge; red complexion and yellow eyes; ghost evil.

Illustrative Point Combinations & Applications: The five malarias with severe chills and even more severe fevers can be treated with PC-5 and BL-11. *(Song More Precious than Jade)*

Stimulation: 0.5-1.0″ perpendicular insertion.
Moxa: 3-5 cones; pole 5-15 min.

Needle Sensation: Distention and numbness, sometimes spreading down to the hands, or upward to the elbow or armpit.

Point Categories & Associations: River-jing (metal) point; 9th of the 13 ghost points.

PC-6
內關

nèi guān

"Inner Pass"

Location: 2″ above the transverse crease of the wrist, between the tendons of the long palmar muscle and the radial flexor muscle of the wrist (m. palmaris longus and m. flexor carpi radialis).

Classical Location: Between the sinews two inches behind the wrist, at the point opposite to TB-5. *(The Great Compendium)*

Local Anatomy: See PC-5.

Functions: Clears heat and eliminates vexation; loosens the chest and rectifies qi; downbears counterflow and stops vomiting; harmonizes the stomach and relieves pain.

Indications: Cardiac pain; palpitations; stomach pain; retching; mania and withdrawal; epilepsy; pain and hypertonicity of the elbow and arm; heat diseases; malarial disease.

Supplementary Indications: Gastric reflux; splenogastric dishar-mony; vomiting; diseases of the chest and ribs; hot, red face; red eyes; prolapse of the rectum; poor memory and derangement; lump glomus; concretions; wind strike.

Illustrative Point Combinations & Applications: CV-11 and PC-6 sweep away bitter thoracic oppression.
(Ode of a Hundred Patterns)

Stimulation: 0.5-2.0″ perpendicular insertion.
Moxa: 3-5 cones; pole 5-15 min.
Needle Sensation: Distention and numbness, sometimes spreading down to the hand or up to the elbow or armpit.

Point Categories & Associations: Connecting-luo point of the pericardium channel connecting to the triple burner channel; confluence-jiaohui point of the eight extraordinary vessels (related to the yin linking vessel).

Location: In the depression in the middle of the transverse crease of the wrist, between the tendons of the long palmar muscle and the radial flexor muscle of the wrist (m. palmaris longus and m. flexor carpi radialis).

Classical Location: In the depression between the two sinews behind the hand. *(The Systematized Canon)*

Local Anatomy: The palmar arterial and venous network of the wrist. At the deeper level, the median nerve.

PC-7
大陵
dà líng
"Great Mound"

Functions: Clears the heart and quiets the spirit; harmonizes the stomach and loosens the chest; clears construction and cools the blood.

Indications: Cardiac pain; palpitations; stomach pain; vomiting; fright palpitations; mania and withdrawal; pain in the chest and lateral costal region.

Supplementary Indications: Blood ejection; pain at the root of the tongue; heat in the palms; reddening or yellowing of the eyes; fire-like body fever; shortness of breath; vexation; joy, sorrow, weeping, fright and fear; incessant laughter; jie, xian, and other sores.

Illustrative Point Combinations & Applications: For abdominal pain with constipation, needle PC-7, TB-5, and TB-6.
(Ode of the Jade Dragon)

Stimulation: 0.3-0.5″ perpendicular insertion.
Moxa: 1-3 cones; pole 5-15 min.
Needle Sensation: Localized numbness or swelling. Sometimes numbness may spread to the fingers.

Point Categories & Associations: Stream-shu (earth) point; source-yuan point; 4th of the 13 ghost points; one of the nine needles for returning yang.

PC-8
勞宮
láo gōng
"Palace of Toil"

Location: On the palm of the hand between the 2nd and 3rd metacarpal bones, proximal to the metacarpophalangeal joint, on the radial side of the 3rd metacarpal bone.
Classical Location: At the pulsating vessel in the palm of the hand, bend the fourth finger to locate. *(The Great Compendium)*

Note: When the finger is bent, the point will be found where the fingertip meets the palm.
Local Anatomy: The common palmar digital artery. The 2nd common palmar digital nerve of the median nerve.

Functions: Clears heart fire; eliminates damp-heat; extinguishes wind and cools the blood; quiets the spirit and harmonizes the stomach.
Indications: Cardiac pain; mania and withdrawal; epilepsy; vomiting; mouth sores; halitosis; goose foot wind.

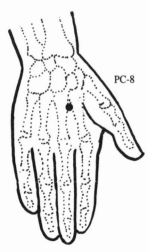
PC-8

Supplementary Indications: Wind strike; irascibility; elation; apprehensiveness; vexation thirst; difficult ingestion; nosebleed; bloody stool or urine; erosion of the gums in infants; lower abdominal accumulations and concretions.
Illustrative Point Combinations & Applications: PC-8 can treat the five epilepsies; the addition of KI-1 makes it even more effective. *(Song of Point Applications for Miscellaneous Disease)*

Stimulation: 0.3-0.5″ perpendicular insertion.
Moxa: 1-3 cones; pole 5-15 min.
Needle Sensation: Distention or pain, and sometimes distention and numbness of the whole hand.

Figure 14.6

Point Categories & Associations: Spring-ying (fire) point.

Location: 0.1 ″ proximal to the corner of the nail on the radial side of the middle finger.

Classical Location: At the tip of the middle finger, in the depression the width of a Chinese leek leaf away from corner of the nail. *(The Great Compendium)*

Local Anatomy: The arterial and venous network formed by the palmar digital proprial artery and vein. The palmar digital proprial nerve of the median nerve.

Functions: Clears the heart and eliminates heat; opens the portals and resuscitates; returns yang and stems counterflow.

Indications: Cardiac pain; vexation and oppression; clouding inversion; stiffness of the tongue impeding speech; heat diseases; summerheat strike; fright inversion; heat in the palm.

Supplementary Indications: Elbow pain; thoracic oppression; pain in the root of the tongue.

Stimulation: 0.1 ″ upward oblique insertion; or bleed.
Moxa: 1 cone; pole 2 min.

Needle Sensation: Localized pain.

Point Categories & Associations: Well-jing (wood) point.

PC-9
中衝
zhōng chōng
"Central Hub"

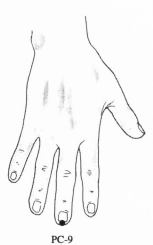

PC-9

Figure 14.7

Hand Jue Yin Pericardium Channel			
Point	**Location**	**Indications**	
		Primary	**Secondary**
*PC-1	Chest	Oppression in the chest axillary swelling	
PC-2	Upper arm	Cardiac pain pain and distention of the chest and lateral costal region	
Chest and upper arm: disorders of the heart and chest			
*PC-3	Elbow	Cardiac pain stomach pain vomiting	Heat Disease
PC-4	Forearm	Cardiac pain palpitations retching of blood	
*PC-5		Cardiac pain vomiting epilepsy mania and withdrawal	
*PC-6		Cardiac pain palpitations oppression in the chest epilepsy	Malarial disease
*PC-7	Wrist	Cardiac pain mania and withdrawal	Sores
*PC-8	Palm	Cardiac pain epilepsy mania and withdrawal	Mouth sores
*PC-9	Finger	Cardiac pain coma	Heat disease
Hand and arm: disorders of the heart, chest, and stomach; mental disorders; heat disease			

15. The Triple Burner Channel System (Hand Shao Yang) 手少陽三焦經

15.1 The Primary Triple Burner Channel

Pathway: The hand shao yang triple burner channel starts at the ulnar side of the tip of the fourth finger and travels up between the fourth and fifth metacarpal bones on the dorsum of the hand to the outside of the wrist. Proceeding up the posterior midline of the forearm between the radius and the ulna, it runs over the olecranon process of the elbow, and then travels up the posterior midline of the upper arm to the shoulder. Here it meets the hand tai yang small intestine channel at SI-12 and then runs over to the back to meet the governing vessel at GV-14. It crosses back over the shoulder to intersect the foot shao yang gallbladder channel at GB-21 before running into the supraclavicular fossa, penetrating to the interior and traveling into the mid-chest region to meet the conception vessel at CV-17, where it links with the pericardium. It then descends internally, homing through each of the three burners successively.

A branch breaks off from the mid-chest region, rises to emerge in the supra-clavicular fossa, then runs up the neck and behind the ear to intersect with the foot shao yang gallbladder channel at GB-6 and GB-4 on the forehead before winding down around the cheek to return to the infraorbital region where it meets the hand tai yang small intestine channel at SI-18.

Another branch separates behind the ear, enters the ear and reemerges in front of it, then intersects with the hand tai yang small intestine channel at SI-19. It then crosses in front of the foot shao yang gallbladder channel at GB-3 and runs along the zygoma to terminate at the outer canthus at TB-23.

The *Spiritual Axis* adds that an internal branch descends from the triple burner to emerge at its lower uniting-he point, BL-39.

Main pathologic signs associated with the external course of the channel: sore throat; pain in the cheeks; reddening of the eyes and pain; deafness; pain behind the ears and on the posterior aspect of the shoulder and upper arm.

Main pathologic signs associated with the internal organ: abdominal distention and fullness; or hardness and fullness in the lower abdomen; urinary frequency and distress; vacuity edema of the skin; water swelling; enuresis.

15.2 The Connecting Vessel of the Triple Burner Channel

Pathway: After separating from the primary channel at TB-5 this vessel winds up the arm, flows into the chest, and unites with the pericardium.

Main pathologic signs:

Repletion: spasms and cramps of the muscles around the elbow.

Vacuity: atony on the muscles around the elbow.

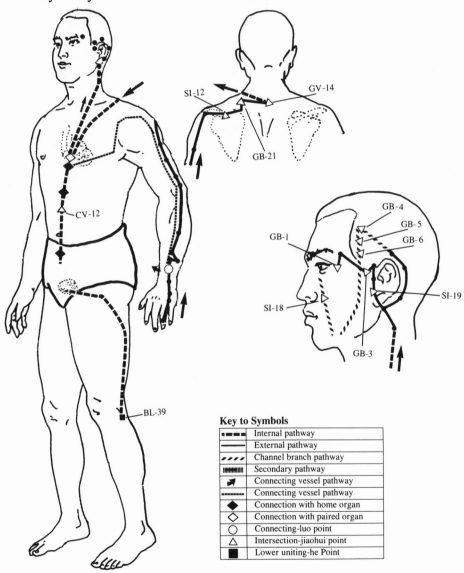

Key to Symbols

▰▰▰▰	Internal pathway
———	External pathway
⫻⫻⫻	Channel branch pathway
▥▥▥▥▥	Secondary pathway
➘	Connecting vessel pathway
▪▪▪▪▪▪	Connecting vessel pathway
◆	Connection with home organ
◇	Connection with paired organ
○	Connecting-luo point
△	Intersection-jiaohui point
■	Lower uniting-he Point

Figure 15.1 - 15.2 Primary channel and connecting vessel of the triple burner.

15.3 The Triple Burner Channel Divergence

Pathway: This divergence leaves the primary channel at the head and branches to the vertex. From there it enters downward through the supraclavicular fossa and down again through each of the three burners. Finally, it disperses over the chest.

15.4 The Triple Burner Channel Sinews

Pathway: These sinews originate at the tip of the ring finger, bind at the wrist and proceed up the forearm to bind at the elbow. They then wind up the lateral aspect of the upper arm onto the shoulder. The sinews then travel up the neck where they unite with the channel sinews of the hand tai yang small intestine.

A branch separates at the angle of the jaw and enters to connect with the root of the tongue. Another branch rises past the jaw, passes in front of the ear and homes to the outer canthus. Finally, it rises across the forehead to bind at the corner of the head.

Main pathologic signs: Tension and cramps along the course of the sinews and curling of the tongue.

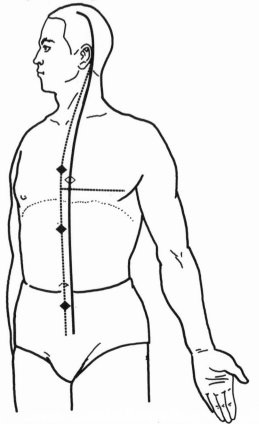

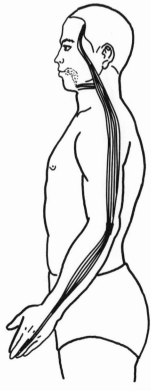

Figure 15.4 The triple burner channel sinews.

Figure 15.3 Channel divergences of the triple burner and pericardium.

279

TB-1
關衝
guān chōng

"Passage Hub"

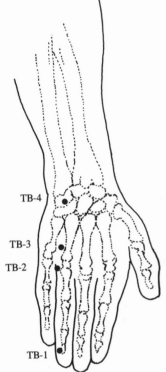

TB-4

TB-3

TB-2

TB-1

Figure 15.5

Location: On the lateral side of the ring finger, about 0.1" posterior to the corner of the nail.

Classical Location: On outer side of the finger next to the little finger, the width of a Chinese leek leaf away from the nail. *(The Great Compendium)*

Local Anatomy: The arterial and venous network formed by the palmar digital proprial artery and vein. The palmar digital proprial nerve derived from the ulnar nerve.

Functions: Dispels wind and dissipates pathogens; resolves triple burner pathogenic heat; courses channel and connecting vessel qi; clears heat and drains fire.

Indications: Headache; reddening of the eyes; sore, swollen throat; stiff tongue; heat diseases; vexation.

Supplementary Indications: Pain in the shoulder and arm; tinnitus; deafness; difficult ingestion; eye screens; pathogenic heat in the triple burner; absence of sweating in heat diseases; throat bi; curled tongue; dry mouth; pain at the root of the tongue.

Illustrative Point Combinations & Applications: Triple-burner heat qi congesting the upper burner with dry tongue and bitter taste in the mouth can be treated by bleeding TB-1, thus letting out toxic blood and causing fluid to wet the mouth.
(Ode of the Jade Dragon)

Stimulation: 0.1" upward oblique insertion.
Moxa: 1-3 cones; pole 5-15 min.
Needle Sensation: Localized pain.

Point Categories & Associations: Well-jing (metal) point.

TB-2
液門
yè mén

"Humor Gate"

Location: Proximal to the margin of the web between the ring and small fingers. The point is located with clenched fist.

Classical Location: In the depression between the little finger and the one next to it. *(The Systematized Canon)*

Local Anatomy: The dorsal digital artery of the ulnar artery. The dorsal branch of the ulnar nerve.

Functions: Courses the channels and quickens the connecting vessels; reduces swelling and relieves pain; clears and drains pathogenic heat in the triple burner.

Indications: Headache; reddening of the eyes; deafness; sore swollen throat; pain of the arm and hand; malarial disease.

Supplementary Indications: Fright palpitations and raving; red complexion and tearing; aching among the upper teeth; shortness of breath; wind-heat and wind-cold; ear pain; tinnitus; pain at the back of the hand; dry eyes.

Illustrative Point Combinations & Applications: TB-2 and LU-10 can treat sore throat. *(Ode of a Hundred Patterns)*

For redness and swelling of the hand and arm, TB-3 and TB-2 are important. *(Ode of the Jade Dragon)*

Stimulation: 0.2-0.5″ perpendicular insertion.
Moxa: 3 cones; pole 5-10 min.

Point Categories & Associations: Spring-ying (water) point.

TB-3
中渚
zhōng zhǔ
"Central Islet"

Location: When the hand is placed with the palm facing downward, the point is on the dorsum of the hand between the 4th and 5th metacarpal bones, in the depression proximal to the metacarpophalangeal joint.

Classical Location: In the depression behind the base joints of the little finger and the one next to it, one inch from TB-2.
(The Great Compendium)

Local Anatomy: The dorsal venous network of the hand and the 4th dorsal metacarpal artery. The dorsal branch of the ulnar nerve.

Functions: Dissipates wind-heat; clears the head and eyes; courses the channels and frees the connecting vessels.

Indications: Headache; reddening of the eyes; deafness; tinnitus; sore, swollen throat; pain in the elbow and arm; inability to bend and stretch the fingers; heat diseases.

Supplementary Indications: Absence of sweating in heat disease; enduring malaria; pain in the spine.

Illustrative Point Combinations & Applications: For shoulder and back pain, needle LI-10 combined with TB-3.
(Wo Yan's Efficacious Point Applications)

Stimulation: 0.3-0.5" perpendicular insertion.
Moxa: 3 cones; pole 5-10 min.

Point Categories & Associations: Stream-shu (wood) point.

TB-4
陽池
yáng chí
"Yang Pool"

Location: At the junction of the ulna and carpal bones, in the depression lateral to the tendon of the digitorum communis extensor muscle (m. extensor digitorum communis).

Classical Location: In a depression on the back of the wrist, from the base joint of the fingers, move straight back to the center of the wrist. *(The Great Compendium)*

Local Anatomy: Inferiorly, the dorsal venous network of the wrist and the posterior carpal artery. The dorsal branch of the ulnar nerve and the terminal branch of the posterior antebrachial cutaneous nerve.

Functions: Dissipates wind and drains heat; frees the channels and connecting vessels.

Indications: Wrist pain; arm and shoulder pain; malarial disease; deafness.

Supplementary Indications: Wasting thirst and dry mouth; vexation and oppression; weak wrist; painful swelling of the eyes; tinnitus; throat bi; absence of sweating in heat disease; swelling of the neck.

Stimulation: 0.3" perpendicular insertion.
Moxa: 3-5 cones; pole 5-15 min.

Point Categories & Associations: Source-yuan point of the triple burner.

TB-5
外關
wài guān
"Outer Pass"

Location: 2" above TB-4, between the radius and ulna.

Classical Location: Between the two bones two inches behind the wrist, opposite PC-6. *(The Great Compendium)*

Local Anatomy: At the deeper level, the posterior and anterior interosseous arteries and veins. The posterior antebrachial cutaneous nerve; deeper, the posterior interosseous nerve of the radial nerve and the anterior interosseous nerve of the median nerve.

Functions: Dissipates wind and resolves the exterior; clears heat and resolves toxin; frees the channels and quickens the connecting vessels.

Indications: Heat diseases; headache; pain in the cheek; lateral costal pain; deafness; tinnitus; inhibited bending and stretching of the arm; pain in the fingers; tremor of the hand; abdominal pain and constipation.

Illustrative Point Combinations & Applications: For abdominal pain with constipation, needle PC-7, TB-5 and TB-6.
(Ode of the Jade Dragon)

TB-5 and KI-6 can bring down the afterbirth.
(Ode to Elucidate Mysteries)

Stimulation: 0.3-1.0″ perpendicular insertion.
Moxa: 2-3 cones; pole 5-15 min.

Needle Sensation: Distention and numbness, sometimes spreading down to the fingers or up to the elbow and shoulder.

Point Categories & Associations: Connecting-luo point of the triple burner channel connecting to the pericardium channel. TB-5 is a confluence-jiaohui point of the eight extraordinary channels (related to the yang linking channel).

Location: 3″ above TB-4, between the ulna and radius.

Classical Location: On the outer face of the arm, three inches back from the wrist, in the depression between the two bones.
(The Great Compendium)

Local Anatomy: See TB-5.

TB-6
支溝
zhī gōu
"Branch Ditch"

Functions: Clears the triple burner; frees bowel qi; downbears counterflow and fire.

Indications: Sudden loss of voice; tinnitus; deafness; pain and heaviness of the shoulder and back; vomiting; constipation.

Supplementary Indications: Painful or red eyes; postpartum blood dizziness; cough; hot face; sudden cardiac pain; counterflow qi; cholera with vomiting; sore pharynx; inability to turn the head; acute pain in the lateral costal or axillary region; absence of sweating in heat disease; saber lumps; jie and xian; ghost attacks.

Illustrative Point Combinations & Applications: For immediate relief from pain in the lower ribs, needle GB-34 combined with TB-6. *(Song More Precious than Jade)*

For vacuity constipation, supplement TB-6 and drain ST-36.
(Song of Point Applications for Miscellaneous Disease)

Stimulation: 0.7-1.0″ perpendicular insertion.
Moxa: 3-5 cones; pole 5-15 min.
Needle Sensation: Distention and numbness that can spread down
to the fingers or up to the elbow and shoulder.

Point Categories & Associations: River-jing (fire) point.

TB-7
會宗
huì zōng

*"Convergence and
Gathering"*

Location: 3″ proximal to the wrist, about one finger's breadth
lateral to TB-6, on the radial side of the ulna.
Classical Location: Three inches behind the wrist, one inch out
from the space between the bones. *(The Great Compendium)*
Local Anatomy: The posterior interosseous artery and vein. The
posterior and medial antebrachial cutaneous nerves; deeper, the
posterior and anterior interosseous nerves.

Functions: Clears and drains pathogenic heat in the triple burner;
soothes the liver and rectifies qi.
Indications: Deafness; pain in the upper limbs; epilepsy.
Supplementary Indications: Muscular pain; hearing loss.

Stimulation: 0.5-1.0″ perpendicular insertion.
Moxa: 3-7 cones; pole 5-15 min.

Point Categories & Associations: Cleft-xi point of the triple
burner channel.

TB-8
三陽絡
sān yáng luò

*"Three Yang
Connection"*

Location: 4″ above TB-4, between the radius and ulna.
Classical Location: Obliquely inward one inch up from TB-7.
(The Golden Mirror)
Local Anatomy: See TB-7.

Functions: Frees the channels and quickens the connecting
vessels; opens the portals and relieves pain.
Indications: Sudden loss of voice; deafness; pain in the arm.
Supplementary Indications: Tooth decay; inability to move the
hand and arm; prostrate exhaustion; lack of desire to move the
four limbs.

Stimulation: Needle contraindication (see contraindication).
Moxa: 5-7 cones; pole 5-20 min.
Needle Sensation: Distention and numbness, sometimes stretching
down to the hand, or up to the elbow, shoulder and chest.

Contraindications: Though traditionally contraindicated for needling, TB-8 in recent years has been combined with (joined by a
single needle to) PC-4 in acuanesthesia for removal of pulmonary
lobes.

Location: 5″ below the olecranon, between the radius and ulna.
Classical Location: Five inches in front of the elbow, in the
depression on the outer side. *(The Great Compendium)*
Local Anatomy: See TB-7.

TB-9
四瀆
sì dú

"Four Rivers"

Functions: Courses the channels and quickens the connecting
vessels; frees and regulates the waterways; disinhibits the throat
and opens the portals.
Indications: Sudden loss of voice; deafness; toothache; pain in the
forearm.
Supplementary Indications: Blocked sensation in the throat.

Stimulation: 0.5-1.0″ perpendicular insertion.
Moxa: 3 cones; pole 5-10 min.
Needle Sensation: Distention and numbness spreading toward the
hand or elbow.

Location: When the elbow is flexed, the point is in the depression
about 1″ superior to the olecranon.
Classical Location: Up one inch from the back of the tip of the
large bone on the outer side of the elbow, in the depression
between two sinews and the bone. The point is located with the
arm bent over the chest. *(The Golden Mirror)*
Local Anatomy: The arterial and venous network of the elbow.
The posterior brachial cutaneous nerve and muscular branch of the
radial nerve.

TB-10
天井
tiān jǐng

"Celestial Well"

285

Functions: Transforms phlegm damp in the channels and connecting vessels; courses fire qi in the triple burner.

Indications: Unilateral headache; pain in the lateral costal region, neck, shoulder, and arm; scrofulous lumps; epilepsy.

Supplementary Indications: Malarial disease; numbness of the flesh at the shoulder; thoracic bi; cardiac pain; qi ascent cough; fright palpitations; clonic spasm; eye pain; deafness; throat bi; spitting of pus; sorrow.

Illustrative Point Combinations & Applications: Scrofulus lumps can be treated with SI-8 and TB-10.

Stimulation: 0.3-0.7" perpendicular insertion.
Moxa: 3 cones; pole 5-10 min.
Needle Sensation: Distention and numbness, spreading down to the hand or over the shoulder.

Point Categories & Associations: Uniting-he (earth) point.

TB-11
清冷淵
qīng lěng yuān
"Clear Cold
Abyss"

Location: 1" above TB-10.

Classical Location: Two inches above the elbow. The point is found with the elbow stretched and the arm raised.
(The Great Compendium)

Local Anatomy: The terminal branches of the median collateral artery and vein. The posterior brachial cutaneous nerve and the muscular branch of the radial nerve.

Functions: Frees channel and connecting vessel qi; clears heat and drains fire.

Indications: Shoulder and arm pain.

Supplementary Indications: Back pain; elbow pain; qi ascent cough; prostrate exhaustion; scrofulous lumps; epilepsy; eye pain; headache; deafness; throat bi; no pleasure in eating.

Stimulation: 0.3-0.5" perpendicular insertion.
Moxa: 3-5 cones; pole 5-10 min.

Location: On the line joining the olecranon and TB-14, midway between TB-11 and TB-13. It is just on the lower end of the bulge of the lateral head of the triceps muscle of the arm (m. triceps brachii) when the forearm is in pronation.

Classical Location: On the outer aspect of the arm, below the shoulder and above the elbow, below the parting of the flesh. *(The Golden Mirror)*

Local Anatomy: The median collateral artery and vein. The posterior brachial cutaneous nerve and the muscular branch of the radial nerve.

Functions: Courses the channels, quickens the connecting vessels, and moves qi; clears and drains depressed heat in the triple burner.

Indications: Headache; pain and stiffness in the neck; pain in the arm.

Supplementary Indications: Toothache; madness; bi pain.

Stimulation: 0.5-0.7″ perpendicular insertion.
Moxa: 3 cones; pole 5-10 min.

TB-12

消濼

xiāo luò

"Dispersing Riverbed"

Location: On the line joining TB-14 and the olecranon, 3″ below TB-14, on the posterior border of the deltoid muscle (m. deltoideus).

Classical Location: On the outer face of the shoulder, in the depression three inches from the tip of the shoulder. *(The Golden Mirror)*

Local Anatomy: The medial collateral artery and vein. The posterior brachial cutaneous nerve, the muscular branch of the radial nerve; deeper, the radial nerve.

Functions: Clears and discharges pathogenic heat; frees the channels and connecting vessels; disinhibits the joints.

Indications: Shoulder and arm pain; goiter.

Supplementary Indications: Fever and chills; swelling of the shoulder causing pain in the shoulder blade.

TB-13

臑會

nào huì

"Upper Arm Convergence"

Stimulation: 0.5-0.8 ″ perpendicular insertion.
Moxa: 3-7 cones; pole 5-15 min.

Point Categories & Associations: Intersection-jiaohui point of the hand shao yang triple burner channel and the yang linking vessel.

TB-14
肩髎
jiān liáo

"Shoulder Bone-Hole"

Location: Posterior and inferior to the acromion, in the depression about 1 ″ posterior to LI-15.
Classical Location: Above TB-13, above the arm at the end of the shoulder. The point is found when the arm is lifted to a slanting position. *(The Golden Mirror)*
Local Anatomy: The muscular branch of the posterior circumflex humeral artery. The muscular branch of the axillary nerve.

Functions: Dispels wind and overcomes damp; moves qi, quickens the blood, and relieves pain.
Indications: Heaviness of the shoulder; arm pain.

Stimulation: 0.7-1.0 ″ perpendicular insertion.
Moxa: 3-5 cones; pole 5-15 min.

Point Categories & Associations: Intersection-jiaohui point of the hand shao yang triple burner channel and the yang linking vessel.

TB-15
天髎
tiān liáo

"Celestial Bone-Hole"

Location: Midway between GB-21 and SI-13, on the superior angle of the scapula.
Classical Location: One inch above TB-14 in the center of the supraclavicular fossa one inch behind GB-21.
(The Golden Mirror)
Local Anatomy: The descending branch of the transverse cervical artery; deeper, the muscular branch of the suprascapular artery. The accessory nerve and the branch of the suprascapular nerve.

Functions: Dispels wind and eliminates damp; frees the channels and quickens the connecting vessels; relieves pain.
Indications: Shoulder and arm pain; pain and stiffness in the neck.
Supplementary Indications: Body fever with absence of sweating; vexation in the chest; tension in the nape and neck; pain in the supraclavicular fossa; fever and chills.

Stimulation: 0.3-0.5″ perpendicular insertion.
Moxa: 3 cones; (see contraindications) pole 5-15 min.

Contraindications: Supplementing stimulus and moxibustion are
contraindicated at this point in many older texts. Moxibustion at
this point is said to cause facial swelling. Modern sources
disagree with this, but suggest avoiding deep needle insertion.

Point Categories & Associations: Intersection-jiaohui point of the
hand shao yang triple burner channel and the yang linking vessel.

TB-16
天牖
tiān yŏu
"Celestial Oriole"

Location: Posterior and inferior to the mastoid process, on the
posterior border of the sternocleidomastoid muscle (m. sternocleidomastoideus), level with SI-17 and BL-10.
Classical Location: At the outer border of the major sinew of the
neck, behind SI-17 and in front of BL-10, below the mastoid process. *(The Great Compendium)*
Local Anatomy: The posterior auricular artery. The lesser occipital nerve.

Functions: Clears heat and drains fire; dispels wind and eliminates damp; reduces swelling and stops pain; frees the channels
and quickens the connecting vessels.
Indications: Dizziness; facial swelling; sudden loss of hearing;
clouded vision; stiff neck.
Supplementary Indications: Scrofulous lumps; eye pain and tearing; clear, runny snivel with nosebleed; throat bi; loss of smell;
derangement of dream sequence; mammary yong; swelling of
supraclavicular fossa; submandibular swelling.

Stimulation: 0.3-0.5″ perpendicular insertion.
Moxa: 3-5 cones; pole 5-10 min.

TB-17
翳風
yì fēng
"Wind Screen"

Location: Posterior to the lobule of the ear, in the depression
between the mandible and mastoid process.
Classical Location: In the depression behind the ear lobe, which
when pressed causes pain in the ear. *(The Great Compendium)*
Local Anatomy: The posterior auricular artery and vein, the external jugular vein. The great auricular nerve; deeper, the site where
the facial nerve issues from the stylomastoid foramen.

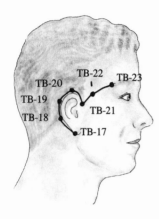

Figure 15.6

Functions: Courses wind and discharges heat; frees the portals and sharpens the hearing; quickens the connecting vessels and relieves pain.

Indications: Tinnitus; deafness; wryness of the eyes and mouth; clenched jaws; swelling of the cheek.

Supplementary Indications: Jaw pain; mania; wryness of the eyes and mouth; clenched jaws preventing speech; red and white eye screens; poor eye sight; all wind diseases.

Illustrative Point Combinations & Applications: Deafness and qi block [in the ears] can both be treated through GB-2 and TB-17. *(Ode of a Hundred Patterns)*

Stimulation: 0.5-1.0″ perpendicular insertion.
Moxa: 3-5 cones; pole 5-10 min.

Needle Sensation: Localized needle stimulus sensation and distention, sometimes spreading into the region of the throat or radiating into the ear.

Point Categories & Associations: Intersection-jiaohui point of the foot shao yang gallbladder and hand shao yang triple burner channels.

TB-18
瘈脈
chì mài
"Spasm Vessel"

Location: In the center of the mastoid process, at the junction of the middle and lower third of the curve formed by TB-17 and TB-20 posterior to the helix.

Classical Location: Behind the base of the ear, at the cyan connecting vessels that resemble a chicken's foot.
(The Great Compendium)

Local Anatomy: The posterior auricular artery and vein. The posterior auricular branch of the great auricular nerve.

Functions: Clears heat and resolves tetany; quickens the connecting vessels and relieves pain; opens the portals.

Indications: Headache; tinnitus; deafness.

Supplementary Indications: Infantile fright epilepsy and clonic spasm; vomiting; diarrhea; head wind; poor eyesight; fright and fear; seminal emission.

Stimulation: 0.1-0.3″ perpendicular insertion or bleed a few drops of blood.
Moxa: 3 cones; pole 5-10 min.

Location: Posterior to the ear, at the junction of the upper and middle third of the curve formed by TB-17 and TB-20.

Classical Location: Between the cyan connecting vessels behind the ear. *(The Great Compendium)*

Local Anatomy: The posterior auricular artery and vein. The anastomotic branch of the great auricular nerve and the lesser occipital nerve.

Functions: Courses wind and quickens the connecting vessels; frees the channels and relieves pain; quiets the spirit and settles fright.

Indications: Headache; tinnitus; ear pain.

Supplementary Indications: Head wind; fright and fear; insomnia; tautness across the chest and lateral costal region; body fever and headache; swelling of the ear with discharge of pus.

Stimulation: 0.1-0.3″ perpendicular insertion.
Moxa: 3 cones; pole 5-10 min.

TB-19
顱息
lú xí
"Skull Rest"

Location: Directly above the ear apex, within the hairline of the temple.

Classical Location: Above the ear, at the place where a hollow appears when the mouth is opened. *(The Golden Mirror)*

Local Anatomy: The branches of the superficial temporal artery and vein. The branches of the auriculotemporal nerve.

Functions: Clears the head and brightens the eyes; courses wind and quickens the connecting vessels.

Indications: Reddening and swelling in the region of the eyes; reddening and swelling of the eyes; toothache.

Supplementary Indications: Swelling of the gums that prevents chewing; eye screens; stiffness in the nape and neck; red, swollen auricle.

Stimulation: 0.1″ perpendicular insertion or 0.2-0.8″ transverse insertion. Moxa: 3 cones; pole 5-10 min.

TB-20
角孫
jiǎo sūn
"Angle Vertex"

291

Point Categories & Associations: Intersection-jiaohui point of the hand shao yang triple burner, hand tai yang small intestine, and foot shao yang gallbladder channels.

TB-21
耳門

ěr mén

"Ear Gate"

Location: In the depression anterior to the supratragic notch and slightly superior to the condyloid process of the mandible. The point is located with the patient's mouth open.

Classical Location: In the depression by the protuberance of the flesh in front of the ear at the notch at the top of the tragus. *(The Great Compendium)*

Local Anatomy: The superficial temporal artery and vein. The branches of the auriculotemporal and facial nerves.

Functions: Courses the channels and quickens the connecting vessels; opens the portals and boosts the hearing.

Indications: Deafness; tinnitus; purulent discharge from the ear; toothache.

Supplementary Indications: Upper tooth decay; ringing in the ears like the sound of cicadas; submandibular swelling.

Illustrative Point Combinations & Applications: TB-21 and TB-23 relieve toothache immediately. *(Ode of a Hundred Patterns)*

Stimulation: 0.3-0.5″ perpendicular insertion.
Moxa: 3 cones; pole 5-10 min.

TB-22
耳和髎

hé liáo

"Harmony Bone-Hole"

Location: Anterior and superior to TB-21, level with the root of the auricle, on the posterior border of the hairline of the temple, where the superficial temporal artery passes.

Classical Location: In front of TB-21 below the sidelock, at the site of the horizontal pulse.

Local Anatomy: The superficial temporal artery and vein. The branch of the auriculotemporal nerve, on the course of the temporal branch of the facial nerve.

Functions: Dispels wind and frees the connecting vessels; opens the portals.

Indications: Tinnitus; headache and heavy-headedness; hypertonicity of the jaws.

Supplementary Indications: Submandibular swelling; runny nose; swelling of the tip of the nose; clonic spasm; wryness of the mouth.

Stimulation: 0.1-0.3″ perpendicular insertion or 0.3-0.5″ oblique insertion. Moxa: 1-2 cones; pole 3-5 min.

Point Categories & Associations: Intersection-jiaohui point of the hand shao yang triple burner, hand tai yang small intestine, and foot shao yang gallbladder channels.

Location: In the depression at the lateral end of the eyebrow.

Classical Location: In the depression behind the eyebrow. *(The Great Compendium)*

Local Anatomy: The frontal branches of the superficial temporal artery and vein. The zygomatic branch of the facial nerve and the branch of the auriculotemporal nerve.

TB-23

絲竹空

sī zhú kōng

"Silk Bamboo Hole"

Functions: Dispels wind and resolves heat; brightens the eyes and relieves pain; frees the channels and quickens the connecting vessels.

Indications: Headache; visual dizziness; pain and swelling of the eyes; twitching of the eyelids.

Supplementary Indications: Unilateral and bilateral headache; ingrown eyelash; toothache; epilepsy; periodic attacks of mania with foaming at the mouth; vexation thirst; unclear vision.

Illustrative Point Combinations & Applications: For unilateral and ambilateral headaches that are difficult to cure, try TB-23, inserting the needle transversely under the skin to join the point to GB-8. *(Song of the Jade Dragon)*

Stimulation: 0.3″ backward transverse insertion.

Contraindications: Moxibustion contraindicated.

Hand Shao Yang Triple Burner Channel			
Point	**Location**	**Indications**	
		Primary	**Secondary**
*TB-1	Finger	Headache red eyes deafness pain and swelling of the throat	Heat disease
TB-2		Headache red eyes deafness pain and swelling of the throat	Malarial disease
*TB-3	Back of hand	Headache red eyes tinnitus deafness pain and swelling of the throat	Heat disease
*TB-4	Wrist	Wrist pain red eyes deafness pain and swelling of the throat	Malarial disease wasting thirst
*TB-5	Forearm	Headache red, swollen, painful eyes tinnitus deafness rib pain bi and pain of the upper limbs	Heat disease
*TB-6		Sudden loss of voice rib pain constipation	Heat disease
TB-7		Deafness	Epilepsy
TB-8		Deafness sudden loss of voice bi and pain of the upper limbs	
TB-9		Deafness toothache sudden loss of voice bi and pain of the upper limbs	

Point	Location	Indications	
Hand Shao Yang Triple Burner Channel			
		Primary	**Secondary**
TB-10	Elbow	Hemilateral headache scrofula	Epilepsy
Hand to elbow: Disorders of the side of the head, ears, eyes, ribs, and throat; heat disease			
TB-11	Upper arm	Bi and pain of the upper limbs	
TB-12		Stiffness and rigidity of the neck	
TB-13		Bi and pain of the upper limbs	
*TB-14	Shoulder	Hypertonicity, pain, and paralysis of the shoulder and upper arm	
TB-15		Pain in the shoulder and upper arm rigidity of the neck	
Upper arm and shoulder: Localized disorders			
TB-16	Neck	Deafness scrofula stiff neck	
*TB-17	Ear	Tinnitus deafness wry mouth and eyes swelling of the cheeks	
TB-18		Headache tinnitus deafness;	
TB-19		Headache tinnitus;	
TB-20		Toothache eye screen	
TB-21	Anterior to ear	Deafness tinnitus toothache	
TB-22		Headache tinnitus clenched jaws	
*TB-23	Eyebrow	Headache eye pain	
Neck and lateral aspect of the head: Disorders of the side of the head, ears, and eyes			

16. The Gallbladder Channel System
(Foot Shao Yang) 足少陽膽經

16.1 The Primary Gallbladder Channel

Pathway: The foot shao yang gallbladder channel starts from the outer canthus of the eye, traverses the temple to TB-22, then rises to the corner of the forehead where it intersects with the foot yang ming stomach channel at ST-8. Descending behind the ear, it passes down the neck in front of the hand shao yang triple burner channel and meets the hand tai yang small intestine channel at SI-17. After reaching the shoulder it turns back and runs behind the triple burner channel to intersect the governing vessel at GV-14. It then moves parallel with the shoulderline outwards to intersect with the hand tai yang small intestine channel at SI-12 before crossing over to ST-12 in the supraclavicular fossa.

A branch separates from the main channel behind the ear and intersects the hand shao yang triple burner channel at TB-17 before entering the ear. It emerges in front of the ear, meeting SI-19 on the hand tai yang small intestine channel and ST-7 on the foot yang ming stomach channel before terminating at the outer canthus of the eye.

Another branch separates from the outer canthus and runs downwards to ST-5 on the mandible. Turning upwards, it crosses the hand shao yang triple burner channel and ascends to the infraorbital region before traveling down the cheek into the neck, where it joins the main channel again at ST-12 in the supraclavicular fossa. From there it submerges in the chest, intersects PC-1 of the hand jue yin pericardium channel, and passes through the diaphragm before connecting with the liver and homing to the gallbladder. It then follows the inside of the false ribs to emerge in the qi thoroughfare in the inguinal region, where it skirts round the genitals and submerges into the hip at GB-30.

Yet another branch separates from the main channel at the supraclavicular fossa at ST-12, descends into the axilla and runs down the lateral jue yin liver channel at LV-13 before turning back to the sacral region to cross the foot tai yang bladder channel at BL-31 and BL-34. From there it passes laterally over to GB-30 on the hip joint, descending down the lateral aspect of the thigh and knee, and passes along the anterior aspect of the fibula to its lower extremity. It crosses in front of the lateral malleolus and runs over the dorsum of the foot, traveling between the fourth and fifth metatarsal bones before terminating at the lateral side of the tip of the fourth toe at GB-44.

Another branch separates on the dorsum of the foot at GB-41 and runs between the first and second metatarsal bones to the end of the great toe and crosses under the toenail to join with the foot jue yin liver channel at LV-1.

Main pathologic signs associated with the external course of the channel: alternating fever and chills; headache; malaria; ashen complexion; ocular pain; pain under the chin; subaxillary swelling; scrofulous swellings; deafness; pain in the lateral knee and fibula.

Main pathologic signs associated with the internal organ: pain in the lateral costal area; vomiting; bitter taste in the mouth; pain in the chest.

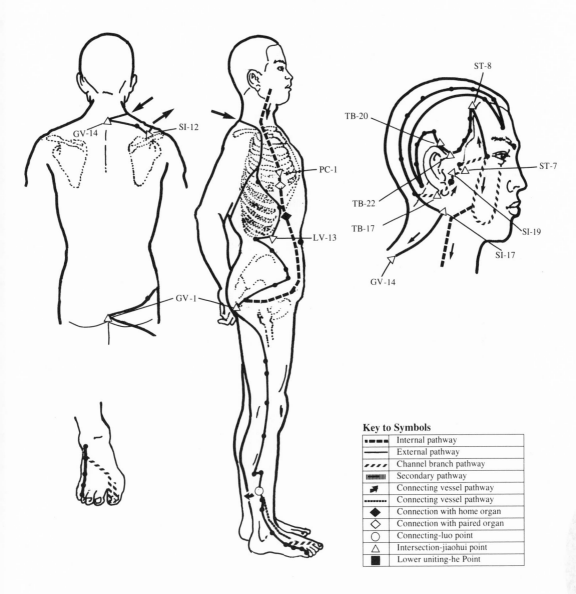

Key to Symbols

▬ ▬ ▬	Internal pathway
───	External pathway
⁄⁄⁄⁄	Channel branch pathway
▥▥▥▥	Secondary pathway
➹	Connecting vessel pathway
▬▬▬▬	Connecting vessel pathway
◆	Connection with home organ
◇	Connection with paired organ
○	Connecting-luo point
△	Intersection-jiaohui point
■	Lower uniting-he Point

Figure 16.1 - 16.2 Primary channel and connecting vessel of the gallbladder.

16.2 The Connecting Vessel of the Gallbladder Channel

Pathway: This vessel separates from the primary channel at GB-37 5″ above the lateral malleolus and branches to the foot jue yin liver channel. It also connects downward to the dorsal aspect of the foot.

Main pathologic signs:

Repletion: inversion.

Vacuity: weakness and atony of the lower limbs (with inability to walk and difficulty standing).

16.3 The Gallbladder Channel Divergence

Pathway: This divergence leaves the primary channel at the thigh and enters the pelvic region at the border of the pubic hair, where it unites with the foot jue yin liver channel divergence. Here the divergence enters into the area of the free ribs, homes to the gallbladder and disperses over the liver. Rising upward the divergence links with the heart, follows along the pharynx, issues at the submandibular region and disperses over the face. The divergence connects to the region behind the eye and unites with the foot shao yang gallbladder channel at the outer canthus.

A branch issues at the axilla, links to the supraclavicular fossa and issues in front of the foot tai yang channel, which it then follows up behind the ear. It then rises to the corner of the forehead, intersects at the vertex, goes downward to the submandibular region and rises slightly to bind at the side of the nose. A sub-branch binds to the outer canthus.

16.4 The Gallbladder Channel Sinews

Pathway: These sinews originate at the fourth toe, rise to bind at the lateral malleolus and follow the lateral aspect of the lower leg up to where they bind at the lateral aspect of the knee. A branch begins at the proximal lateral aspect of the fibia and ascends along the thigh binding above the "crouching rabbit" on the front of the body and at the sacro-coccygeal region in the rear.

The main sinew group rises up the lateral aspect of the thigh and past the ribs to the axilla connecting to the breast region and binding at the supraclavicular fossa.

A branch issues at the axilla, links to the supraclavicular fossa and issues in front of the foot tai yang channel, which it then follows up behind the ear. It then rises to the corner of the forehead, intersects at the vertex, goes downward to the submandibular region and rises slightly to bind at the side of the nose. A sub-branch binds to the outer canthus.

Main pathologic signs:

Inability to support the fourth toe; strain and sprains of the outer aspect of the knee; inability to extend and bend the knee; spasm of the popliteal fossa; strains in the pelvic region in the front or the sacro-coccygeal region in the rear, with pain extending up to the lateral costal region or the area just below the lateral costal region. Pain in the supraclavicular fossa, the side of the chest or neck. If one looks to the right, the right eye can not remain open, and vice versa.

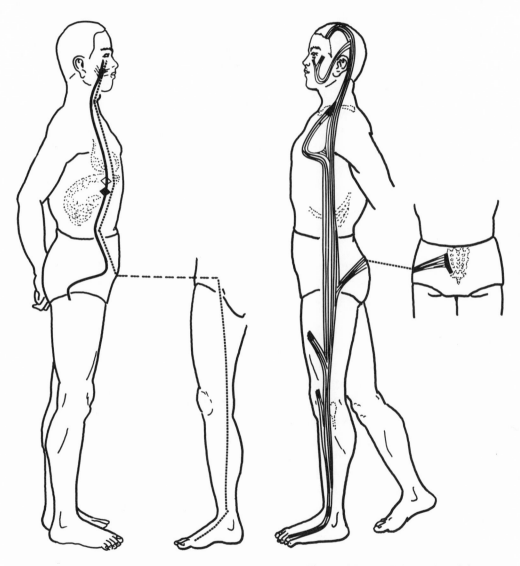

Figure 16.3 Channel divergences of the gallbladder and liver.   **Figure 16.4** The gallbladder channel sinews.

GB-1

瞳子髎

tóng zǐ liáo

"Pupil Bone-Hole"

Location: Lateral to the outer canthus, in the depression on the lateral side of the orbit.

Classical Location: Five fen out from the outer canthus. *(The Great Compendium)*

Local Anatomy: The zygomaticoorbital artery and vein. The zygomaticofacial and zygomaticotemporal nerves, the temporal branch of the facial nerve.

Functions: Dispels wind and discharges heat; courses the channels and frees qi; relieves pain and brightens the eyes.

Indications: Headache; eye pain; loss of visual acuity; reddening of the eyes and tearing.

Supplementary Indications: Blindness; nearsightedness; eye screens; painful reddening of the outer canthus; itching of the inner canthus.

Illustrative Point Combinations & Applications: GB-1 with SI-1 can treat mammary swelling in women. *(Illustrated Supplement)*

Stimulation: 0.2-0.3″ backward transverse insertion.
Moxa: 8 cones; 5-15 pole min.

Point Categories & Associations: Intersection-jiaohui point of the hand tai yang small intestine, hand shao yang triple burner and foot shao yang gallbladder channels.

GB-2

聽會

tīng huì

"Auditory Convergence"

Location: Anterior to the intertragic notch, directly below SI-19, at the posterior border of the condyloid process of the mandible. The point is located with the mouth open.

Classical Location: In the depression in front of the ear, where a pulsating vessel can be felt, one inch below GB-3. The point is found when the mouth is opened. *(The Great Compendium)*

Local Anatomy: The superficial temporal artery. The great auricular nerve and facial nerve.

Functions: Courses the liver and gallbladder; dispels wind, moves qi and opens the ears.

Indications: Tinnitus; deafness; toothache.

Supplementary Indications: Purulent discharge from the ear; tearing; dislocation of the jaw; swelling of the cheeks; wryness of eyes and mouth and paralysis of the limbs due to wind strike.

Illustrative Point Combinations & Applications: With BL-63 and GB-2, deafness due to cold damage is gone like the wind.
(Ode of Xi Hong)

For deafness and qi block [in the ears], needle GB-2 and TB-17.
(Ode of a Hundred Patterns)

Stimulation: 0.5-0.7″ perpendicular insertion.
Moxa: 3 cones; pole 5-15 min.

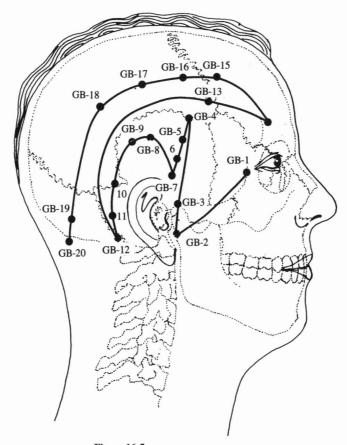

Figure 16.5

Location: On the side of the face anterior to the ear, on the upper border of the zygomatic arch, in the depression directly above ST-7.

Classical Location: Above the bone in front of the ear, where a hollow appears when the mouth is opened.
(The Great Compendium)

GB-3
上關
shàng guān

"Upper Gate"

Local Anatomy: The zygomaticoorbital artery and vein. The zygomatic branch of the facial nerve and the zygomaticofacial nerve.

Functions: Frees the channels and quickens the connecting vessels; opens the portals and boosts the hearing.
Indications: Headache; deafness; tinnitus; toothache; wryness of the eyes and mouth.
Supplementary Indications: Visual dizziness; aversion to wind and cold; painful upper tooth decay; unilateral headache; fever and chills; tetany with bone pain.

Stimulation: 0.3″ perpendicular insertion.
Moxa: 3 cones; pole 3-5 min.
Contraindications: Originally needling was contraindicated at this point. The *Essential Questions* explains that puncturing of the vessels can cause internal bleeding leading to deafness. Nowadays, the point is needled, but care is taken not to exceed a depth of 0.3″.

Point Categories & Associations: Intersection-jiaohui point of the foot shao yang gallbladder, hand shao yang triple burner, and foot yang ming stomach channels.

GB-4
頷厭
hàn yàn
"Forehead Fullness"

Location: Within the hairline of the temporal region, one quarter of the distance between ST-8 and GB-7.

Classical Location: Diagonally up from GB-3 on the upper border of the tai yang area. *(The Golden Mirror)*

Local Anatomy: The parietal branches of the superficial temporal artery and vein. Just on the temporal branch of the auriculotemporal nerve.

Functions: Courses wind and quickens the connecting vessels; clears heat, settles fright and relieves pain.
Indications: Unilateral headache; visual dizziness; pain in the outer canthus; tinnitus.
Supplementary Indications: Sneezing; toothache; pain in the wrist; articular wind with sweating.
Illustrative Point Combinations & Applications: Needling GB-4 and GB-5 stops unilateral headache. *(Ode of a Hundred Patterns)*

Stimulation: 0.3-0.5″ backward transverse insertion.
Moxa: 3 cones; pole 5-10 min.

Point Categories & Associations: Intersection-jiaohui point of the
foot shao yang gallbladder, hand shao yang triple burner, and foot
yang ming stomach channels.

Location: Within the hairline of the temporal region, midway
along a line connecting ST-8 and GB-7.
Classical Location: In the middle of the temporal hairline.
(The Systematized Canon)
Local Anatomy: See GB-4.

GB-5
懸顱
xuán lú
"Suspended Skull"

Functions: Courses wind and quickens the connecting vessels;
disperses swelling and relieves pain.
Indications: Unilateral headache; pain in the outer canthus.
Supplementary Indications: Vexation and fullness with absence of
sweating in heat diseases; toothache; facial swelling.
Illustrative Point Combinations & Applications: Needling GB-4
and GB-5 relieves unilateral headache.
(Ode of a Hundred Patterns)

Stimulation: 0.3-0.5″ backward transverse insertion.
Moxa: 3 cones; pole 3 min.

Point Categories & Associations: Intersection-jiaohui point of the
foot shao yang gallbladder, hand shao yang triple burner, foot
yang ming stomach, and hand yang ming large intestine channels.

Location: Within the hairline of the temporal region, midway
between GB-5 and GB-7.
Classical Location: Behind GB-5 above the upper corner of the ear
on the lower border of the tai yang region. *(The Golden Mirror)*
Local Anatomy: See GB-4.

GB-6
懸厘
xuán lí
"Suspended Tuft"

Functions: Courses wind and quickens the connecting vessels;
frees the portals and moves qi.
Indications: Headache; pain in the outer canthus.
Supplementary Indications: Tinnitus; sneezing; painful reddening
of the outer canthus; absence of sweating in heat diseases; facial
swelling and reddening; unilateral headache.

Stimulation: 0.2-0.3 ″ backward transverse insertion.
Moxa: 3 cones; pole 5-10 min.

Point Categories & Associations: Intersection-jiaohui point of the foot shao yang gallbladder, hand shao yang triple burner, and foot yang ming stomach channels.

GB-7
曲鬢

qū bìn

"Temporal Hairline Curve"

Location: Within the hairline of the temporal region, anterior and superior to the auricle, level with and roughly a finger's breadth anterior to TB-20.

Classical Location: In a depression behind GB-6 in front of the ear behind the curved hairline. A space can be felt when the jaw is moved. *(The Golden Mirror)*

Local Anatomy: See GB-4.

Functions: Clears heat and disperses swelling; extinguishes wind and relieves pain.

Indications: Pain in the temporal region; swelling of the cheek and submandibular region; clenched jaws.

Supplementary Indications: Eye diseases; retching and vomiting; stiff neck; toothache; infantile convulsions.

Stimulation: 0.2-0.3 ″ backward transverse insertion.
Moxa: 3-5 cones; pole 3-5 min.

Point Categories & Associations: Intersection-jiaohui point of the foot shao yang gallbladder and foot tai yang bladder channels.

GB-8
率谷

shuài gǔ

"Valley Lead"

Location: Superior to the apex of the auricle, 1.5 ″ within the hairline.

Classical Location: In the depression one and one half inches within the hairline above the ear. Bite and the point can be felt. *(The Great Compendium)*

Local Anatomy: The parietal branches of the superficial temporal artery and vein. The anastomotic branch of the auriculotemporal nerve and great occipital nerve.

Functions: Courses wind and quickens the connecting vessels; relieves pain.

Indications: Unilateral headache.

Supplementary Indications: Stomach cold; vexation and fullness after eating; persistent retching and vomiting; chronic infantile fright wind; cough; expectoration of phlegm; eye disorders; head wind with pain at the corners of the forehead.

Stimulation: 0.2-0.3″ transverse insertion.
Moxa: 3 cones; pole 5-15 min.

Point Categories & Associations: Intersection-jiaohui point of the foot shao yang gallbladder and foot tai yang bladder channels.

Location: Posterior and superior to the auricle, 2″ within the hairline, about 0.5″ posterior to GB-8.
Classical Location: Approximately three fen behind GB-8, two inches within the hairline . *(The Golden Mirror)*
Local Anatomy: The posterior auricular artery and vein. The branch of the great occipital nerve.

Functions: Clears and disinhibits gallbladder heat; settles and calms the spirit.
Indications: Headache; swelling of the gums; epilepsy.
Supplementary Indications: Madness; wind tetany; susceptibility to fright and fear.

Stimulation: 0.3″ transverse insertion.
Moxa: 3 cones; pole 5-15 min.

Point Categories & Associations: Intersection-jiaohui point of the foot shao yang gallbladder and foot tai yang bladder channels.

GB-9
天衝
tiān chōng
"Celestial Hub"

Location: Posterior to the ear and superior to the mastoid process, in the middle of a line drawn from GB-9 to GB-11.
Classical Location: Behind the ear, one inch within the hairline. *(The Great Compendium)*
Local Anatomy: See GB-9.

Functions: Courses and disinhibits the liver and gallbladder; dissipates wind and frees the connecting vessels.
Indications: Headache; tinnitus; deafness.
Supplementary Indications: Fever and chills; wind headache; heavy headedness; toothache; throat bi; thoracic fullness and dyspnea; painful swelling of the neck; goiter; counterflow cough with phlegm and foam; atony of the legs that prevents walking.

GB-10
浮白
fú bái
"Floating White"

Stimulation: 0.3″ transverse insertion.
Moxa: 3 cones; pole 5-15 min.

Point Categories & Associations: Intersection-jiaohui point of the foot shao yang gallbladder and foot tai yang bladder channels.

GB-11
頭竅陰
tóu qiào yīn

"Head Portal Yin"

Location: Posterior to the ear and superior to the mastoid process, about midway between GB-10 and GB-12.
Classical Location: Above GB-12 and below [in front of] the occipital bone, in a depression felt when the head is turned. *(The Great Compendium)*
Local Anatomy: The branches of the posterior auricular artery and vein. The anastomotic branch of the great and lesser occipital nerves.

Functions: Clears heat and disinhibits gallbladder channel damp-heat; frees the ears and disinhibits the throat.
Indications: Headache and pain in the neck; ear pain; deafness; tinnitus.
Supplementary Indications: yong and ju; vexatious heat in the hands and feet; stiff tongue; throat bi; taxation ju; goiter; nauseatingly bitter taste in the mouth.

Stimulation: 0.3″ transverse insertion.
Moxa: 5 cones; pole 5-15 min.

Point Categories & Associations: Intersection-jiaohui point of the foot shao yang gallbladder and foot tai yang bladder channels.

GB-12
完骨
wán gǔ

"Completion Bone"

Location: In the depression posterior and inferior to the mastoid process.
Classical Location: Four fen into the hair at the back of the ear. *(The Systematized Canon)*
Local Anatomy: The posterior auricular artery and vein. The lesser occipital nerve.

Functions: Rouses the brain and opens the portals; dissipates wind and clears heat.
Indications: Headache; insomnia; pain and stiffness in the neck; swelling of the cheek; toothache; wryness of the eyes and mouth.

Supplementary Indications: Atony of the lower extremities with inability to walk; pain in the neck and nape; head wind with pain behind the ear; vexation; dark-colored urine; throat bi; tooth decay; clenched jaws.

Stimulation: 0.3-0.5 " downward oblique insertion.
Moxa: 3-7 cones; pole 5-15 min.

Point Categories & Associations: Intersection-jiaohui point of the foot shao yang gallbladder and foot tai yang bladder channels.

Location: 0.5 " within the hairline of the forehead, two-thirds of the distance from GV-24 to ST-8.
Classical Location: One inch and five fen to the side of BL-4, directly above the ears, four fen within the hairline.
(The Great Compendium)
Local Anatomy: The frontal branches of the superficial temporal artery and vein, the lateral branches of the frontal artery and vein. The lateral branch of the frontal nerve.

Functions: Clears and drains the liver and gallbladder; calms the liver and extinguishes wind; settles epilepsy and quiets the spirit.
Indications: Headache; visual dizziness; epilepsy.
Supplementary Indications: Stiff neck and nape; lateral costal pain; infantile fright epilepsy; hemilateral wind.

Stimulation: 0.3-0.5 " backward transverse insertion.
Moxa: 3-5 cones; pole 5-15 min.

Point Categories & Associations: Intersection-jiaohui point of the foot shao yang gallbladder channel and the yang linking vessel.

GB-13
本神
běn shén
"Root Spirit"

Location: On the forehead, 1 " above the midpoint of the eyebrow, approximately at one third of the distance from the eyebrow to the anterior hairline.
Classical Location: One inch above the eyebrow, on a line with the pupil. *(The Great Compendium)*
Local Anatomy: The lateral branches of the frontal artery and vein. On the lateral branch of the frontal nerve.

GB-14
陽白
yáng bái
"Yang White"

Functions: Dispels wind and clears heat; perfuses qi and brightens the eyes.

Indications: Frontal headache; visual dizziness; tearing on exposure to wind; pain in the outer canthus; twitching of the eyelids.

Supplementary Indications: Itching and painful pupils; upward-looking eyes; nearsightedness; inability to see at dusk or night; eye pain; eye discharge; aversion to cold in the back.

Stimulation: 0.3-0.5″ downward transverse insertion.
Moxa: 3 cones; pole 3-5 min.

Point Categories & Associations: Intersection-jiaohui point of the foot shao yang gallbladder, hand yang ming large intestine, foot yang ming stomach channels and the yang linking vessel.

GB-15
頭臨泣

tóu lín qì

"Head Overlooking Tears"

Location: Directly above GB-14, 0.5″ within the hairline, midway between GV-24 and ST-8.

Classical Location: In the depression five fen into the hair, directly above the eyes. The point is found by having the patient look straight forward. *(The Great Compendium)*

Local Anatomy: The frontal artery and vein. The anastomotic branch of the medial and lateral branches of the frontal nerve.

Functions: Clears the brain and brightens the eyes; frees the nose.

Indications: Headache; visual dizziness; tearing on exposure to wind; pain in the outer canthus; nasal congestion.

Supplementary Indications: Eye screens; loss of consciousness due to wind strike; thoracic bi.

Illustrative Point Combinations & Applications: To treat tearing needle GB-15 and ST-8. *(Ode of a Hundred Patterns)*

Stimulation: 0.3-0.5″ upward transverse insertion.
Moxa: 3 cones; pole 2-5 min.

Point Categories & Associations: Intersection-jiaohui point of the foot shao yang gallbladder and foot tai yang bladder channels and the yang linking vessel.

Location: 1.5″ posterior to GB-15, on the line connecting GB-15 and GB-20.

Classical Location: One and a half inches behind GB-15. *(The Great Compendium)*

Local Anatomy: The frontal branches of the superficial temporal artery and vein. The anastomotic branch of the medial and lateral branches of the frontal nerve.

Functions: Courses the channels and connecting vessels; clears the head and brightens the eyes.

Indications: Headache; visual dizziness; painful reddening of the eyes.

Supplementary Indications: Nearsightedness; aching among the upper teeth; aversion to cold and nasal congestion; fever and chills without sweating.

Stimulation: 0.3-0.5″ backward transverse insertion.
Moxa: 3-5 cones; pole 5-15 min.

Point Categories & Associations: Intersection-jiaohui point of the foot shao yang gallbladder channel and the yang linking vessel.

GB-16
目窗
mù chuāng
"Eye Window"

Location: 1.5″ posterior GB-16, on the line joining GB-15 and GB-20.

Classical Location: One and one half inches behind GB-16. *(The Great Compendium)*

Local Anatomy: The anastomotic plexus formed by the parietal branches of the superficial temporal artery and vein and the occipital artery and vein. The anastomotic branch of the frontal and great occipital nerves.

Functions: Clears heat and drains the gallbladder; soothes the sinews and quickens the connecting vessels.

Indications: Unilateral headache; visual dizziness.

Supplementary Indications: Unilateral headache and stiffness of the neck; aversion to wind and cold; toothache; nausea; retching and vomiting; stiff lips.

GB-17
正營
zhèng yíng
"Upright Construction"

Stimulation: 0.3-0.5″ backward transverse insertion.
Moxa: 5 cones; pole 5-15 min.

Point Categories & Associations: Intersection-jiaohui point of the foot shao yang gallbladder channel and yang linking vessel.

GB-18
承靈
chéng líng
"Spirit Support"

Location: 1.5″ posterior to GB-17, on the line connecting GB-15 and GB-20.

Classical Location: One inch and five fen behind GB-17.
(The Great Compendium)

Local Anatomy: The branches of the occipital artery and vein. The branch of the great occipital nerve.

Functions: Clears the gallbladder and drains heat; diffuses the lung and frees the portals.

Indications: Headache; deep-source nasal congestion; nosebleed.

Supplementary Indications: Brain wind headache; fever and aversion to cold; clear, runny snivel and nosebleed; nasal congestion; dizziness; eye pain.

Stimulation: 0.3-0.5 ″ backward transverse insertion.
Moxa: 3-5 cones; pole 5-15 min.

Point Categories & Associations: Intersection-point of the foot shao yang gallbladder channel and yang linking vessel.

GB-19
腦空
nǎo kōng
"Brain Hollow"

Location: Directly above GB-20, level with GV-17, on the lateral side of the external occipital protuberance.

Classical Location: One inch and five fen behind GB-18, in the depression on either side beneath the occipital bone.
(The Great Compendium)

Local Anatomy: See GB-18.

Functions: Clears the gallbladder and drains fire; soothes the sinews and quickens the connecting vessels; rouses the brain and frees the portals.

Indications: Headache; pain and stiffness of the neck.

Supplementary Indications: Wind dizziness; palpitations; stiff neck; manic disorders.

Stimulation: 0.3-0.5″ downward transverse insertion.
Moxa: 3-5 cones; pole 5-15 min.

Point Categories & Associations: Intersection-jiaohui point of the
foot shao yang gallbladder channel and the yang linking vessel.

Location: On the posterior aspect of the neck, below the occipital
bone, in the depression between the sternocleidomastoid muscle
(m. sternocleidomastoideus) and trapezius muscle (m. trapezius).
Classical Location: In the depression within the hairline behind
the temporal region. *(The Systematized Canon)*
Local Anatomy: The branches of the occipital artery and vein.
The branch of the lesser occipital nerve.

Functions: Courses wind and clears heat; clears the head and
opens the portals; brightens the eyes and sharpens the hearing;
frees the channels and quickens the connecting vessels; harmonizes qi and blood.
Indications: Headache; visual dizziness; pain and stiffness of the
neck; painful reddening of the eyes; deep-source nasal congestion;
pain in the shoulder and back; heat diseases; common cold;
epilepsy.
Supplementary Indications: Clear, runny snivel and nosebleed;
tinnitus; deafness; wind-strike loss of speech; lumbar and back
pain; unilateral and ambilateral headache; insomnia; goiter; madness; absence of sweating in cold damage or thermic disease.
Illustrative Point Combinations & Applications: Zhang Zhong-
Jing says if Cinnamon Twig Decoction (guì zhī tāng) prescribed
for initial-stage tai yang disease gives rise to persistent vexation,
needle GB-20 and GV-16 and again prescribe Cinnamon Twig
Decoction to bring about recovery. *(Treatise on Cold Damage)*

Stimulation of GB-20 and GB-39 treats stoop.
(Ode of the Jade Dragon)

Stimulation: 0.5-1.0″ perpendicular insertion.
Moxa: 3-7 cones; pole 5-20 min.

Point Categories & Associations: Intersection-jiaohui point of the
foot shao yang gallbladder and hand shao yang triple burner channels with the yang linking and yang motility vessels.

GB-20
風池
fēng chí
"Wind Pool"

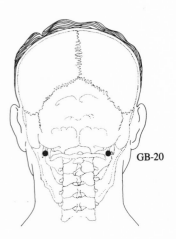

GB-20

Figure 16.6

GB-21
肩井
jiān jǐng

"Shoulder Well"

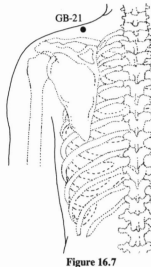

GB-21

Figure 16.7

Location: Midway between C7 (GV-14) and the bony prominence above LI-16, at the highest point of the shoulder.

Classical Location: In the depression above ST-12, in front of the great bone. *(The Systematized Canon)*

Local Anatomy: The transverse cervical artery and vein. The lateral branch of the supraclavicular nerve, the accessory nerve.

Functions: Frees the channels and quickens the connecting vessels; sweeps phlegm and opens the portals.

Indications: Stiff neck; shoulder and back pain; inability to move the arm; mammary yong; wind strike; difficult delivery.

Supplementary Indications: Dizziness; fever and chills; inversion cold in the limbs; counterflow qi ascent cough; shortness of breath; miscarriage with loss of blood.

Illustrative Point Combinations & Applications: The pain of foot qi is treated by first needling GB-21 and then ST-36 and GB-34. *(The Celestial Emperor's Secret)*

Stimulation: 0.5 " perpendicular insertion.
Moxa: 3-7 cones; pole 10-30 min.

Contraindications: 1) Needling contraindicated in pregnancy since it may cause abortion. 2) After needling GB-21 it is necessary to needle ST-36 to assure qi regulation. *(Ode of Xi Hong)*

Point Categories & Associations: Intersection-jiaohui point of the foot shao yang gallbladder, the hand shao yang triple burner, and the foot yang ming stomach channels and the yang linking vessel.

GB-22
淵腋
yuān yè

"Armpit Abyss"

Location: On the midaxillary line, 3 " below the axilla.

Classical Location: In the depression three inches below the armpit. The point is found with the arm raised.
(The Great Compendium)

Local Anatomy: The thoracoepigastric vein, the lateral thoracic artery and vein, the 5th intercostal artery and vein. The lateral cutaneous branch of the 5th intercostal nerve, the branch of the long thoracic nerve.

Functions: Loosens the chest and normalizes qi; soothes the sinews and quickens the connecting vessels.
Indications: Lateral costal pain; swelling of the axillary region.
Supplementary Indications: Thoracic fullness; cough.

Stimulation: 0.3-0.5″ perpendicular insertion.
Moxa: pole 5-10 min.

Location: 1″ anterior to GB-22, approximately level with the nipple.
Classical Location: Three inches down from the armpit and one inch forward. *(The Systematized Canon)*
Local Anatomy: The lateral thoracic artery and vein, the 5th intercostal artery and vein. The lateral cutaneous branch of the 5th intercostal nerve.

Functions: Courses the liver and rectifies qi; calms dyspnea and downbears counterflow.
Indications: Vomiting; acid regurgitation; hiccough; jaundice.
Supplementary Indications: Fulminant fullness in the chest; insomnia.

Stimulation: 0.3-0.5″ oblique insertion.
Moxa: 3-5 cones; pole 10-20 min.

Point Categories & Associations: Intersection-jiaohui point of the foot shao yang gallbladder and foot tai yang bladder channel.

Note: According to *The Great Compendium* this point is the alarm-mu point of the gallbladder. Most other sources list GB-24 as the alarm-mu point.

GB-23
輒筋
zhé jīn
"Sinew Seat"

Location: Inferior to the nipple, between the cartilage of the 7th and 8th ribs, one rib space below and slightly lateral to LV-14.
Classical Location: Five fen below LV-14
Local Anatomy: The 7th intercostal artery and vein. The 7th intercostal nerve.

GB-24
日月
rì yuè
"Sun and Moon"

313

Functions: Courses gallbladder and qi; transforms damp-heat; harmonizes the central burner.

Indications: Borborygmi; diarrhea; abdominal distention; lumbar and lateral costal pain.

Supplementary Indications: Pain in the ribs; pain in the venter; retching and vomiting; acid regurgitation; jaundice; eructation; abdominal distention; somnolence; sighing and sorrowfulness; heat in the lower abdomen.

Stimulation: 0.3-0.5″ oblique insertion.
Moxa: 5 cones; pole 10-20 min.

Point Categories & Associations: Alarm-mu point of the gallbladder; intersection-jiaohui point of the foot shao yang gallbladder and foot tai yang bladder channels, and the yang linking vessel.

GB-25
京門
jīng mén

"Capital Gate"

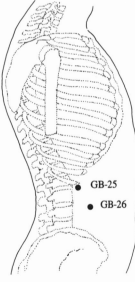

GB-25

GB-26

Figure 16.8

Location: At the inferior border of the free end of the 12th rib.

Classical Location: From GB-24 towards the ilium, in the low back, in the region of the free ribs on either side of the spine, five fen above and nine and a half inches either side of the navel. The patient should lie on his side, bend the top leg, straighten the bottom leg, and raise the arm to facilitate point location.
(The Golden Mirror)

Local Anatomy: The 11th intercostal artery and vein. The 11th intercostal nerve.

Functions: Warms kidney cold; abducts water-damp; downbears stomach counterflow; soothes the sinews and quickens the connecting vessels; promotes free flow through the waterways.

Indications: Borborygmi; diarrhea; abdominal distention; lumbar and lateral costal pain.

Supplementary Indications: Fever and chills; opisthotonos; pain in the hip joint; throughflux diarrhea; facial swelling and reduced urine; vomiting; lower abdominal pain; abdominal urgency; stoppage of the waterways.

Stimulation: 0.3-0.5″ perpendicular insertion.
Moxa: 3-5 cones; pole 20-30 min.

Point Categories & Associations: Alarm-mu point of the kidney.

Location: Below the free end of the 11th rib (LV-13), level with the umbilicus.

Classical Location: In the depression one inch and eight fen below the region of the free ribs, two inches above the navel, seven and a half inches either side of the midline. *(The Great Compendium)*

Local Anatomy: The subcostal artery and vein. The subcostal nerve.

Functions: Frees the channels and quickens the connecting vessels; clears and disinhibits damp-heat; regulates the menses and stops vaginal discharge.

Indications: Irregular menses; vaginal discharge; hernia; lumbar and lateral costal pain.

Supplementary Indications: Lower abdominal pain in women; intestinal shan pain; abdominal urgency; clonic spasm.

Illustrative Point Combinations & Applications: GB-26 and CV-4 should be investigated in cases of kidney debilitation [of yin or yang]. *(Ode of the Jade Dragon)*

Stimulation: 0.5-1.0″ perpendicular insertion.
Moxa: 5-7 cones; pole 10-30 min.

Point Categories & Associations: Intersection-jiaohui point of the foot shao yang gallbladder channel and the girdling vessel.

GB-26
帶脈
dài mài
"Girdling Vessel"

Location: On the lower abdomen, just medial to the anterior superior iliac spine, 3″ below the level of the umbilicus.

Classical Location: Three inches below GB-26, five inches and five fen to the side of ST-28. *(The Great Compendium)*

Local Anatomy: The superficial and deep circumflex iliac arteries and veins. The iliohypogastric nerve.

Functions: Strengthens the lumbus and boosts the kidney; courses the liver and rectifies qi; treats vaginal discharge.

Indications: Vaginal discharge; lumbar and hip pain; hernia.

Supplementary Indications: Cold shan in males; lumbar and back pain; abdominal pain; constipation; abdominal urgency; clonic spasm.

GB-27
五樞
wǔ shū
"Fifth Pivot"

Illustrative Point Combinations & Applications: For shoulder and spine pain, needle GB-27 and *bèi fēng* (back seam) [an extra point located superior to the posterior axillary fold approximately level with the fourth thoracic spinous process].
(Ode of the Jade Dragon)

Stimulation: 0.5-1.0″ perpendicular insertion.
Moxa: 5-10 cones; pole 10-30 min.

Point Categories & Associations: Intersection-jiaohui point of the foot shao yang gallbladder channel and the girdling vessel.

GB-28
維道
wéi dào

"Linking Path"

Location: 0.5″ inferior and slightly medial to GB-27.

Classical Location: Five inches and three fen below LV-13.
(The Great Compendium)

Local Anatomy: The superficial and deep circumflex iliac arteries and vein. The ilioinguinal nerve.

Functions: Courses stagnant qi; rectifies the two intestines; leashes the girdling vessel.

Indications: Lumbar and hip pain; vaginal discharge; lower abdominal pain; prolapse of the uterus.

Supplementary Indications: Water swelling; intestinal yong; cold shan; vomiting; no thought of food.

Stimulation: 0.5-1.0″ perpendicular insertion.
Moxa: 5-10 cones; pole 5-20 min.

Point Categories & Associations: Intersection-jiaohui point of the foot shao yang gallbladder channel and the girdling vessel.

GB-29
居髎
jū liáo

"Squating Bone-Hole"

Location: Midway between the anterior superior iliac spine and the greater trochanter. Locate this point in lateral recumbent posture.

Classical Location: Eight inches and three fen below LV-13, in the depression above the iliac bone. *(The Golden Mirror)*

Local Anatomy: Branches of the superficial circumflex iliac artery and vein, the ascending branches of the lateral circumflex femoral artery and vein. The lateral femoral cutaneous nerve.

Functions: Soothes the sinews and quickens the connecting vessels; strengthens the lumbus and legs.

Indications: Bi pain in the lumbus and thigh; paralysis.

Supplementary Indications: Diarrhea; cold shan.

Illustrative Point Combinations & Applications: GB-29, with GB-30 and BL-40 treat wind-damp thigh pain.
(Ode of the Jade Dragon)

Stimulation: 0.5-1.0 ″ perpendicular insertion.
Moxa: 5-10 cones; pole 10-30 min.

Needle Sensation: Numbness and distention that can spread to the hip joint.

Point Categories & Associations: Intersection-jiaohui point of the foot shao yang gallbladder channel and the yang motility vessel.

Location: One third of the distance from the greater trochanter to the sacral hiatus (GV-2). When locating the point, the patient should be in lateral recumbent posture with the thigh flexed.

Classical Location: With the patient lying on his side with his bottom leg stretched out and his top leg bent the point is found in the hip joint. The left hand shakes the leg as the right hand feels for the point. *(The Great Compendium)*

Local Anatomy: Medially, the inferior gluteal artery and vein. The inferior cluneal cutaneous nerve, the inferior gluteal nerve; deeper, the sciatic nerve.

Functions: Dissipates wind-damp in the channels and connecting vessels; disinhibits the lumbus and hip; strengthens the lumbus and legs.

Indications: Lumbar and hip pain; bi and atony of the lower limbs; hemiplegia.

Supplementary Indications: Pain in the lumbus and crotch; bi pain in the legs and knees; wind strike hemiplegia; foot qi; water swelling; wind papules.

Illustrative Point Combinations & Applications: When lumbar pain extending down the thighs defies treatment, needle GB-30, GB-31, and LV-2.
(Song of Point Applications for Miscellaneous Disease)

For cold-wind-damp bi, first needle GB-30 and then GB-34.
(The Celestial Emperor's Secret)

GB-30
環跳
huán tiào
"*Jumping Round*"

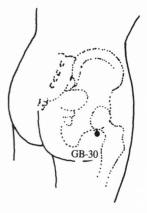

GB-30

Figure 16.9

317

Stimulation: 1.5-3.0" perpendicular insertion.

Moxa: 10-20 cones; pole 20-50 min.

Needle Sensation: Distention and numbness that sometimes spreads down the channel to the foot.

Point Categories & Associations: Intersection-jiaohui point of the foot shao yang gallbladder and foot tai yang bladder channels.

GB-31
風市

fēng shì

"Wind Market"

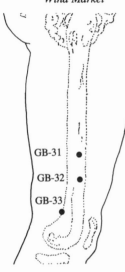

GB-31 •

GB-32 •

GB-33 •

Figure 16.10

Location: On the lateral aspect of the thigh, 7" above the transverse popliteal crease.

Classical Location: Between the two sinews on the outer side above knee, at the end of the middle finger when the hand is placed on the thigh. *(The Great Compendium)*

Local Anatomy: The muscular branches of the lateral circumflex femoral artery and vein. The lateral femoral cutaneous nerve, the muscular branch of the femoral nerve.

Functions: Dispels wind and dissipates cold; strengthens the sinews and bones; regulates qi and the blood.

Indications: Hemiplegia; atony, bi, and numbness of the lower limbs; general itching.

Supplementary Indications: Wind bi pain; small intestine qi pain: vacuity rumbling in the abdomen; scrotal swelling; headache.

Illustrative Point Combinations & Applications: GB-31 and ST-33 eliminates lack of strength in the legs and feet. *(Ode of the Jade Dragon)*

Stimulation: 0.7-1.2" perpendicular insertion.

Moxa: 5-7 cones; pole 5-20 min.

GB-32
中瀆

zhōng dú

"Central River"

Location: On the lateral aspect of the thigh, 5" above the transverse popliteal crease, between the lateral vastus muscle of the femur (m. vastus lateralis) and the biceps muscle of the femur (m. biceps femoris).

Classical Location: On the thigh, five inches above the knee, in the parting of the flesh.

Local Anatomy: See GB-31.

Functions: Soothes the sinews and quickens the connecting vessels; expels wind and dissipates cold.

Indications: Atony, bi, and numbness of the lower limbs; hemiplegia.

Stimulation: 0.5-0.8″ perpendicular insertion.
Moxa: 5-7 cones; pole 5-20 min.

Location: 3.0″ above GB-34, in the depression between the tendon of the biceps muscle of the femur (m. biceps femoris) and the lateral condyle of the femur. This point is easily located posterior to the joint when the knee is bent.

Classical Location: Three inches above GB-34, in the depression lateral to ST-35. *(The Great Compendium)*

Local Anatomy: The superior lateral genicular artery and vein. The terminal branch of the lateral femoral cutaneous nerve.

Functions: Dispels wind and dissipates cold; soothes the sinews, quickens the connecting vessels, and relieves pain.

Indications: Pain and swelling of the knee; hypertonicity of the popliteal sinews; numbness of the lower leg.

Supplementary Indications: Foot qi; crane's knee wind.

Stimulation: 0.5″ perpendicular insertion.
Moxa: 3-7 cones; pole 5-15 min.

GB-33
膝陽關
(xī) yáng guān

"(Knee) Yang Joint"

Location: In the depression anterior and inferior to the head of the fibula.

Classical Location: One inch below the knee, in the depression on the outer face of the shin. The point is found in squatting posture. *(The Great Compendium)*

Local Anatomy: The inferior lateral genicular artery and vein. Just where the common peroneal nerve bifurcates into the superficial and deep peroneal nerves.

Functions: Soothes the sinews and vessels; clears gallbladder heat; expels wind from the knee and legs; courses damp and stagnation in the channels and connecting vessels.

Indications: Hemiplegia; atony, bi and numbness of the lower limbs; pain and swelling of the knee; lateral costal pain; bitter taste in the mouth; vomiting; jaundice.

GB-34
陽陵泉
yáng líng quán

"Yang Mound Spring"

Supplementary Indications: Fullness in the chest and lateral costal region; bitter taste in the mouth; sighing; urinary incontinence; constipation; headache; wind-strike hemiplegia; swelling of the mouth, tongue, throat, head or face; disorders of the sinews.

Illustrative Point Combinations & Applications: For hemiplegia, use GB-34 and LI-11. *(Ode of a Hundred Patterns)* ⬧

Cold-wind-damp bi can be treated by needling GB-30 and warming the tail of the needle at GB-34 and ST-36.
(Song of Point Applications for Miscellaneous Disease)

Stimulation: 0.8-1.2 ″ perpendicular insertion.
Moxa: 5-7 cones; pole 20-30 min.

Point Categories & Associations: Uniting-he (earth) point; meeting-hui point of the sinews.

GB-35
陽交
yáng jiāo

"Yang Intersection"

Location: 7 ″ above the tip of the external malleolus, on the posterior border of the fibula, level with GB-36 and BL-58.

Classical Location: Seven inches above the outer ankle, in the parting of the flesh among the three yang channels.
(The Great Compendium)

Local Anatomy: The branches of the peroneal artery and vein. The lateral sural cutaneous nerve.

Functions: Disinhibits the gallbladder and quiets the spirit; soothes the sinews, quickens the blood, and relieves pain.

Indications: Distention and fullness in the chest and lateral costal region; knee pain; weakness and atony of the lower extremities.

Supplementary Indications: Fever and chills; dyspnea; throat bi; cold inversion; fright mania; foot qi; swelling of the face.

Stimulation: 0.5-0.8 ″ perpendicular insertion.
Moxa: 5-7 cones; pole 5-15 min.

Point Categories & Associations: Cleft-xi point of the yang linking channel; intersection-jiaohui point of the foot shao yang gallbladder channel and the yang linking vessel.

Location: 7″ above the tip of the external malleolus, on the anterior border of the fibula level with GB-35 and ST-39.

Classical Location: Seven inches above the outer ankle bone. *(The Great Compendium)*

Local Anatomy: The branches of the anterior tibial artery and vein. The superficial peroneal nerve.

Functions: Disinhibits the liver and gallbladder; dispels wind, resolves toxin and clears heat.

Indications: Neck pain; pain in the chest and lateral costal region.

Supplementary Indications: Fever and aversion to cold; bitter fullness in the chest and lateral costal region; fever and chills due to rabid dog bite; madness; pigeon chest in infants.

Illustrative Point Combinations & Applications: GB-36 constringes the large intestine [i.e., treats prolapse of the rectum]. *(Ode of a Hundred Patterns)*

Stimulation: 0.5-0.8″ perpendicular insertion.
Moxa: 3-5 cones; pole 5-20 min.

Point Categories & Associations: Cleft-xi point of the gallbladder channel.

GB-36
外丘
wài qiū
"Outer Hill"

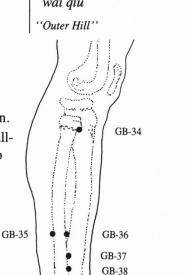

Figure 16.11

Location: 5.0″ above the tip of the external malleolus, on the anterior border of the fibula. (Note: The bone lies deep here, so it is not the best landmark. GB-36, GB-37 and GB-38 are situated between the m. peroneus longus and the m. flexor digitorum longus.)

Classical Location: Five inches above the outer ankle. *(The Great Compendium)*

Local Anatomy: The branches of the anterior tibial artery and vein. The superficial peroneal nerve.

Functions: Regulates the liver and brightens the eyes; dispels wind and disinhibits damp.

Indications: Knee pain; loss of locomotive ability of the lower extremities; eye pain; night blindness; pain and distention of the breast.

GB-37
光明
guāng míng
"Bright Light"

Supplementary Indications: Fever and chills without sweating; madness; itching of the eyes; retention of rabid dog bite toxin; pigeon chest in infants; grinding of the teeth.

Illustrative Point Combinations & Applications: If BL-1 is not effective in treating the eyes, combine it with GB-37.
(Ode of Xi Hong)

For failure of rabid dog bite toxin to come out, with fever and chills, burn three cones of moxa on the bite wound and at the connecting-luo point of the shao yang (GB-37).
(The Great Compendium)

Stimulation: 0.7-1.0 ″ perpendicular insertion.
Moxa: 3-5 cones; pole 5-20 min.

Point Categories & Associations: Connecting-luo point of the gallbladder channel connecting to the liver channel.

GB-38
陽輔
yáng fú

"Yang Assistance"

Location: 4 ″ above and slightly anterior to the tip of the external malleolus, on the anterior border of the fibula, between the long extensor muscle of the toes (m. extensor digitorum longus) and the short peroneal muscle (m. peroneus brevis).

Classical Location: Four inches above the outer ankle, in front of the fibula three fen from the edge of the bone seven inches above GB-40.

Local Anatomy: See GB-37.

Functions: Harmonizes the shao yang; dissipates cold and eliminates heat; soothes the liver and resolves depression; quickens the connecting vessels and relieves pain.

Indications: Unilateral headache; pain in the outer canthus; pain in the supraclavicular fossa; axillary pain; scrofulous lumps; pain in the chest, lateral costal region, and lateral aspect of the lower extremities; malarial disease.

Supplementary Indications: Foot qi; sinew-vascular hypertonicity; throat bi; hemilateral wind.

Stimulation: 0.3-0.7 ″ perpendicular insertion.
Moxa: 3-7 cones; pole 5-20 min.

Point Categories & Associations: River-jing (fire) point.

Location: 3 ″ above the tip of the external malleolus, in the depression between the posterior border of the fibula and the tendon of the long peroneus muscle (m. peroneus longus) and the short peroneus muscle (m. peroneus brevis).

Classical Location: At the pulsating vessel three inches above the outer ankle; feel for the tip of the bone. *(The Great Compendium)*

Local Anatomy: See GB-37.

Functions: Discharges gallbladder fire; clears marrow heat; expels wind damp from the channels and connecting vessels.

Indications: Hemiplegia; stiffness; abdominothoracic distention and fullness; lateral costal pain; pain in the knee and thigh; foot qi.

Supplementary Indications: Heat in the stomach; dry nose; nosebleed; throat bi; stiff neck; counterflow cough; hypertonicity of the sinews; the five stranguries; saber lumps; axillary swelling; generalized heaviness due to wind taxation; inability to lift the limbs; anxiety and anger.

Illustrative Point Combinations & Applications: In cold damage supplement GB-39; if there is heat, drain it.
(Song to Keep Up Your Sleeve)

For pain in the ankle bone burn moxa at BL-60, adding GB-39 and GB-40. *(Song More Precious than Jade)*

Stimulation: 0.4-0.5 ″ perpendicular insertion.
Moxa: 3-5 cones; pole 5-20 min.

Needle Sensation: Distention and numbness spreading toward the foot.

Point Categories & Associations: Meeting-hui point of the marrow.

GB-39
懸鐘
xuán zhōng
"Suspended Bell"
often called
絕骨
jué gǔ
"(Severed Bone)"

Location: Anterior and inferior to the external malleolus, in the depression on the lateral side of the tendon of the long extensor muscle of the toes (m. extensor digitorum longus).

Classical Location: In the depression below the lower outer ankle bone, three inches from GB-41.
(The Systema.ized Canon)

Local Anatomy: The branch of the anterolateral malleolar artery. The branches of the intermediate dorsal cutaneous nerve and superficial peroneal nerve.

GB-40
丘墟
qiū xū
"Hill Ruins"

Functions: Dispels midstage pathogens; clears the liver and gallbladder; transforms damp-heat; courses inversion qi.

Indications: Neck pain; axillary pain; thoracic and lateral costal pain; vomiting and acid eructation; loss of locomotive ability of the lower extremities; pain and swelling of the external malleolus; malarial disease.

Supplementary Indications: Foot qi; fever and chills; swelling of the neck; cough and rapid breathing; poor eyesight; intestinal qi pain; lower abdominal pain; sighing; axillary swelling; atony; inversion cold; inability to move the wrist.

Illustrative Point Combinations & Applications: Use SP-5, ST-41 and GB-40 for pain in the feet. *(Ode of the Jade Dragon)*

Stimulation: 0.3-0.5″ perpendicular or oblique insertion. Moxa: 3 cones; pole 5-25 min.

Point Categories & Associations: Source-yuan point of the gallbladder channel.

GB-41
足臨泣

(zú) lín qì

"*(Foot) Overlooking Tears*"

Location: In the depression distal to the junction of the 4th and 5th metatarsal bones, on the lateral side of the tendon of the short extensor muscle of the small toe (m. extensor digitorum brevis).

Classical Location: In the depression behind and between the base joints of the little toe and the one next to it, one inch and five fen from GB-43. *(The Great Compendium)*

Local Anatomy: The branch of the intermediate dorsal cutaneous nerve of the foot.

Functions: Clears fire and extinguishes wind; brightens the eyes and sharpens the hearing; courses liver and gallbladder qi stagnation; transforms obstructing phlegm-heat.

Indications: Pain in the outer canthus; visual dizziness; pain in the lateral costal region; pain and swelling of the dorsum of the foot; pain and distention of the breasts; malarial disease.

Supplementary Indications: Axillary swelling; dyspnea; dry eyes; fever and chills; thoracic bi; pain in the supraclavicular fossa; mammary yong; menstrual disorders; saber and pearl-string lumps; migratory wind pain; damp swelling of the dorsum of the feet; pain at the vertex; fullness and pain in the region of the free ribs.

Illustrative Point Combinations & Applications: ST-44 and GB-41 rectify lower abdominal distention. *(Ode of the Jade Dragon)*

Stimulation: 0.3-0.5 ″ perpendicular insertion.
Moxa: 3 cones; pole 3-5 min.

Point Categories & Associations: Stream-shu (wood) point.
Confluence-jiaohui point of the 8 extraordinary vessels; related to
the girdling vessel.

Location: Between the 4th and 5th metatarsal bones, on the
medial side of the tendon of the short extensor muscle of the small
toe (m. extensor digitorum brevis).
Classical Location: In the depression behind and between the base
joints of the little toe and the one next to it, one inch from GB-43.
(The Great Compendium)
Local Anatomy: See GB-41.

GB-42
地五會
dì wǔ huì
"Earth
Five-Fold"

Functions: Clears the liver and drains the gallbladder; brightens
the eyes and sharpens the hearing.
Indications: Painful reddening of the eye; axillary swelling;
reddening and swelling dorsum of the foot; pain and distention of
the breast.
Supplementary Indications: Tinnitus; itching eye; spitting of blood
due to internal injury; lumbar pain.
Illustrative Point Combinations & Applications: For painful or
itching eyes, needle GB-37 and GB-42.
(Ode to Elucidate Mysteries)

Stimulation: 0.3-0.4 ″ perpendicular insertion.
Moxa: 2-3 cones; pole 5-10 min.

Location: Between the 4th and 5th toes, proximal to the margin of
the web.
Classical Location: In the depression in front of the base joints of
the little toe and the one next to it, in the depression in the fork of
the bones. *(The Great Compendium)*
Local Anatomy: The dorsal digital artery and vein. The dorsal
digital nerve.

GB-43
俠溪（俠谿）
jiá xī
"Pinched Ravine"

Functions: Clears heat; extinguishes wind; relieves pain.

Indications: Pain in the outer canthus; visual dizziness; tinnitus; pain in the cheek and submandibular region; pain in the lateral costal region; heat disease.

Supplementary Indications: Absence of sweating in heat diseases; tearing; deafness; expectoration of blood; pain in the chest that prevents turning sides; mania; absence of menstrual periods; swollen or burst mammary yong.

Stimulation: 0.2-0.3″ upward oblique or perpendicular insertion. Moxa: 2-3 cones; pole 3-5 min.

Point Categories & Associations: Spring-ying (water) point.

GB-44
足竅陰

(zú) qiào yīn

"(Foot) Portal Yin"

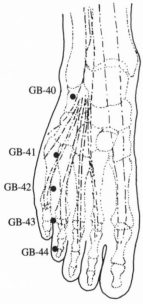

GB-40

GB-41

GB-42

GB-43

GB-44

Figure 16.12

Location: On the lateral side of the 4th toe, about 0.1″ proximal to the corner of the nail.

Classical Location: On the outer side of the toe next to the little toe, the width of a Chinese leek leaf away from the corner of the nail. *(The Great Compendium)*

Local Anatomy: The arterial and venous network formed by the dorsal digital artery and vein and plantar digital artery and vein. The dorsal digital nerve.

Functions: Extinguishes wind and courses the liver and gallbladder; clears heat and drains fire.

Indications: Unilateral headache; visual dizziness; tinnitus; lateral costal pain; excessive dreaming; heat diseases.

Supplementary Indications: Cough; cramp in the limbs; eye pain; throat bi; headache; vexation; dry curled tongue; deafness; menstrual disorders; pain and swelling of the dorsum of the foot; pain in the outer canthus.

Stimulation: 0.1-0.2″ oblique insertion. Moxa: 2-3 cones; pole 3-5 min.

Point Categories & Associations: Well-jing (metal) point.

		Foot Shao Yang Gallbladder Channel		
Point	**Location**	**Indications**		
		Primary		**Secondary**
*GB-1	Outer canthus	Headache eye disease		
*GB-2	Anterior to ear	Tinnitus deafness toothache		
GB-3		Unilateral headache tinnitus deafness toothache wryness of the mouth and eyes		
GB-4	Side of head	Unilateral headache visual dizziness tinnitus		
GB-5		Unilateral headache red, swollen, painful eyes		
GB-6		Unilateral headache red, swollen, painful eyes		
GB-7		Temporal headache clenched jaws		
*GB-8		Headache		
GB-9		Headache pain and swelling of the gums		
GB-10	Back of head	Headache tinnitus deafness		
GB-11		Headache ear disease		
GB-12		Headache stiffness and rigidity of the neck		
GB-13	Front of head	Headache visual dizziness		Epilepsy
*GB-14		Frontal headache eye disease		
*GB-15		Headache eye disease nasal congestion		
GB-16		Headache eye disease nasal congestion		

		Indications	
Point	**Location**		
		Primary	**Secondary**
GB-17	Front of head	Unilateral headache visual dizziness	
GB-18	Back of head	Headache deep source nasal congestion	
GB-19		Headache stiffness and rigidity of the neck	Mania and withdrawal
Head: Disorders of the head, neck, and sensory organs			
*GB-20	Neck	Headache eye disease deep source nasal congestion pain and stiffness of the neck	Common cold epilepsy
*GB-21	Shoulder	Pain and stiffness of the head and neck pain in the shoulders and back	Mammary yong delayed labor
Neck and shoulders: Disorders of the head, neck and shoulders			
GB-22	Lateral costal region	Fullness in the chest lateral costal pain	
GB-23		Fullness in the chest dyspnea	
*GB-24	Free rib region	Lateral costal pain vomiting eructation	Jaundice
Chest and lateral costal region: Localized disorders			
GB-25	Lumbus	Inhibited urination water swelling pain in the lumbar and lateral costal regions	
*GB-26	Lateral abdomen	Abdominal pain menstrual disorders vaginal discharge	
GB-27		Abdominal pain vaginal discharge	
GB-28	Pubis	Abdominal pain vaginal discharge hernia prolapse of the uterus	
Free ribs to pubis: Gynecologic, genital and intestinal disorders			

Foot Shao Yang Gallbladder Channel (continued)

Foot Shao Yang Gallbladder Channel (continued)			
Point	**Location**	Indications	
		Primary	**Secondary**
GB-29	Hip joint	Lumbar pain paralysis of the lower limbs	
*GB-30		Lumbar pain paralysis of the lower limbs	
*GB-31	Upper leg	Paralysis of the lower limbs	Unilateral itching
GB-32		Paralysis of the lower limbs	
GB-33	Knee joint	Pain and swelling of the knee	
Hip joint to knee: Disorders of the lumbus and leg			
*GB-34	Lower leg	Lateral costal pain paralysis of the lower limbs	Jaundice
GB-35		Distention and pain in the chest and lateral costal region paralysis of the lower limbs	Mania and with-drawal
GB-36		Distention and pain in the chest and lateral costal region paralysis of the lower limbs	Madness
*GB-37		Eye disease knee pain	
GB-38		Unilateral headache paralysis of the lower limbs	
*GB-39		Lateral costal pain pain in the thigh and knee	Stiff neck
*GB-40	Back of foot	Distention and pain in the chest and lateral costal region paralysis of the lower limbs	
*GB-41		Eye disease lateral costal pain mammary yong menstrual disorders	
GB-42		Red, swollen, painful eyes mammary yong pain and swelling of the dorsum of the foot	

Point	Location	Indications	
		Primary	**Secondary**
GB-43	Toe	Eye disease tinnitus deafness, lateral costal pain	Heat disease
*GB-44		Headache red, swollen, painful eyes throat bi	Heat disease
Lower leg and foot: Disorders of the head, eyes, ears, throat, and lateral costal region; mental disorders; heat disease			

Table header: **Foot Shao Yang Gallbladder Channel** (continued)

17. The Liver Channel System (Foot Jue Yin) 足厥陰肝經

17.1 The Primary Liver Channel

Pathway: The foot jue yin liver channel starts on the dorsum of the great toe and runs up the foot between the first and second metatarsal bones to a point one body-inch in front of the medial malleolus. It then proceeds upward to SP-6, where it intersects the foot tai yin spleen channel. Continuing up the medial tai yin spleen channel eight body-inches above the medial malleolus, it then runs posterior to that channel over the knee and thigh. Once again it crosses the foot tai yin spleen channel at SP-12 and SP-13, and then skirts around the genitals and penetrates the lower abdomen where it meets the conception vessel at CV-2, CV-3, and CV-4. It then ascends, moving toward the lateral aspect of the trunk to home to the liver and connect with the gallbladder. Continuing its upward course through the diaphragm, it disperses over the costal region, then runs up to the neck posterior to the pharynx, enters the nasopharynx, and meets the tissues surrounding the eyes. The channel finally runs up the forehead to meet the governing vessel at the vertex.

A branch breaks off below the eye and runs through the cheeks to contour the inside of the lips.

Another branch separates from the liver, passes through the diaphragm, and enters the lung.

Main pathologic signs associated with the external course of the channel: headache; dizziness; blurred vision; tinnitus; fever; spasm of the limbs.

Main pathologic signs associated with the internal organ: fullness; distention and pain in the costal region with lump glomus; fullness and thoracic oppression in the venter; abdominal pain; vomiting; jaundice; swill diarrhea; lower abdominal pain; shan qi; enuresis; urinary block; yellow urine.

17.2 The Connecting Vessel of the Liver Channel

Pathway: This vessel separates from the primary channel at LV-5 and connects to the foot shao yang gallbladder. A branch follows the primary channel up to bind at the genitals.

Main pathologic signs:

Qi counterflow: testicular swelling.

Repletion: frequent erection.

Vacuity: fulminant genital itching.

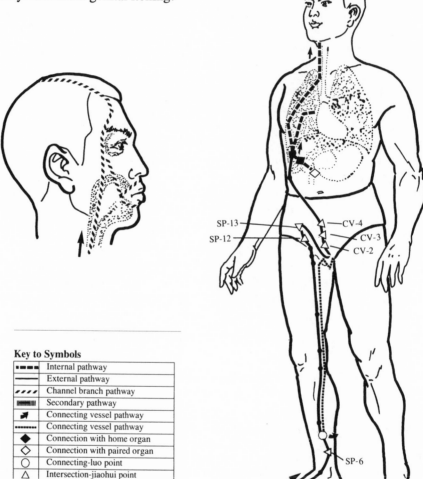

Key to Symbols

▪▬▬▪	Internal pathway
▬▬	External pathway
▰▰▰▰	Channel branch pathway
▨▨▨▨	Secondary pathway
↗	Connecting vessel pathway
▪▪▪▪▪▪	Connecting vessel pathway
◆	Connection with home organ
◇	Connection with paired organ
○	Connecting-luo point
△	Intersection-jiaohui point
■	Lower uniting-he Point

Figure 17.1 - 17.2 Primary channel and connecting vessel of the liver.

17.3 The Liver Channel Divergence

Pathway: This divergence leaves the primary channel at the dorsal aspect of the foot and rises up to the border of the pubic hair where it unites with the foot shao yang gallbladder channel divergence.

17.4 The Liver Channel Sinews

Pathway: These sinews originate on the top of the large toe and bind at the front of the medial malleolus. They run up the lower leg and bind at the medial aspect of the knee. Continuing up the yin side of the thigh they bind at the genitals and at that point connect with other sinews.

Main pathologic signs:

Inability to support the large toe; pain anterior to the medial malleolus; pain at the medial aspect of the knee; pain or spasm of the medial aspect of the thigh; dysfunction of the genitals; hindered erectile function due to internal damage; retraction of the genitals due to cold damage; frequent erection due to heat damage.

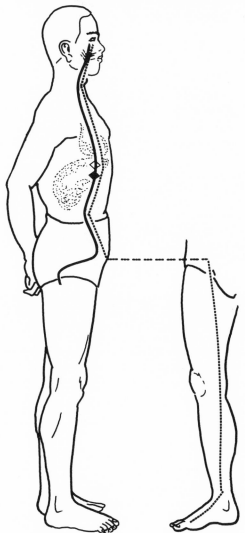

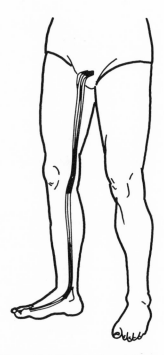

Figure 17.4 The liver channel sinews.

Figure 17.3 Channel divergences of the liver and gallbladder.

333

LV-1
大敦
dà dūn

"Large Pile"

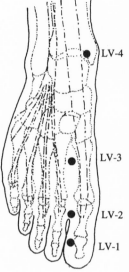

Figure 17.5

Location: On the lateral side of the great toe, 0.1″ proximal to the dorsum of the terminal phalanx of the great toe, midway between the lateral corner of the nail and interphalangeal joint.

Classical Location: On the great toe, about the width of a Chinese leek leaf away from the nail, on the lateral side amid the "three hairs." *(The Golden Mirror)*

Local Anatomy: The dorsal digital artery and vein. The dorsal digital nerve derived from the deep peroneal nerve.

Functions: Courses inversion qi; regulates menstruation; harmonizes construction qi; rectifies the lower burner; returns yang and stems inversion counterflow; clears the spirit-disposition; frees the channels; opens the spirit portals.

Indications: Prolapse of the uterus; hernia; metrorrhagia; enuresis.

Supplementary Indications: Profuse, incessant uterine bleeding; absence of menstruation; genital retraction; swelling of one testicle; pain in the glans penis; the five stranguries; the seven shans; epilepsy; urinary incontinence in children; worried oppression; excessive perspiration; umbilical pain.

Stimulation: 0.3″ perpendicular insertion.
Moxa: 3 cones; pole 5-7 min.

Needle Sensation: Localized pain.

Illustrative Point Combinations & Applications: For small intestine qi pain, first needle GV-1, then needle LV-1.
(The Celestial Emperor's Secret)

Point Categories & Associations: Well-jing (wood) point.

LV-2
行間
xíng jiān

"Moving Between"

Location: Between the first and second toe, proximal to the margin of the web, distal to the MTP (metatarsal phalange) joint.

Classical Location: On the web of the great toe, in the depression where the pulsating vessel may be sensed through palpation. *(The Great Compendium)*

Local Anatomy: The dorsal venous network of the foot and the first dorsal digital artery and vein. The site where the dorsal digital nerves split from the deep peroneal nerve.

Functions: Drains liver fire; cools blood heat; clears the lower burner; extinguishes wind; courses the vessels and quickens the connecting vessels; clears heat and drains fire; rectifies qi.

Indications: Incessant menorrhagia; urinary tract pain; enuresis; urinary stoppage; hernia; wryness of the mouth; red, swollen, painful eyes; pain in the lateral costal region; headache; visual dizziness; epilepsy; convulsive spasms; insomnia.

Supplementary Indications: White turbid urethral discharge; wasting thirst; bitter fullness below the lateral costal region; counterflow retching; throughflux diarrhea; counterflow cough; swollen knees; lumbar pain; abdominal pain; fullness below the heart; retching of blood; chest and back pain; throat bi; liver disease; fecal incontinence in children and the elderly; lower abdominal swelling; shan pain.

Illustrative Point Combinations & Applications: LV-2 and KI-1 treat kidney exhaustion associated with wasting thirst. *(Ode of a Hundred Patterns)*

Stimulation: 0.3-0.6″ perpendicular insertion, or oblique insertion angled slightly towards the heel.
Moxa: 3 cones; pole 5-15 min.
Needle Sensation: Localized distention.

Point Categories & Associations: Spring-ying (fire) point.

LV-3
太衝
tài chōng

"Supreme Surge"

Location: In the depression distal to the junction of the 1st and 2nd metatarsal bones.

Classical Location: One and a half to two inches below the base of the great toe, in the depression where the pulsating vessel may be sensed through palpation. *(The Great Compendium)*

Local Anatomy: The dorsal venous network of the foot, and the first dorsal metatarsal artery. The branch of the deep peroneal nerve.

Functions: Extinguishes liver fire and clears liver yang; discharges damp-heat in the lower burner; soothes the liver; rectifies qi; courses the connecting vessels and quickens the blood.

Indications: Metrorrhagia; hernia; enuresis; urinary stoppage; pain immediately anterior to the medial malleolus; distention of the lateral costal region; wryness of the mouth; infantile fright wind; epilepsy patterns; headache; dizziness; insomnia.

Supplementary Indications: Genital pain; genital retraction; saber and pearl-string lumps; fright wind; swill diarrhea; sore throat; dryness of the upper esophageal opening; lateral knee pain; weakness and aching in the lower leg; red, painful eyes; lumbar pain; lower abdominal fullness; pain in the umbilical region; cold feet; difficult evacuation; jaundice; thunderous rumbling in the abdomen; counterflow retching with no food intake; strangury; vacuity taxation edema; profuse, incessant postpartum perspiration; absence of menstruation.

Illustrative Point Combinations & Applications: When walking is difficult or impossible, needle ST-36, LV-4, and LV-3.
(Ode of the Jade Dragon)

HT-7 relieves the stupefied mind when used in conjunction with LV-3. *(Wo Yan's Efficacious Point Applications)*

Stimulation: 0.3-0.5″ perpendicular insertion.
Moxa: 3 cones; pole 3-7 min.
Needle Sensation: Localized numbness and distention.

Point Categories & Associations: Stream-shu (earth) and source-yuan point.

LV-4
中封
zhōng fēng
"Mound Center"

Location: 1″ anterior to the medial malleolus, midway between SP-5 and ST-41, in the depression on the medial side of the tendon of the anterior tibial muscle (m. tibialis anterior).
Classical Location: One inch in front of the inner ankle bone, in the depression between the sinews. *(The Great Compendium)*
Local Anatomy: The dorsal venous network of the foot and the anterior medial malleolar artery. The branch of the medial dorsal cutaneous nerve of the foot and the saphenous nerve.

Functions: Courses the liver and frees the connecting vessels.
Indications: Pain in the genital region; seminal emission; urinary stoppage; hernia.
Supplementary Indications: Genital retraction into the lower abdomen and associated pain; the five stranguries; difficult urination; cold shan; lumbar pain; no pleasure in eating; genital pain.

Stimulation: 0.3″ downward oblique or perpendicular insertion.
Moxa: 3 cones; pole 5-15 min.

Needle Sensation: Localized numbness and distention.

Point Categories & Associations: River-jing (metal) point.

Location: 5.0″ above the tip of the medial malleolus, in a small depression on the medial aspect of the tibia.

Classical Location: Five inches above the inner ankle bone. *(The Great Compendium)*

Local Anatomy: Posteriorly, the great saphenous vein. The branch of the saphenous nerve.

Functions: Courses the liver and rectifies qi; disinhibits damp-heat.

Indications: Irregular menstruation; inhibited urination; hernia; aching and pain in the lower leg.

Supplementary Indications: Scant uterine bleeding; testicular pain and swelling; frequent erection; cold shan; aching and cold in the feet and lower leg; lumbar pain; frequent eructation; swelling and pain in the lower abdomen; white vaginal discharge; vaginal protrusion.

Stimulation: 0.2-0.5″ backward oblique insertion. Moxa: 3 cones; pole 5-10 min.

Needle Sensation: Localized numbness and distention, sometimes extending up to the knee or the external reproductive organs.

Point Categories & Associations: Connecting-luo point of the liver channel, connecting with the gallbladder channel.

LV-5
蠡溝
lǐ gōu
"Woodworm Canal"

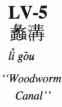

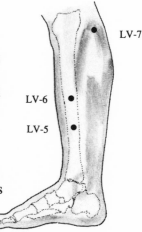

Figure 17.6

Location: 7″ above the tip of the medial malleolus, or 2″ above LI-5, on the medial aspect and near the medial border of the tibia.

Classical Location: Two inches directly above LV-5, at the midpoint on the length of the tibia. *(The Great Compendium)*

Local Anatomy: The great saphenous vein. The branch of the saphenous nerve.

Functions: Frees the channels and connecting vessels; regulates qi and blood; relieves pain.

Indications: Metrorrhagia; hernia.

Supplementary Indications: Profuse uterine bleeding; abdominal pain; continual discharge of lochia; cold in the lower leg; damp bi with an inability to walk; fulminant pain of the genitalia.

LV-6
中都
zhōng dū
"Central Metropolis"

Stimulation: 0.2-0.5 ″ backward oblique insertion.
Moxa: 5 cones; pole 5-10 min.

Point Categories & Associations: Cleft-xi point of the liver
channel.

LV-7
膝關
xī guān

"Knee Joint"

Location: Inferior to the medial condyle of the tibia, in the upper
portion of the medial head of the gastrocnemius muscle (m. gas-
trocnemius), 1 ″ posterior to SP-9.
Classical Location: In the depression two inches below the Inner
Eye of the Knee (M-LE-16). *(The Great Compendium)*
Local Anatomy: At the deeper level, the posterior tibial artery.
The branch of the medial sural cutaneous nerve; deeper, the tibial
nerve.

Functions: Frees the channels and connecting vessels; disinhibits
the joints; dispels wind and relieves pain.
Indications: Medial knee pain.
Supplementary Indications: Pain in the medial aspect of the knee
causing an inability to bend or extend the leg; lower abdominal
pain accompanied by pharyngeal pain; wind bi.
Illustrative Point Combinations & Applications: A red swollen
knee causing an inability to walk requires the needling of
M-LE-16 and LV-7. *(Song of the Jade Dragon)*

Stimulation: 0.3-0.6 ″ perpendicular insertion.
Moxa: 3-5 cones; pole 5 min.

LV-8
曲泉
qū quán

*"Spring at
the Bend"*

Location: On the medial side of the knee joint. When the knee is
bent, the point is posterior to the medial condyle of the tibia and
superior to the border of the tendons of those muscles attaching at
the medial side of the knee.
Classical Location: Above LV-7 at the inside of the knee . . . in
the depression above the larger sinew and below the smaller
sinew. When the knee is flexed the point is found at the [medial]
end of the horizontal crease. *(The Great Compendium)*

Local Anatomy: Anteriorly, the great saphenous vein, on the pathway of the genu suprema artery. The saphenous nerve.

Functions: Clears damp-heat; disinhibits the bladder; drains liver fire; frees the lower burner; soothes the sinews and quickens the connecting vessels; disinhibits the lower burner.

Indications: Prolapse of the uterus; lower abdominal pain; urinary stoppage; genital itch; seminal emission; genital pain; pain in the knee and medial aspect of the upper leg; fright mania.

Supplementary Indications: Swelling and itching of the genitalia; impotence; difficult urination; female blood conglomeration; kui shan; blood block infertility; no pleasure in eating; thin stool diarrhea.

Illustrative Point Combinations & Applications: In treating wind bi or atonic inversion, BL-11 and LV-8 work wonders.
(Song to Keep Up Your Sleeve)

Stimulation: 0.5-0.8″ perpendicular insertion.
Moxa: 3 cones; pole 5-20 min.

Point Categories & Associations: Uniting-he (water) point.

Figure 17.7

Location: 4″ above the medial epicondyle of the femur, between the vastus medialis muscle and the sartorius muscle (m. vastus medialis and m. sartorius).

Classical Location: Four inches above the knee, between the two sinews on the inner face of the thigh.   When the foot is flexed, the groove in which the point is located may be observed.
(The Great Compendium)

Local Anatomy: Deeper, on the lateral side, the femoral artery and vein, the superficial branch of the medial circumflex femoral artery. The anterior femoral cutaneous nerve, on the pathway of the anterior branch of the obturator nerve.

Functions: Courses the liver and rectifies qi; adjusts the penetrating and conception vessels; clears and disinhibits the lower burner.

Indications: Irregular menstruation; inhibited urination; lumbosacral pain referring to the lower abdomen.

Supplementary Indications: Urinary incontinence; lumbar pain accompanied by lower abdominal swelling.

LV-9
陰包
yīn bāo

"Yin Bladder"

Stimulation: 0.6″ perpendicular insertion.
Moxa: 3-7 cones; pole 5-7 min.

LV-10
足五里
(zú) wǔ lǐ

"(Foot) Five Li"

Location: 3″ below ST-30, on the anterior border of the long adductor muscle (m. adductor longus).
Classical Location: Below LV-12 where a pulsating vessel can be felt in the groin, three inches below ST-30.
(The Great Compendium)
Local Anatomy: The superficial branches of the medial circumflex femoral artery and vein. The genitofemoral nerve, the anterior femoral cutaneous nerve; deeper, the anterior branch of the obturator nerve.

Functions: Soothes the sinews and quickens the connecting vessels; clears and disinhibits lower burner damp-heat.
Indications: Lower abdominal distention; inhibited urination.
Supplementary Indications: Wind taxation; cough; respiratory difficulty.

Stimulation: 0.6″ perpendicular insertion.
Moxa: 5 cones; pole 5-10 min.

LV-11
陰廉
yīn lián

"Yin Corner"

Location: 2″ below ST-30, on the anterior border of the long adductor muscle (m. adductor longus).
Classical Location: Below LV-12, two inches below ST-30, located at the pulsating vessel. *(The Great Compendium)*
Local Anatomy: The branches of the medial circumflex femoral artery and vein. The genitofemoral nerve, the branch of the medial femoral cutaneous nerve; deeper, the anterior branch of the obturator nerve.

Functions: Soothes the sinews and quickens the connecting vessels; regulates the penetrating and conception vessels.
Indications: Irregular menstruation; pain in the leg.
Illustrative Point Combinations & Applications: The Great Compendium recommends burning three cones of moxa at this point for infertility in women who have never had children.

Stimulation: 0.5-0.8″ perpendicular insertion.
Moxa: 3 cones; pole 3-5 min.

Location: Lateral to the pubic symphysis, 2.5" from the conception vessel. At the inguinal groove it is lateral and inferior to ST-30.

Classical Location: Above LI-11 and the genitals, two and a half inches either side of the midline. A hardness can be dimly felt under pressure and hard pressure will produce pain that radiates up and down. *(The Golden Mirror)*

Local Anatomy: The branches of the external pudendal artery and vein, the pubic branches of the inferior epigastric artery and vein; laterally, the femoral vein. The ilioinguinal nerve; deeper, in the inferior aspect, the anterior branch of the obturator nerve.

Functions: Frees the channels and dissipates cold.

Indications: Pain in the external genitalia; hernia.

Supplementary Indications: Pain in the penis; shan; prolapse of the uterus; pain in the lower abdomen.

Stimulation: 0.3-0.5" perpendicular insertion.
Moxa: 3-5 cones; pole 5-15 min.

LV-12
急脈
jí mài
"Urgent Pulse"

Location: Below the free end of the eleventh floating rib.

Classical Location: In the region of the free ribs, two inches above the navel and six inches either side of the midline. The point is selected with the patient on his side and the upper leg bent and the lower leg extended. Also; the point is located where the tip of the elbow touches. *(The Great Compendium)*

Local Anatomy: The sixth intercostal artery and vein. The sixth intercostal nerve.

Functions: Courses the liver and rectifies qi; quickens the blood and transforms stasis.

Indications: Vomiting; abdominal swelling; diarrhea; untransformed digestate; lumbar pain; pain in the costal region.

Supplementary Indications: Cold strike throughflux diarrhea; copious urine and white turbid urethral discharge; cold and pain in the back and lumbar region; pain in the lateral costal region;

LV-13
章門
zhāng mén
*"Camphorwood
Gate"*

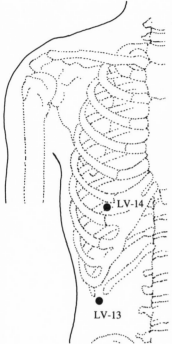

branching fullness in the chest and lateral costal region; all types of accumulations, gatherings, and lump glomi; stone water swelling; yellowing of the body and marked emaciation; heat vexation with no pleasure in eating; dyspnea; cardiac pain and retching; irascibility; diminished qi inversion counterflow; inability to raise the arms and shoulders; saber scrofula; twitching of the body; fetal pressure causing an inability to urinate; enduring jaundice developing into black jaundice; yellowing of the body with darkening of the forehead.

Stimulation: 0.6-1.0" perpendicular insertion.
Moxa: 3 cones; pole 20-50 min.
Needle Sensation: Localized distention, sometimes extending towards the rear abdominal wall.

Point Categories & Associations: Alarm-mu point of the spleen; intersection-jiaohui point of the foot jue yin liver and foot shao yang gallbladder channels; meeting-hui point of the five viscera.

Figure 17.8

LV-14
期門
qí mén

"Cycle Gate"

Location: On the mammillary line, two ribs below the nipple, in the sixth intercostal space.

Classical Location: Two ribs directly below the nipple, one inch and five fen to the side of ST-19. *(The Great Compendium)*

Local Anatomy: The sixth intercostal artery and vein. The sixth intercostal nerve.

Functions: Dispels pathogens and heat from the blood chamber; harmonizes mid-stage patterns; transforms phlegm and disperses stasis; calms the liver and disinhibits qi;

Indications: Pain in the chest and lateral costal region; abdominal distention; thoracic fullness; vomiting; hiccough.

Supplementary Indications: Heat in the chest; swelling of the lateral costal region; cardiac pain; running piglet pattern and abdominal hardness; malarial disease; cold damage with heat entering the blood chamber and excessive menstrual flow; abdominal tightness with respiratory difficulty; postpartum illness; desire to eat despite difficult ingestion; visual dizziness.

Illustrative Point Combinations & Applications: LI-7 and LV-14 govern the treatment of neck stiffness due to cold damage. *(Ode of a Hundred Patterns)*

Stimulation: 0.4″ outward oblique insertion.
Moxa: 5 cones; pole 10-20 min.

Point Categories & Associations: Alarm-mu point of the liver,
intersection-jiaohui point of the foot tai yin spleen channel with the
foot jue yin liver channels and yin linking vessel.

Foot Jue Yin Liver Channel			
Point	**Location**	**Indications**	
		Primary	**Secondary**
*LV-1	Great toe	Hernia enuresis metrorrhagia prolapse of the uterus	Epilepsy
*LV-2	Toe web	Metrorrhagia inhibited urination Headache red, swollen, painful eyes	Wry mouth lateral costal pain epilepsy
*LV-3	Back of foot	Metrorrhagia enuresis hernia headache	Dizziness wry mouth lateral costal pain epilepsy
LV-4	Ankle	Hernia seminal emission inhibited urination	
LV-5	Lower leg	Menstrual disorders vaginal discharge inhibited urination	
LV-6		Hernia metrorrhagia abdominal pain	
LV-7		Knee pain	
*LV-8	Knee	Abdominal pain inhibited urination hernia seminal emission	
LV-9	Upper leg	Enuresis inhibited urination menstrual disorder	
LV-10		Urinary stoppage	
LV-11		Menstrual disorders	
Lower limb: Primarily gynecologic and genital disorders; secondarily intestinal disorders			

Foot Jue Yin Liver Channel (continued)			
Point	**Location**	Indications	
		Primary	**Secondary**
LV-12	Abdomen	Hernia lower abdominal pain	
*LV-13	Free rib region	Abdominal distention diarrhea lateral costal pain	
LV-14	Ribs	Pain and distention of the chest and lateral costal region vomiting	
Abdomen and lateral costal region: Primarily gastric and intestinal disorders; secondarily gynecologic disorders			

18. The Conception Vessel System 任脉

18.1 The Primary Conception Vessel Channel

Pathway: The conception vessel originates in the pelvic cavity, connects with the internal genito-urinary organs, and emerges in the perineum at CV-1. It ascends through the region of the pubic hair and then runs up the midline of the abdomen, chest, and neck to the mentolabial groove beneath the lower lip. Here it splits into two branches that contour the mouth and ascend to the infraorbital region.

A second course arises in the pelvic cavity, enters the spine and ascends up the back.

Basic functions:

The conception vessel is the sea of the yin channels. The three yin channels of the foot all join the conception vessel, allowing their bilateral courses to communicate. In this way, the conception vessel has a regulating effect on the yin channels, for which reason it is said that it regulates all the yin channels of the body.

The conception vessel regulates menstruation and nurtures the fetus. Thus it is said, "The conception vessel governs the fetus."

Main pathologic signs:

Menstrual irregularities, menstrual block, white vaginal discharge, miscarriage, sterility, shan qi, enuresis, and abdominal masses.

18.2 The Connecting Vessel of the Conception Vessel

This connecting vessel separates from the primary channel at CV-15 and disperses downward over the abdomen.

Main pathologic signs:

Repletion: abdominal stasis pain.

Vacuity: itching.

345

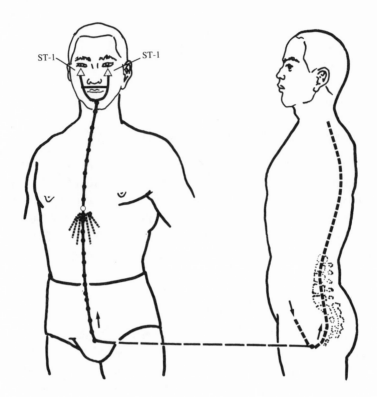

Figure 18.1 - 18.2 Primary channel and connecting vessel of the conception vessel.

Key to Symbols

▪▪▪▪	Internal pathway
────	External pathway
⁄⁄⁄⁄	Channel branch pathway
▮▮▮▮▮	Secondary pathway
◢	Connecting vessel pathway
▪▪▪▪▪▪▪	Connecting vessel pathway
◆	Connection with home organ
◇	Connection with paired organ
○	Connecting-luo point
△	Intersection-jiaohui point
■	Lower uniting-he Point

Location: In the center of the perineum.   It is between the anus and the scrotum in males and between the anus and the posterior labial commissure in females.

Classical Location: Midway between the genitals and the anus. *(The Great Compendium)*

Local Anatomy: The branches of the perineal artery and vein. The branch of the perineal nerve.

Functions: Strengthens the lumbus and boosts the kidney; regulates the penetrating and conception vessels; clears heat and disinhibits damp.

Indications: Genital itch; irregular menstruation; pain and swelling of the anus; urinary stoppage; enuresis; seminal emission; mania and withdrawal.

Supplementary Indications: Genital sweating; pain at the head of the penis; postpartum stupor; vaginal protrusion; pain and swelling of the vagina; enduring hemorrhoids; inability to urinate and defecate; cold at the end of the penis; heat in the portals; sudden infantile epilepsy; shan qi; connecting vessel repletion: abdominal skin pain; connecting vessel vacuity; itch.

Stimulation: 0.5-1.0″ perpendicular insertion.
Moxa: 3 cones; pole 10-20 min.

Point Categories & Associations: Intersection-jiaohui point of the conception, governing, and penetrating vessels.

CV-1
會陰
huì yīn
"Meeting of Yin"

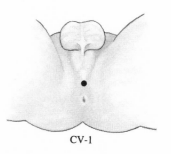

CV-1

Figure 18.3

Location: On the anterior midline just above the pubic symphysis, 5.0″ below the umbilicus.

Classical Location: Directly above CV-1, above the transverse bone, in the depression at the pubic hairline where the pulsating vessel may be sensed through palpation, five inches below the navel. *(The Golden Mirror)*

Local Anatomy: The branches of the inferior epigastric artery and the obturator artery. The branch of the iliohypogastric nerve.

CV-2
曲骨
qū gǔ
"Curved Bone"

347

Functions: Warms yang and supplements the kidney; regulates the menses and stops vaginal discharge.

Indications: Seminal emission; impotence; vaginal discharge; urinary block; hernia.

Supplementary Indications: Seminal loss; vacuity exhaustion of the five viscera; red and white vaginal discharge; impotence; dribbling urination; shan pain; distention and fullness of the lower abdomen; lower abdominal pain; fetal pressure causing an inability to urinate; dryness and pain in the genitals; water swelling; cholera with cramps.

Stimulation: 0.3-1.5″ perpendicular insertion.
Moxa: 3-10 cones; pole 10-20 min.

Needle Sensation: Aching and distention extending down towards the external reproductive organs.

Point Categories & Associations: Intersection-jiaohui point of the foot jue yin liver channel and the conception vessel.

CV-3
中極
zhōng jí
"Central Pole"

Location: On the anterior midline, 4″ below the umbilicus, 1″ above the upper border of the pubic symphysis.

Classical Location: Directly above CV-2, four inches below the navel. *(The Golden Mirror)*

Local Anatomy: The branches of the superficial epigastric and inferior epigastric arteries and veins. The branch of the iliohypogastric nerve.

Functions: Regulates the blood chamber; warms the palace of essence; disinhibits the bladder; rectifies the lower burner.

Indications: Seminal emission; enuresis; urinary stoppage; urinary frequency; lower abdominal pain; irregular menstruation; metrorrhagia; vaginal discharge; prolapse of the uterus; genital pain; genital itch.

Supplementary Indications: Menstrual block; profuse uterine bleeding; red and white vaginal discharge; persistent flow of lochia; retention of afterbirth; shan; water swelling; running piglet rushing up to the heart (if severe, causing respiratory difficulty) ; vacuity exhaustion of yang qi; white turbid urethral discharge; heat and pain in the abdomen; deathlike inversion; pain and vexation in the heart; hunger with inability to eat; swelling and pain of the cervical canal (child gate); lower origin vacuity and cold; infertility.

Stimulation: 0.5-1.5 ″ perpendicular insertion.
Moxa: 7-15 cones; pole 10-20 min.
Needle Sensation: Aching and distention following the course of
the conception vessel down to the external reproductive organs.

Point Categories & Associations: Alarm-mu point of the bladder;
intersection-jiaohui point of the three yin channels of the foot and
the conception vessel.

Location: On the anterior midline of the abdomen, 3 ″ below the
umbilicus.

Classical Location: Three inches below the navel.
(The Great Compendium)

Local Anatomy: The branches of the superficial epigastric and
inferior epigastric arteries and veins. The anterior cutaneous
nerve of the subcostal nerve.

CV-4
關元
guān yuǎn
"Origin Pass"

Functions: Banks the kidney and secures the root; supplements qi
and returns yang; warms and regulates the blood chamber and the
palace of essence; dispels cold damp and eliminates cold in the
genitals; separates the clear and turbid; regulates original qi and
dissipates pathogens; safeguards health and prevents disease.

Indications: Seminal emission; enuresis; urinary frequency; urinary stoppage; menstrual disorders; menalgia; painful menstruation, menstrual block and other menstrual disorders; vaginal
discharge; scant metrorrhagia; prolapse of the uterus; postpartum
hemorrhage; hernia; lower abdominal pain; diarrhea; wind strike
desertion patterns; impotence.

Supplementary Indications: Sudden strike desertion patterns; all
forms of vacuity detriment; conglomerations and gatherings; infertility; persistent flow of lochia; subumbilical gripping pain gradually extending to the genitals; hematuria; rough urination with
dark-colored urine; kidney inversion headache; summerheat
strike; dizziness and headache; running piglet pattern; cold qi
entering the lower abdomen; water swelling; fulminant disruption;
kidney vacuity dyspnea; bowstring and elusive masses; hemafecia;
wasting thirst disease.

Illustrative Point Combinations & Applications: In cases of strain
leading to damage of kidney qi [shan qi], needle CV-4 and LV-1.
(Song of the Jade Dragon)

Infertility is treated through CV-7, CV-5, and CV-4.
(Ode of a Hundred Patterns)

Stimulation: 0.5-1.5″ perpendicular insertion.
Moxa: 7-14 cones; pole 20-30 min.
Needle Sensation: Generally characterized by distention and numbness following the course of the conception vessel downward to the perineum and the external reproductive organs; may also extend laterally above or below the point.

Contraindications: This point is contraindicated for acupuncture during pregnancy.

Point Categories & Associations: Alarm-mu point of the small intestine; intersection-jiaohui point of the three foot yin channels (spleen, liver and kidney) and the conception vessel.

CV-5
石門
shí mén

"Stone Gate"

Location: On the anterior midline, 2″ below the umbilicus.
Classical Location: Directly above CV-4, two inches below the navel. *(The Golden Mirror)*
Local Anatomy: The branches of the superficial epigastric and inferior epigastric arteries and veins. The anterior cutaneous branch of the eleventh intercostal nerve.

Functions: Warms the kidney and invigorates yang; regulates the menses and treats vaginal discharge.
Indications: Scant metrorrhagia; vaginal discharge; amenorrhea; postpartum hemorrhage; hernia; abdominal pain; diarrhea; urinary stoppage; enuresis; edema.
Supplementary Indications: Concretions and conglomerations; no desire for food; untransformed stool; scrotal retraction; counterflow vomiting; constipation; mammary disease.

Note: *The Great Compendium, Bronze Statue* and *The Glorious Anthology of Acupuncture* all state that this point "may not be needled on women, if it is needled they will be rendered incapable of bearing children for life." There are, however, patterns for which it is appropriate to needle women at this point, and it may be used in such cases.

Stimulation: 0.5-0.8″ perpendicular insertion.
Moxa 7 cones; pole 20-30 min.

Needle Sensation: Generally characterized by distention extending along the course of the conception vessel to the genital area.

Contraindications: This point is contraindicated for acupuncture during pregnancy.

Point Categories & Associations: Alarm-mu point of the triple burner.

Location: On the anterior midline, 1.5″ below the umbilicus.
Classical Location: In the depression one inch and five fen below the navel. *(The Great Compendium)*
Local Anatomy: See CV-5.

CV-6
氣海
qì hǎi
"Sea of Qi"

Functions: Regulates qi and boosts the origin; banks the kidney and supplements vacuity; harmonizes construction-blood; treats menstrual disorders and vaginal discharge; warms the lower burner; dispels damp turbidity.

Indications: Metrorrhagia; vaginal discharge; irregular menstruation; postpartum hemorrhage; hernia; enuresis; abdominal pain; diarrhea; constipation; edema; wind-strike desertion patterns.

Supplementary Indications: Cold damage periumbilical pain; yin pattern testicular retraction; yang desertion; inversion frigidity of the limbs; organ qi vacuity fatigue; insufficiency of true qi; lumbar pain; urinary incontinence in children; cardialgia; sudden strike desertion patterns; pain throughout the organs and viscera; rough micturition with dark urine; infertility; summerheat strike.

Illustrative Point Combinations & Applications: For rapid, dyspneic breathing that hampers sleep, and causes worry day and night, drain CV-21 and also treat the sea of qi (CV-6) and all will be right. *(Song of the Jade Dragon)*

Stimulation: 0.8-1.2″ perpendicular insertion.
Moxa: 5-14 cones; pole 20-30 min.
Needle Sensation: Generally characterized by a sensation of distention following the course of the conception vessel down to the external reproductive organs, or upward or downward lateral extension.

351

Figure 18.4   Points on the **Conception Vessel** Channel

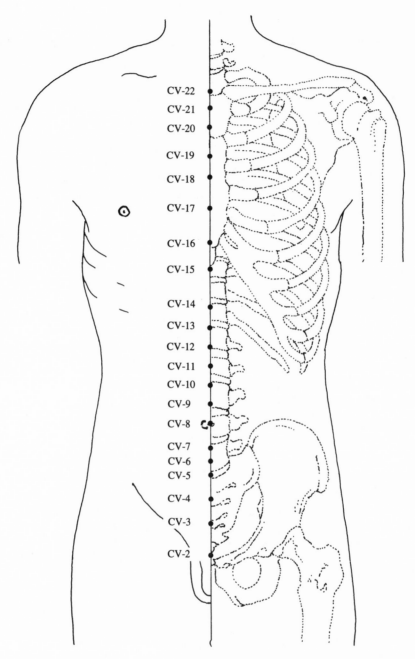

Figure 18.6

Location: On the anterior midline, 1 ″ below the umbilicus.

Classical Location: One inch below the umbilicus, even with the upper border of the bladder. *(The Great Compendium)*

Local Anatomy: The branches of the superficial epigastric and inferior epigastric arteries and veins. The anterior cutaneous branch of the tenth intercostal nerve.

Functions: Warms and supplements kidney yang; regulates the menses and the blood.

Indications: Metrorrhagia; vaginal discharge; irregular menstruation; genital itch; periumbilical pain; hernia; postpartum hemorrhage.

Supplementary Indications: Running piglet pattern; vacuity desertion; fecal and urinary stoppage; water swelling; nosebleed; postpartum non-contraction of the delivery gate; non-closure of the fontanels in infants.

Illustrative Point Combinations & Applications: Infertility is treated through CV-7 and KI-18. *(Ode of a Hundred Patterns)*

For glomus and fullness in the chest and diaphragm, needle first CV-7, then BL-57, and ingestion of food and drink will again be a pleasure. *(The Secrets of the Celestial Star)*

Stimulation: 0.8-1.2 ″ perpendicular insertion.
Moxa: 5 cones; pole 20-30 min.

Needle Sensation: Generally characterized by a sensation of distention and numbness following the course of the conception vessel downward to the external reproductive organs, or lateral extensions.

Point Categories & Associations: Intersection-jiaohui point of the conception and penetrating vessels.

CV-7
陰交
yīn jiāo
"Yin Intersection"

Location: In the center of the umbilicus.

Classical Location: In the center of the navel.
(The Great Compendium)

Local Anatomy: The inferior epigastric artery and vein. The anterior cutaneous branch of the tenth intercostal nerve.

CV-8
神闕
shén què
"Spirit Tower Gate"

353

Functions: Warms and frees the original yang; opens the portals and restores consciousness; moves gastrointestinal qi; transforms cold-damp accumulating stagnations.

Indications: Wind strike desertion patterns; borborygmi; abdominal pain; incessant diarrhea; prolapse of the rectum.

Supplementary Indications: The five stranguries; vacuity desertion; infantile diarrhea after breast feeding; water swelling and drum distention; periumbilical pain; heat-bind urinary stoppage.

Illustrative Point Combinations & Applications: In treating yin patterns and extreme cold, when hot drugs are to no avail, and when the patient presents with inversion frigidity of the hands and feet, scrotal retraction, and tightly clenched jaws, and death appears imminent, burn a large cone of moxa at the center of the umbilicus. *(Recovery from the Myriad Illnesses)*

Stimulation: Moxa: 7-14 cones moxibustion on salt; pole 20-30 min.

Contraindications: This point is contraindicated for acupuncture.

CV-9
水分
shuǐ fēn
"Water Divide"

Location: On the anterior midline, 1″ above the umbilicus.
Classical Location: Directly above CV-8, one inch above the navel. *(The Golden Mirror)*
Local Anatomy: See CV-8.

Functions: Moves spleen-earth and disinhibits water-damp.

Indications: Intestinal rumbling; abdominal pain; edema.

Supplementary Indications: Gastric reflux food vomiting; through-flux diarrhea; tetany; choleraic cramps; prolapse of the rectum; inhibited defecation and urination; failure of the fontanel to close.

Illustrative Point Combinations & Applications: For intolerable water-related diseases that present with abdominal fullness and vacuity swelling that refuses to abate, first moxa CV-9 and ST-28, then needle ST-36 and CV-7. *(Song of the Jade Dragon)*

SP-9 and CV-9 relieve the umbilical fullness associated with water swelling. *(Ode of a Hundred Patterns)*

Stimulation: 0.5-1.0″ perpendicular insertion.
Moxa: 5-7 cones; pole 10-20 min.

Contraindications: In older texts, this point is contraindicated for acupuncture in cases of swelling and distention (use moxa).

Location: On the anterior midline, 2″ above the umbilicus.

Classical Location: Directly above CV-9, two inches above the navel. *(The Golden Mirror)*

Local Anatomy: See CV-8.

CV-10
下脘
xià guǎn
"Lower Venter"

Functions: Assists movement and transformation in the stomach and intestines; disperses digestate accumulations and qi stagnation.

Indications: Stomach pain; abdominal distention; dysenteric disease; borborygmi; vomiting; untransformed digestate.

Supplementary Indications: No pleasure in eating; dark-colored urine; abdomen hardness; lump glomi; cold bowel qi.

Illustrative Point Combinations & Applications: CV-12 and CV-10 treat abdominal hardness. *(Ode of Spiritual Light)*

Stimulation: 0.8-1.2″ perpendicular insertion.
Moxa: 5-7 cones; pole 20-30 min.

Needle Sensation: Generally characterized by a sensation of distention or heaviness; sometimes localized, sometimes extending upwards or downwards, and sometimes extending laterally to both sides.

Contraindications: This point is contraindicated for moxibustion in cases of pregnancy.

Point Categories & Associations: Intersection-jiaohui point of the foot tai yin spleen channel and the conception vessel.

Location: On the anterior midline, 3″ above the umbilicus.

Classical Location: Directly above CV-10, three inches above the navel. *(The Great Compendium)*

Local Anatomy: The branches of the superior and inferior epigastric arteries. The anterior cutaneous branch of the eighth intercostal nerve.

CV-11
建里
jiàn lǐ
*"Interior
    Strengthening"*

Functions: Moves the spleen and rectifies qi; harmonizes the stomach and disperses accumulation; transforms damp and loosens the center.

Indications: Stomach pain; vomiting; loss of appetite; abdominal distention; edema.

Supplementary Indications: Abdominal distention with counter-flow qi ascent; true cardiac pain; counterflow retching; no desire for food; abdominal pain and intestinal rumbling; fullness of the venter.

Illustrative Point Combinations & Applications: CV-11 and PC-6 sweep away bitterness in the chest. *(Ode of a Hundred Patterns)*

Stimulation: 0.5-1.0″ perpendicular insertion.
Moxa: 5-7 cones; pole 20-30 min.

CV-12
中脘
zhōng guǎn

"Central Venter"

Location: On the anterior midline, 4″ above the umbilicus.

Classical Location: Directly above CV-11, four inches above the navel. *(The Golden Mirror)*

Local Anatomy: The superior epigastric artery and vein. The anterior cutaneous branch of the seventh intercostal nerve.

Functions: Harmonizes the stomach and downbears counterflow; fortifies the spleen and disinhibits damp.

Indications: Stomach pain; abdominal distention; gastric reflux and acid regurgitation; vomiting; diarrhea; dysenteric disease; untransformed digestate.

Supplementary Indications: Abdominal pain; abdominal fullness; abdominal rumbling; stomach pain; scorched stench in the nose; difficult defecation; yellow or dark-colored urine; loss of taste; cholera; deathlike inversion; urgent or chronic fright wind; damage due to preoccupation; cardiac pain; generalized swelling; vacuity taxation and blood ejection; mania and withdrawal; jaundice; running piglet pattern; postpartum blood dizziness; endogenous damage to the spleen and stomach.

Illustrative Point Combinations & Applications: For sudden abdominal fullness that does not give under pressure, choose the connecting-luo point of the hand tai yang stomach channel (ST-40) and the alarm-mu point of the stomach (CV-12).
(Essential Questions)

CV-13 and CV-12 treat the nine types of cardiac pain.
(Song of the Jade Dragon)

To treat phlegm, first needle CV-12, then ST-36.
(Song of Needle Practice)

Stimulation: 0.8-1.5″ perpendicular insertion.
Moxa: 7-14 cones; pole 20-30 min.
Needle Sensation: Generally characterized by a sensation of distention, numbness, or heat following the course of the conception vessel upward and downward, or laterally downward.

Point Categories & Associations: Intersection-jiaohui point of the hand tai yang small intestine, hand shao yang triple burner, and foot yang ming stomach channels, and the conception vessel; alarm-mu point of the stomach; one of the nine needles for returning yang; meeting-hui point of the six bowels.

Location: On the anterior midline, 5″ above the umbilicus.
Classical Location: Directly above CV-12, five inches above the navel. *(The Golden Mirror)*
Local Anatomy: See CV-12.

CV-13
上脘
shàng guǎn
"Upper Venter"

Functions: Rectifies the spleen and the stomach; transforms phlegm turbidity; courses qi; stabilizes the spirit-disposition.
Indications: Stomach pain; gastric reflux; vomiting; epilepsy.
Supplementary Indications: Abdominal distention qi fullness; fright palpitations; inability to eat; periodic retching of blood; copious phlegm and drool; running piglet pattern; sudden cardiac pain; wind epilepsy heat disease; visual dizziness; headache and dizziness; body fever with or without perspiration; cholera; accumulations and gatherings; abdominal fullness and intestinal rumbling; heat vexation in the heart; jaundice; stomach vacuity fullness and distention.
Illustrative Point Combinations & Applications: Manic running amok is treated through CV-13 and HT-7.
(Ode of a Hundred Patterns)

Stimulation: 0.8-1.5″ perpendicular insertion.
Moxa: 5-7 cones; pole 20-30 min.
Needle Sensation: Generally characterized by distention and numbness extending up and down along the course of the conception vessel, or extending laterally.

Point Categories & Associations: Intersection-jiaohui point of the foot yang ming stomach and hand tai yang small intestine channels and the conception vessel.

CV-14

巨闕

jù què

"Great Tower Gate"

Location: On the anterior midline, 6″ above the umbilicus.

Classical Location: Directly above the umbilicus, two inches below the joining of the ribs. *(The Golden Mirror)*

Local Anatomy: See CV-12.

Functions: Disperses congealed phlegm in the chest and diaphragm; transforms damp stagnation in the central burner; clears the heart and stabilizes the spirit; rectifies qi and frees the center.

Indications: Cardiothoracic pain; gastric reflux and acid regurgitation; esophageal constriction; nausea; vomiting; mania and withdrawal; epilepsy; palpitations .

Supplementary Indications: Qi ascent counterflow cough; fullness in the chest and shortness of breath; back pain; chest pain; stoppage glomus; cholera; fright palpitations; abdominal distention with fulminant pain; vexation in cold damage; phlegm-rheum water ejection; cold in the stomach; periodic spitting of blood; clonic spasm accompanied by abdominal pain; vulpine shan; raving and manic rage; chest pain extending to the lateral costal region; jaundice; impaired memory.

Illustrative Point Combinations & Applications: For diaphragmatic pain accompanied by rheum accumulations, needle CV-17 and CV-14. *(Ode of a Hundred Patterns)*

Stimulation: 0.3-0.8″ perpendicular insertion.

Moxa: 5-9 cones; pole 20-30 min.

Needle Sensation: Generally characterized by distention and numbness extending up and down along the course of the conception vessel, or extending laterally.

Point Categories & Associations: Alarm-mu point of the heart.

CV-15

鳩尾

jiū wěi

"Turtledove Tail"

Location: On the anterior midline, 7″ above the umbilicus, ideally below the xiphoid process. (In the case of a long xiphoid, CV-14 is used as the reference.)

Classical Location: One inch above CV-14. *(The Golden Mirror)*

Local Anatomy: See CV-12.

Functions: Loosens the chest and rectifies qi; transforms phlegm and suppresses cough; harmonizes the stomach and downbears counterflow; clears heat and extinguishes wind.

Indications: Cardiothoracic pain; gastric reflux; mania and withdrawal; epilepsy.

Supplementary Indications: Fullness in the chest; counterflow cough; blood ejection; wheezing and dyspnea; gripping pain in the heart; epilepsy; manic disease; abdominal swelling; unilateral headache extending to the outer canthus; fright palpitations; adolescent sexual taxation; shortness of breath; diminished qi; throat bi; difficult ingestion of fluids; prolapse of the rectum; sudden unchecked blood ejection; cold damage chest bind.

Illustrative Point Combinations & Applications: SI-3, CV-15 and HT-7 treat the five epilepsies. *(Song More Precious than Jade)*

Stimulation: 0.3-0.5″ perpendicular insertion (avoid deep insertion). Moxa: 3-5 cones; pole 10-30 min.

Point Categories & Associations: Connecting-luo point of the conception vessel.

Location: On the midline, level with the fifth intercostal space.

Classical Location: In the depression one inch directly above CV-15. *(The Golden Mirror)*

Local Anatomy: The perforating branches of the internal mammary artery and vein. The anterior cutaneous branch of the sixth intercostal nerve.

CV-16
中庭

zhōng tíng

"Central Palace"

Functions: Loosens the chest and rectifies qi; downbears counterflow and harmonizes the center.

Indications: Distention and fullness in the chest; esophageal constriction.

Supplementary Indications: Fullness in the chest and lateral costal region; sore pharynx; difficult ingestion; esophageal blockage; vomiting and gastric reflux; vomiting of breast milk; cardiac pain.

Stimulation: 0.3″ downward oblique insertion.
Moxa: 3-5 cones; pole 5-20 min.

CV-17
膻中
shān zhōng

"Chest Center"

Location: On the anterior midline, between the nipples, level with the fourth intercostal space.

Classical Location: One inch and six fen directly above CV-16. *(The Golden Mirror)*

Local Anatomy: The perforating branches of the internal mammary artery and vein. The anterior cutaneous branch of the fourth intercostal nerve.

Functions: Regulates qi and downbears counterflow; clears the lung and transforms phlegm; loosens the chest and disinhibits the diaphragm.

Indications: Dyspnea; hiccough; chest pain; lactation insufficiency.

Supplementary Indications: Wheezing dyspnea and shortness of breath; cough and blood ejection; spitting of blood; chest pain; goiter; vomiting of foamy drool; deathlike inversion; sudden pain and vexation; heart palpitations with sorrow and fear.

Illustrative Point Combinations & Applications: CV-22 and CV-17 treat dyspnea and cough. *(Song of the Jade Dragon)*

Stimulation: 0.3-0.5″ downward oblique insertion.
Moxa: 5-9 cones; pole 3-5 min.

Note: When needling this point it is best to insert the needle horizontally just under the skin; in most cases moxibustion is used rather than acupuncture.

Needle Sensation: Generally characterized by localized distention.

Point Categories & Associations: Meeting-hui point of the qi; intersection-jiaohui point of the foot tai yin spleen, foot shao yin kidney, hand tai yang small intestine, and hand shao yang triple burner channels and the conception vessel; alarm-mu point of the pericardium.

CV-18
玉堂
yù táng

"Jade Hall"

Location: On the anterior midline, level with the third intercostal space.

Classical Location: In the depression one inch and six fen directly above CV-17.

Local Anatomy: The perforating branches of the internal mammary artery and vein. The anterior cutaneous branch of the third intercostal nerve.

Functions: Loosens the chest and rectifies qi; suppresses cough and dispels phlegm.

Indications: Cough; dyspnea; chest pain.

Supplementary Indications: Vomiting and vexation; pain in the anterior chest; dyspnea with fullness; vomiting and phlegm congestion; qi ascent; pain in the lateral costal region.

Stimulation: 0.2-0.3″ downward oblique insertion.
Moxa: 5 cones; pole 5-20 min.

CV-19
紫宮
zǐ gōng
"Purple Palace"

Location: On the anterior midline, level with the second intercostal space.

Classical Location: In the depression one inch and six fen directly above CV-18. *(The Golden Mirror)*

Local Anatomy: The perforating branches of the internal mammary artery and vein. The anterior cutaneous branch of the second intercostal nerve.

Functions: Loosens the chest and rectifies qi; suppresses cough and disinhibits the throat.

Indications: Cough; dyspnea; chest pain.

Supplementary Indications: Fullness and pain in the chest and lateral costal region; vexation; blood ejection; glue-like spittle; difficult ingestion of food and drink.

Stimulation: 0.3″ downward oblique insertion.
Moxa: 5 cones; pole 5-20 min.

CV-20
華蓋
huá gài
"Florid Canopy"

Location: On the anterior midline, at the level of the first intercostal space.

Classical Location: In the depression one inch and six fen directly above CV-19. *(The Golden Mirror)*

Local Anatomy: The perforating branches of the internal mammary artery and vein. The anterior cutaneous branch of the first intercostal nerve.

Functions: Loosens the chest, disinhibits the diaphragm; clears the lung and stops cough.

Indications: Dyspnea; cough; chest pain.

Supplementary Indications: Fullness and pain in the chest and lateral costal region; counterflow cough and qi ascent; blood ejection; throat bi; swollen pharynx; difficult ingestion of fluids.

Illustrative Point Combinations & Applications: For pain amongst
the ribs; ST-13 and CV-20 work miracles.
(Ode of a Hundred Patterns)

Stimulation: 0.3″ downward oblique insertion.
Moxa: 5 cones; pole 5-20 min.

CV-21
璇璣

xuán jī

"Jade Pivot"

Location: On the anterior midline, midway between CV-22 and
CV-20. At the center of the manubrium.

Classical Location: In the depression one inch directly above
CV-20. *(The Golden Mirror)*

Local Anatomy: The perforating branches of the internal mammary artery and vein. The medial supraclavicular nerve and the
anterior cutaneous branch of the first intercostal nerve.

Functions: Loosens the chest and rectifies qi; suppresses cough
and downbears counterflow.

Indications: Cough; dyspnea; chest pain.

Supplementary Indications: Fullness and pain in the chest and
lateral costal region; laryngeal bi; swollen pharynx; difficult
ingestion of fluids; hot, red facial skin in infants; pulmonary yong.

Illustrative Point Combinations & Applications: For accumulations within the stomach, needling CV-21 and ST-36 is more
effective than people think. *(Ode of Xi Hong)*

Stimulation: 0.3″ downward oblique insertion.
Moxa: 5 cones; pole 5-20 min.

Location: On the anterior midline in the center of the suprasternal notch.

Classical Location: One inch directly above CV-21. *(The Golden Mirror)*

Local Anatomy: Superficially, the jugular arch and the branch of the inferior thyroid artery; deeper, the trachea; inferiorly, at the posterior aspect of the sternum, the inominate vein and aortic arch.

Functions: Diffuses the lung and transforms phlegm; disinhibits the pharynx and restores the voice.

Indications: Cough; dyspnea; sudden loss of voice; sore, swollen throat; hiccough.

Supplementary Indications: Fulminant dyspnea and counterflow cough; expectoration of pus and blood; pharyngeal swelling; esophageal constriction; frog rattle in the throat; early stages of goiter; vomiting; swelling at the back of the neck and shoulder pain; cardiac pain; dormant papules; generalized insensitivity of the flesh; pulmonary yong.

Illustrative Point Combinations & Applications: CV-22 and CV-17 treat dyspnea and cough. *(Ode of the Jade Dragon)*

Stimulation: 0.5-1.0″ downward oblique insertion following along the inner surface of the sternum. Perpendicular insertion is contraindicated to avoid damage to the trachea.

Moxa: 3-5 cones, pole 5-20 min.

Needle Sensation: Generally characterized by a sensation of heaviness extending downwards along the posterior aspect of the sternum.

Point Categories & Associations: Intersection-jiaohui point of the yin linking and conception vessels.

CV-22
天突
tiān tú
"Celestial Chimney"

CV-23
廉泉
lián quán
''Ridge Spring''

Location: On the anterior midline of the throat, above the Adam's apple, in the depression at the upper border of the hyoid bone.

Classical Location: When the head is tilted back, the point is directly above CV-22, midway between the chin and the Adam's apple, below the root of the tongue. *(The Golden Mirror)*

Local Anatomy: The anterior jugular vein. The branch of the cutaneous cervical nerve, the hypoglossal nerve, and the branch of the glossopharyngeal nerve.

Functions: Disinhibits the throat and eliminates phlegm; clears fire and downbears counterflow.

Indications: Subglossal swelling; sluggish tongue and drooling; stiffness of the tongue with inability to speak; sudden loss of voice; difficulty in swallowing.

Supplementary Indications: Cough and qi ascent; dyspnea and retching of foam; swelling of the subglossal region with difficulty in speech; contraction of the root of the tongue; drooling; wasting thirst; mouth sores; clenched jaws.

Illustrative Point Combinations & Applications: CV-23 and PC-9 may be needled in cases of sublingual swelling and pain.
(Ode of a Hundred Patterns)

Stimulation: With the head tilted back, 0.3-1.0″ upward oblique insertion (with the needle pointed towards GV-17).
Moxa: pole 5-20 min.

Needle Sensation: Generally characterized by a sensation of numbness and distention at the root of the tongue.

Contraindications: Direct moxibustion is contraindicated at this point.

Point Categories & Associations: Intersection-jiaohui point of the yin linking and conception vessels.

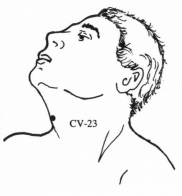

CV-23

Figure 18.5

Location: On the anterior midline, in the depression in the center of the mentolabial groove.

Classical Location: When the mouth is open, the point is in the center of the depression beneath the protrusion of the lower lip. *(The Great Compendium)*

Local Anatomy: The branches of the inferior labial artery and vein. The branch of the facial nerve.

Functions: Dispels wind and frees the connecting vessels; relieves pain and settles tetany; eliminates wind and disperses swelling.

Indications: Wryness of the eyes and mouth; facial swelling; swelling of the gums; toothache; drooling; mania and withdrawal.

Supplementary Indications: Sudden loss of voice; wasting thirst; hemilateral wind.

Illustrative Point Combinations & Applications: For toothache, first supplement or drain at CV-24 [depending on the nature of the pain], then needle GV-16. *(Song of the Jade Dragon)*

Stimulation: 0.2-0.3″ upward oblique insertion.
Moxa: 3-5 cones; pole 5-20 min.

Needle Sensation: Generally characterized by localized aching and distention.

Point Categories & Associations: Intersection-jiaohui point of the foot yang ming stomach and hand yang ming large intestine channels and the conception and governing vessels; 8th of the 13 ghost points.

CV-24
承漿
chéng jiāng
"Sauce Receptacle"

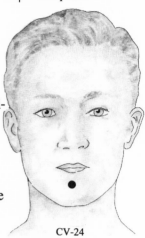

CV-24

Figure 18.7

Conception Vessel			
Point	**Location**	Indications	
		Primary	**Secondary**
CV-1	Perineum	Inhibited urination seminal emission menstrual disorders	Coma
CV-2	Lower abdomen	Inhibited urination enuresis impotence vaginal discharge	
*CV-3		Enuresis inhibited urination seminal emission menstrual disorders	Prolapse of the uterus
*CV-4		Enuresis urinary block diarrhea impotence menstrual disorders	Vacuity taxation
CV-5		Abdominal pain edema diarrhea menstrual block	
*CV-6		Abdominal pain diarrhea enuresis metrorrhagia	Vacuity desertion
CV-7		Abdominal pain edema menstrual disorders	
Lower abdomen: Gynecologic, genital, and intestinal disorders (CV-4 and CV-6 also have a general strengthening effect)			
*CV-8	Umbilicus	Abdominal pain diarrhea	Vacuity desertion
CV-9	Upper abdomen	Urinary stoppage edema diarrhea	
CV-10		Abdominal pain diarrhea vomiting	
CV-11		Stomach pain vomiting loss of appetite	Edema

Point	Location	Indications Primary	Secondary
*CV-12	Upper abdomen	Stomach pain vomiting abdominal distention diarrhea	Mania and withdrawal
CV-13		Stomach pain vomiting	Epilepsy
CV-14		Chest pain palpitations vomiting	Epilepsy mania and withdrawal
CV-15		Chest pain abdominal distention	Epilepsy mania and withdrawal

Conception Vessel (continued)

Upper abdomen: Primarily disorders of the stomach and intestines; secondarily mental disorders

Point	Location	Indications Primary	Secondary
CV-16	Chest	Distention and fullness of the chest and lateral costal region cardiac pain	
*CV-17		Dyspnea chest pain palpitations vomiting	Shortage of breast milk
CV-18		Cough dyspnea chest pain	
CV-19		Cough dyspnea chest pain	
CV-20		Cough dyspnea chest pain	Difficult ingestion
CV-21		Cough dyspnea chest pain	Digestate Accumulation

Chest: Primarily disorders of the chest, heart, and lung; secondarily disorders of the esophagus

Point	Location	Indications	
Conception Vessel (continued)			
Point	**Location**	**Indications**	
*CV-22	Neck	Cough dyspnea sudden loss of voice pain and swelling of the throat	Esophageal constriction
*CV-23		Stiff tongue with inability to speak pain and swelling of the throat	
Neck: Disorders of the tongue and throat			
*CV-24	Chin	Wry mouth toothache	
Chin: Disorders of the mouth and teeth			

19. The Governing Vessel System 督脈

19.1 The Primary Governing Vessel Channel

Pathway: The governing vessel has four courses. According to the *Spiritual Axis,* the main course of this channel originates in the pelvic cavity. Emerging in the perineum at CV-1, it then passes posteriorly to GV-1 at the tip of the coccyx. From this point, it ascends along the spine to GV-16 at the nape of the neck. It enters the brain and ascends to the vertex, emerging at GV-20, continuing forward along the midline to the forehead, running down the nose and across the philtrum to terminate in the upper gum.

The second channel starts in the lower abdomen, and runs down through the genitals into the perineal region. From here it passes through the tip of the coccyx, where it diverts into the gluteal region. Here it intersects both the leg shao yin kidney channel and the leg tai yang bladder channel before returning to the spinal column. It then travels up the spine and links through to the kidney.

A third path starts at the same two bilateral points as the foot tai yang bladder channel at the inner canthi of the eyes. The branches rise up over the forehead to meet at the vertex. The channel then enters the brain and splits into two channels that descend along opposite sides of the spine to the waist, to join with the kidney.

The fourth path starts in the lower abdomen, travels up past the navel, continues upward to join with the heart, then enters the throat, crosses the cheek, splits into two and rounds the lips, and runs up the cheek to the center of the infraorbital region.

Basic functions:

The governing vessel is the sea of the yang channels. All six yang channels converge at the point GV-14. The governing vessel has a regulating effect on the yang channels, so it is said that it governs all the yang channels of the body.

The governing vessel homes to the brain and connects to the kidney. The kidney engenders marrow, and the brain is known as the "sea of marrow." Therefore, the governing vessel reflects the physiology and pathology of the brain and the spinal fluid, and their relationship with the reproductive organs.

Main pathologic signs:

Opisthotonos, malaria, pain and stiffness in the back, child fright-wind, heavy sensation in the head, hemorrhoids, sterility, essence-spirit disorders.

19.2 The Connecting Vessel of the Governing Vessel

Pathway: Breaking from the governing vessel at GV-1 the connecting vessel forms two branches that ascend on either side of the spine to the nape of the neck. These branches then disperse over the head.

In the region of the scapula branches of the connecting vessel connect to the foot tai yang bladder channel and also penetrate into the paravertebral sinews.

Main pathologic signs:

Repletion: stiffness at the spine.

Vacuity: heavy headedness.

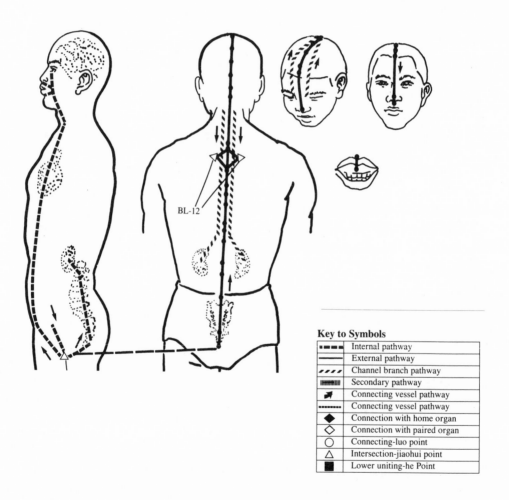

Key to Symbols

▪▪▪▪	Internal pathway
———	External pathway
⁄⁄⁄⁄	Channel branch pathway
▐▟▌	Secondary pathway
➚	Connecting vessel pathway
--------	Connecting vessel pathway
◆	Connection with home organ
◇	Connection with paired organ
○	Connecting-luo point
△	Intersection-jiaohui point
■	Lower uniting-he Point

Figure 19.1 - 19.2 Primary channel and connecting vessel of the governing vessel.

Location: Midway between the coccyx and the anus.

Classical Location: Three fen below the tip of the tail bone. The point is found in prostrate posture. *(The Great Compendium)*

Local Anatomy: The branches of the inferior hemorrhoid artery and vein. The posterior ramus of the coccygeal nerve, the hemorrhoid nerve.

Functions: Courses and regulates localized channel qi; harmonizes yin and yang; rectifies intestinal qi and arrests diarrhea; disperses swelling and relieves pain.

Indications: Hemafecia; diarrhea; constipation; hemorrhoids; prolapse of the rectum; pain in the lumbar spine.

Supplementary Indications: Throughflux diarrhea; bloody stool and the five types of hemorrhoids; seminal emission; fright epilepsy; clonic spasm; mania and withdrawal; retching of blood; turbid strangury; low back pain and stiffness of the spine; difficult defecation and urination; red and white dysentery.

Illustrative Point Combinations & Applications: Moxibustion applied at GV-1 and BL-57 gives miraculous results in treating hemorrhoids. *(Song of the Jade Dragon)*

GV-20 and GV-1 treat dysenteric disease. *(Ode of Spiritual Light)*

Stimulation: 0.5-1.0″ upward oblique or perpendicular insertion. Moxa: 3-15 cones; pole 10-30 min.

Needle Sensation: Localized pain and distention, sometimes extending down to the anus.

Point Categories & Associations: Connecting-luo point of the governing vessel connects to the conception vessel; intersection-jiaohui point of the foot shao yin kidney and foot shao yang gallbladder channels and the governing vessel.

GV-1

長强

cháng qiáng

"Long Strong"

Location: On the posterior midline at the sacral hiatus.

Classical Location: Below the twenty-first vertebra. *(The Golden Mirror)*

Local Anatomy: The branches of the median sacral artery and vein. The branch of the coccygeal nerve.

GV-2

腰俞

yāo shū

"Lumbar Shu"

Functions: Warms the lower burner; expels wind-damp and strengthens the knees and lumbus.

Indications: Irregular menstruation; pain and stiffness of the lumbar spinal column; epilepsy patterns; hemorrhoids; loss of locomotive ability of the lower limbs.

Supplementary Indications: Turbid strangury; enuresis; dark-colored urine; bloody stool; thermic malaria; adiaphoretic fever; pain in the lateral costal region.

Illustrative Point Combinations & Applications: For cold-wind and cold-bi diseases that are difficult to cure, apply acupuncture and moxibustion at GB-30 and GV-2. *(Ode of Xi Hong)*

Stimulation: 0.5-1.0″ upward oblique or perpendicular insertion. Moxa: 3-15 cones; pole 10-30 min.

GV-3
腰陽關

(yāo) yáng guān

"(Lumbar) Yang Pass"

Location: Below the spinous process of the fourth lumbar vertebra.

Classical Location: Below the sixteenth vertebra. *(The Golden Mirror)*

Local Anatomy: The posterior branch of the lumbar artery. The medial branch of the posterior ramus of the lumbar nerve.

Functions: Warms the blood chamber and the palace of essence; dispels cold damp in the lower burner.

Indications: Pain in the lumbosacral region; loss of locomotive ability of the lower limbs; irregular menstruation; seminal emission; impotence.

Supplementary Indications: Red and white vaginal discharge; turbid strangury; intestinal shan pain; dysentery; incessant vomiting; copious drool; knee pain; numbness and insensitivity in the lower limbs.

Stimulation: 0.5-0.8″ insertion slanting slightly to one side. Moxa: 3-7 cones; pole 10-20 min.

GV-4
命門

mìng mén

"Life Gate"

Location: Below the spinous process of the second lumbar vertebra.

Classical Location: Below the fourteenth vertebra. *(The Golden Mirror)*

Local Anatomy: See GV-3.

Functions: Banks the origin and supplements the kidney; secures essence and stops vaginal discharge; soothes the sinews and harmonizes the blood; courses the channels and regulates qi.

Indications: Stiffness of the spinal column; lumbar pain; vaginal discharge; irregular menstruation; impotence; seminal emission; diarrhea.

Supplementary Indications: Headache; tinnitus; aversion to cold and fever without sweating; lumbar and abdominal pain; malarial disease; epilepsy in children; clonic spasm; intestinal shan pain; red and white vaginal discharge; profuse uterine bleeding; white turbid urethral discharge; intestinal wind bleeding; inhibited urination; bleeding hemorrhoids and fistulae; prolapse of the rectum; no food intake.

Illustrative Point Combinations & Applications: For fecal and urinary incontinence in the elderly, apply moxibustion at GV-4 and BL-23. *(Ode of Jade Dragon)*

Stimulation: 0.5-0.8″ sideways and upward oblique insertion. Moxa: 3-15 cones; pole 20-30 min.

Contraindications: This point is contraindicated for moxibustion on patients less than 20 years of age.

Location: Below the spinous process of the first lumbar vertebra.
Classical Location: Below the thirteenth vertebra.
(The Golden Mirror)
Local Anatomy: See GV-3.

GV-5
懸樞
xuán shū
"Suspended Pivot"

Functions: Fortifies the spleen and harmonizes the stomach; strengthens the lumbus and knees.

Indications: Splenogastric vacuity diarrhea; pain and stiffness of the lumbar spine.

Supplementary Indications: Red and white dysentery in children; prolapse of the rectum; abdominal pain; untransformed digestate.

Stimulation: 0.3-0.5″ sideways and upward oblique insertion. Moxa: 3-5 cones; pole 20-30 min.

Figure 19.3　　　　　　　　　　　　　　　　Points on the **Governing Vessel** Channel

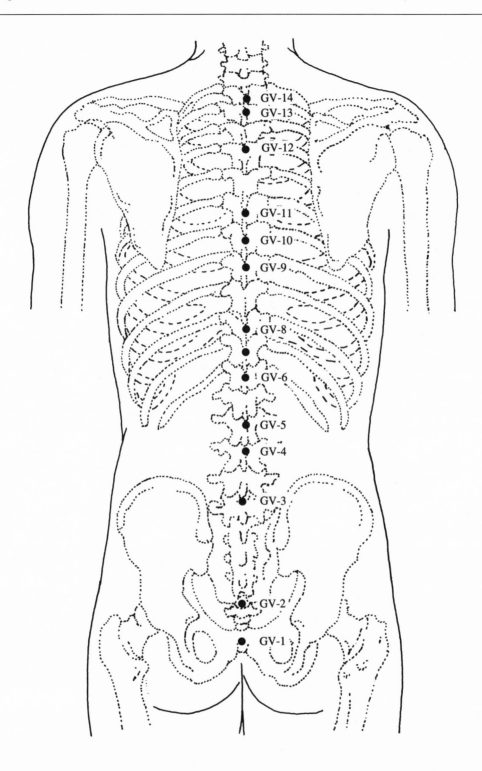

Figure 19.3

Location: Below the spinous process of the eleventh thoracic vertebra.

Classical Location: Below the eleventh vertebra.
(The Golden Mirror)

Local Anatomy: The posterior branch of the eleventh intercostal artery. The medial branch of the posterior ramus of the eleventh thoracic nerve.

Functions: Fortifies the spleen and disinhibits damp; supplements the kidney and stems desertion; strengthens the lumbus.

Indications: Jaundice; diarrhea; epilepsy patterns.

Supplementary Indications: Prolapse of the rectum in children; stomach pain; drum distention; five types of hemorrhoids.

Stimulation: 0.3-0.5″ sideways and upward oblique insertion.

Contraindications: This point is contraindicated for moxibustion.

GV-6
脊中
jǐ zhōng
"Spinal Center"

Location: Below the spinous process of the tenth thoracic vertebra.

Classical Location: Below the tenth vertebra.
(The Golden Mirror)

Local Anatomy: The posterior branch of the tenth intercostal artery. The medial branch of the posterior ramus of the tenth thoracic nerve.

Functions: Supplements the kidney and strengthens the lumbus; harmonizes the stomach and relieves pain.

Indications: Pain in the venter; lumbar pain; stiffness of the spinal column.

Supplementary Indications: Fever and chills; lumbar pain with inability to stoop or bend back; yellowing of the body; abdominal fullness; vomiting with no thought of food; rigidity of the tongue; loss of visual acuity.

Stimulation: 0.3-0.5″ sideways and upward oblique insertion.
Moxa: 3-5 cones; pole 10-20 min.

GV-7
中樞
zhōng shū
"Central Pivot"

GV-8
筋縮
jīn suō

*"Sinew
    Contraction"*

Location: Below the spinous process of the ninth thoracic vertebra.

Classical Location: Below the ninth vertebra.
(The Golden Mirror)

Local Anatomy: The posterior branch of the ninth intercostal artery. The medial branch of the posterior ramus of the ninth thoracic nerve.

Functions: Fortifies the spleen and harmonizes the stomach; strengthens the lumbar and boosts the kidney; relieves pain and quiets the spirit.

Indications: Epilepsy patterns; stiffness of the spinal column; stomach pain.

Supplementary Indications: Madness; dizziness; loss of speech; visceral agitation; pain in the venter; fright epilepsy in children; clonic spasm.

Stimulation: 0.3-0.5 ″ sideways and upward oblique insertion. Moxa: 3-7 cones; pole 5-10 min.

GV-9
至陽
zhì yáng

*"Extremity
    of Yang"*

Location: Below the spinous process of the seventh thoracic vertebra, approximately at the level of the inferior angle of the scapula.

Classical Location: Below the seventh vertebra.
(The Golden Mirror)

Local Anatomy: The posterior branch of the seventh intercostal artery. The medial branch of the posterior ramus of the seventh thoracic nerve.

Functions: Rectifies qi and loosens the chest; clears heat and disinhibits damp; frees the channels and quickens the connecting vessel.

Indications: Cough; dyspnea; jaundice; chest and back pain; stiffness of the spinal column.

Supplementary Indications: Stomach cold; intestinal rumbling; fatigued limbs; fever and chills; aching in the lower legs; diminished qi with difficulty in speaking; branching fullness in the chest and lateral costal region; marked emaciation.

Stimulation: 0.5-0.6" sideways and upward oblique insertion.
Moxa: 3-5 cones; pole 10-20 min.

Needle Sensation: Aching and distention extending laterally
downward, or towards the front of the chest.

Location: Below the spinous process of the sixth thoracic vertebra.

Classical Location: Below the sixth vertebra.
(The Golden Mirror)

Local Anatomy: The posterior branch of the sixth intercostal
artery. The medial branch of the posterior ramus of the sixth
thoracic nerve.

Functions: Diffuses the lung and suppresses cough; frees the
channels and quickens the connecting vessels.

Indications: Cough; dyspnea; back pain and stiffness of the neck;
clove sores.

Supplementary Indications: Wheezing dyspnea and enduring
cough; splenic heat.

Stimulation: 0.3-0.5" sideways and upward oblique insertion.
Moxa: 3-5 cones; pole 10-20 min.

Contraindications: This point is contraindicated for acupuncture
in many texts.

GV-10
靈臺
líng tái
"Spirit Tower"

Location: Below the spinous process of the fifth thoracic vertebra.
Classical Location: Below the fifth vertebra. *(The Golden Mirror)*
Local Anatomy: The posterior branch of the fifth intercostal
artery. The medial branch of the posterior ramus of the fifth
thoracic nerve.

Functions: Settles tetany and extinguishes wind; quiets the heart
and spirit; dispels wind and relieves pain.

Indications: Impaired memory; fright palpitations; cardiac pain;
pain and stiffness in the back and spinal column; cough.

Supplementary Indications: Body fever and headache; impaired
memory; wind epilepsy and clonic spasm in children; malaria; dis-
traction, sorrow, and worry.

GV-11
神道
shén dào
"Spirit Path"

Stimulation: 0.3-0.5″ sideways and upward oblique insertion. Moxa: 3-7 cones; pole 5-10 min.

Contraindications: In many texts this point is contraindicated for acupuncture.

GV-12
身柱
shēn zhù
''Body Pillar''

Location: Below the spinous process of the third thoracic vertebra.

Classical Location: Below the third vertebra. *(The Golden Mirror)*

Local Anatomy: The posterior branch of the third intercostal artery. The medial branch of the posterior ramus of the third thoracic nerve.

Functions: Dispels pathogens and abates fever; clears the heart and stabilizes the disposition; supplements the lung and clears construction.

Indications: Cough; dyspnea; epilepsy patterns; pain and stiffness of the lumbar spinal column; clove sores.

Supplementary Indications: Clonic spasm; vacuity taxation cough; upper portal bleeding; body fever with raving; wind strike with inability to speak; heat in the chest.

Stimulation: 0.3-0.5″ sideways and upward oblique insertion. Moxa: 3-5 cones; pole 20-50 min.

Needle Sensation: Aching and distention extending downward.

GV-13
陶道
táo dào
''Kiln Path''

Location: Below the spinous process of the first thoracic vertebra.

Classical Location: Below the first vertebra. *(The Golden Mirror)*

Local Anatomy: The posterior branch of the first intercostal artery. The medial branch of the posterior ramus of the first thoracic nerve.

Functions: Courses exterior pathogens; clears lung heat; supplements vacuity detriment.

Indications: Stiffness of the spinal column; headache; malaria; heat disease.

Supplementary Indications: Fever and chills; absence of sweating; heavy-headedness and visual dizziness; vacuity taxation; steaming bones.

Stimulation: 0.5 ″ upward oblique insertion.
Moxa: 3-7 cones; pole 10-20 min.

Needle Sensation: Aching and distention, heat, or coolness;
extending downward, upward and toward the shoulders.

Point Categories & Associations: Intersection-jiaohui point of the
governing vessel and the foot tai yang bladder channel.

GV-14
大椎
dà zhuī
"Great Hammer"

Location: Between the spinous processes of the seventh cervical
vertebra and the first thoracic vertebra, approximately at the level
of the shoulder.

Classical Location: Above the first vertebra. *(The Golden Mirror)*

Local Anatomy: The branch of the transverse cervical artery. The
posterior ramus of the eighth cervical nerve and the medial branch
of the posterior ramus of the first thoracic nerve.

Functions: Courses exterior pathogens in the yang channels;
frees yang qi of the whole body; clears the heart and quiets the
spirit; clears lung heat and regulates qi.

Indications: Heat disease; malaria; common cold; steaming bone
tidal fever; cough; dyspnea; stiffness of the neck; tension and stiffness of the spinal column; epilepsy.

Supplementary Indications: Vexation and retching in cold damage
with pronounced fever; fever and chills; cough; pulmonary distention and pain in the lateral costal region; stiffness of the neck;
throat bi; qi fullness and dyspnea; the five taxations and the seven
forms of damage; wind taxation; acute and chronic infantile fright
wind; vacuity perspiration.

Stimulation: 0.5 ″ sideways and upward oblique insertion.
Moxa: 3-15 cones; pole 15-30 min.

Needle Sensation: Aching and distention, heat, or coolness
extending downward, upward and toward the shoulders.

Point Categories & Associations: Intersection-jiaohui point of the
six yang channels and the governing vessel.

GV-15
啞門
yǎ mén
"Mute's Gate"

Location: On the posterior midline, 0.5" below GV-16 in the depression 0.5" within the hairline.

Classical Location: In the depression at the center of the back of the neck, five fen within the hairline. *(The Great Compendium)*

Local Anatomy: The branches of the occipital artery and vein. The third occipital nerve.

Functions: Disinhibits the joints; frees the portals and connecting vessels; clears the spirit-disposition.

Indications: Mania and withdrawal; epilepsy; sudden loss of voice; wind strike with stiffness of the tongue with loss of speech; occipital headache; stiffness of the neck; nosebleed.

Supplementary Indications: Sluggish tongue with loss of speech; dizziness; clonic spasm; deathlike inversion; large scrofulous lumps; phlegm nodules; wind strike.

Illustrative Point Combinations & Applications: GV-15 and TB-1 are important in treating sluggish tongue and inability to speak. *(Ode of a Hundred Patterns)*

Stimulation: 0.4-0.5" perpendicular insertion. This point should not be deeply probed. Moxa: pole 3-5 min.

Needle Sensation: Localized distention and heaviness. If probed deeply into the spinal column, there will be a sensation of electric shock extending to the limbs when the spinal cord is reached.

Contraindications: This point is contraindicated for direct moxibustion.

Point Categories & Associations: Intersection-jiaohui point of the governing vessel and the yang linking vessel; one of the nine points for returning yang.

GV-16
風府
fēng fǔ
"Wind Mansion"

Location: Directly below the external occipital protuberance, in the depression between the attachments of the trapezius muscle (m. trapezius).

Classical Location: One inch above the hairline at the back of the neck; in the depression between the two large sinews. The flesh at the point rises when the patient speaks and sinks back when he ceases talking. *(The Great Compendium)*

Local Anatomy: The branch of the occipital artery. The branches of the third occipital nerve and the great occipital nerve.

Functions: Dispels wind pathogens and dissipates cold; clears the spirit-disposition; disinhibits the joints and drains fire.

Indications: Headache; stiffness of the neck; visual dizziness; nosebleed; sore, swollen throat; wind strike with loss of speech; mania and withdrawal; hemiplegia.

Supplementary Indications: Headache with aversion to cold; loss of voice; jaundice; running amok; head wind and dizziness; wind-cold exterior patterns; lack of sensation in the legs.

Illustrative Point Combinations & Applications: For tai yang disease, first administer Cinnamon Twig Decoction *(guì zhī tāng).* If the agitation is not relieved, then needle GB-20 and GV-16. *(A Treatise on Cold Damage)*

Diseases of the feet and legs are treated through GV-16. *(Song to Keep Up Your Sleeve)*

Stimulation: With the head tilted back, 0.4-0.6″ perpendicular (level, from back to front) insertion. Moxa: pole 3-5 min.

Needle Sensation: Localized distention and heaviness, sometimes extending upward or downward, sometimes causing a sensation of numbness throughout the body.

Contraindications: This point is contraindicated for direct moxibustion.

Point Categories & Associations: Intersection-jiaohui point of the yang linking and governing vessels; the sixth of the thirteen ghost points.

GV-17

腦戶

nǎo hù

"Brain's Door"

Location: 1.5″ above GV-16, superior to the external occipital protuberance.

Classical Location: 1.5″ directly above GV-16, above the occipital bone. *(The Golden Mirror)*

Local Anatomy: The branches of the occipital arteries and veins of both sides. The branch of the great occipital nerve.

Functions: Dispels wind and clears heat; disperses swelling and settles tetany; rouses the brain and opens the portals.

Indications: Epilepsy; dizziness; pain and stiffness of the neck.

Supplementary Indications: Facial swelling with red complexion; yellow eyes; swelling of the head; pain and swelling of the neck; jaundice; bleeding at the root of the tongue; reddening of the eyes; eye pain with unclear vision; loss of voice; clonic spasm.

Stimulation: 0.3″ perpendicular insertion. (See contraindication.) Moxa: pole 2-3 min.

Contraindications: This point is contraindicated for acupuncture in some texts and for direct moxibustion in most.

Point Categories & Associations: Intersection-jiaohui point of the foot tai yang bladder channel and the governing vessel.

GV-18
強間
qiáng jiān
"Unyielding Space"

Location: 1.5″ above GV-17, midway between GV-16 and GV-20.
Classical Location: 1.5″ directly above GV-17.
(The Golden Mirror)
Local Anatomy: See GV-17.

Functions: Calms the liver and extinguishes wind; soothes the sinews and quickens the connecting vessel.
Indications: Mania and withdrawal; headache; visual dizziness; stiffness of the neck.
Supplementary Indications: Vomiting of foamy drool; epilepsy; clonic spasm; pain and stiffness of the neck; insomnia.
Illustrative Point Combinations & Applications: GV-18 and ST-40 treat insufferable headache. *(Ode of a Hundred Patterns)*

Stimulation: 0.2-0.3″ backward transverse insertion.
Moxa: 3-5 cones; pole 5-15 min.

GV-19
後頂
hòu dǐng
"Behind the Vertex"

Location: 1.5″ above GV-18. Or, 1.5″ posterior to GV-20.
Classical Location: One inch and five fen directly above GV-18.
(The Golden Mirror)
Local Anatomy: See GV-17.

Functions: Calms the liver and subdues yang; quiets the heart and spirit.
Indications: Mania and withdrawal; epilepsy; headache; visual dizziness.
Supplementary Indications: Vertex headache; unilateral headache; common cold; clouded or dizzy head.

Stimulation: 0.3 ″ backward transverse insertion.
Moxa: 5-7 cones; pole 5-20 min.

Location: On the mid-saggital line 7 ″ above the posterior hairline, on the midpoint of a line connecting the earlobe and the ear apex, 5 ″ behind the anterior hairline.

Classical Location: One inch and five fen directly above GV-19, in the depression that is in line with the apexes of the ears.
(The Golden Mirror)

Local Anatomy: The anastomotic network formed by the superficial temporal arteries and veins and the occipital arteries and veins of both sides. The branch of the great occipital nerve.

GV-20
百會
bǎi huì
"Hundred Convergences"

Functions: Extinguishes liver wind and subdues liver yang; clears the spirit-disposition and returns inversion; lifts fallen yang qi and discharges blazing heat in the yang channels.

Indications: Mania and withdrawal; wind strike; headache; dizziness; tinnitus; visual dizziness; nasal congestion; prolapse of the rectum.

Supplementary Indications: Fright palpitations; impaired memory; epilepsy; deathlike inversion; deafness; wind dizziness and heavy-headedness; blindness; vertex headache; vaginal protrusion; hemorrhoidal disease; tetany; clenched jaws; hemiplegia; vexation and oppression in the heart; loss of taste.

Illustrative Point Combinations & Applications: For prolapse of the rectum, make haste to GV-20 and GV-1.
(Ode of a Hundred Patterns)

GV-16 and GV-20 are primary points for treating wind disorders.
(Song of Needle Practice)

Stimulation: 0.3 ″ backward transverse insertion.
Moxa: 5-7 cones; pole 5-20 min.

Needle Sensation: Localized distention with numbness or heaviness, extending to the forehead.

Point Categories & Associations: Intersection-jiaohui point of the six yang channels and the governing vessel.

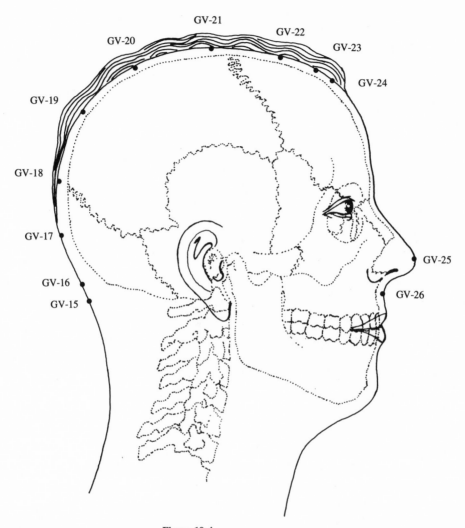

Figure 19.4

GV-21

前頂

qián dǐng

*"Before
  the Vertex"*

Location: On the midline, 1.5″ anterior to GV-20.

Classical Location: One inch and five fen directly in front of
GV-20. *(The Golden Mirror)*

Local Anatomy: The anastomotic network formed by the right and
left superficial temporal arteries and veins. On the communicating
site of the branch of the frontal nerve with the branch of the great
occipital nerve.

Functions: Extinguishes wind and relieves tetany; frees the connecting vessels and disperses swelling; stabilizes the spirit.

Indications: Epilepsy; dizziness; visual dizziness; headache at the top of the head; deep source nasal congestion.

Supplementary Indications: Head wind; facial swelling with red complexion; water swelling; infantile fright epilepsy; clonic spasm; nasal congestion with copious snivel.

Stimulation: 0.3″ backward transverse insertion.
Moxa: 3 cones; pole 5-20 min.

Location: 3″ anterior to GV-20, 2″ posterior to the anterior hairline.

Classical Location: One inch and five fen directly in front of GV-21. *(The Golden Mirror)*

Local Anatomy: The anastomotic network formed by the superficial temporal artery and vein and the frontal artery and vein. The branch of the frontal nerve.

Functions: Calms the liver and extinguishes wind; opens the portals and settles fright.

Indications: Headache; visual dizziness; deep source nasal congestion.

Supplementary Indications: Sudden epilepsy in children; fright epilepsy; swelling of the head and face; nosebleed; nasal congestion; nasal polyps; insomnia or excessive sleeping; headache due to excessive drinking.

Illustrative Point Combinations & Applications: For sudden wind strike, needle GV-22 and GV-20. *(Song of the Jade Dragon)*

Stimulation: 0.3″ backward transverse insertion.
Moxa: 3-5 cones; pole 3-5 min.

Contraindications: This point is contraindicated for acupuncture on children whose fontanels have not yet closed.

GV-22
顖會
xìn huì
"Fontanel Meeting"

Location: 1″ within the anterior hairline, 4″ anterior to GV-20.

Classical Location: Behind GV-24 in the depression one inch within the hairline; it can contain a bean.
(The Great Compendium)

GV-23
上星
shàng xīng
"Upper Star"

385

Local Anatomy: The branches of the frontal artery and vein, the branches of the superficial temporal artery and vein. The branch of the frontal nerve.

Functions: Courses and regulates localized channel qi; dispels wind and brightens the eyes; clears heat and stops bleeding; dissipates pathogens and frees the portals.

Indications: Headache; eye pain; deep source nasal congestion; nosebleed; mania and withdrawal.

Supplementary Indications: Head wind; vacuity swelling of the head and face; nasal polyps; loss of smell; visual dizziness; nearsightedness; absence of sweating in heat diseases.

Illustrative Point Combinations & Applications: For nasal congestion with an inability to smell, LI-20 may be used in conjunction with GV-23. *(Wo Yan's Efficacious Point Applications)*

Stimulation: 0.3-0.4″ backward transverse insertion.
Moxa: 3 cones; pole 5-10 min.

Point Categories & Associations: The tenth of the thirteen ghost points.

GV-24
神庭

shén tíng

"Spirit Court"

Location: On the midsagittal line of the head, 0.5″ within the anterior hairline.

Classical Location: Directly above the nose, five fen within the hairline. *(The Great Compendium)*

Local Anatomy: The branches of the frontal artery and vein. The branch of the frontal nerve.

Functions: Calms the liver and extinguishes wind; quiets the heart and spirit.

Indications: Epilepsy; fright palpitations; insomnia; headache; visual dizziness; deep source nasal congestion.

Supplementary Indications: Dizziness; swelling of the eyes; eye screens; tearing; nosebleed; opisthotonos; protrusion of the tongue; madness; wind epilepsy; hemiplegia.

Stimulation: 0.2-0.3″ backward transverse insertion. (see contraindications) Moxa: 3-5 cones; pole 5-10 min.

Needle Sensation: Localized heaviness and distention.

Contraindications: Some classical texts say that this point is contraindicated for acupuncture and that mania or damage to the eyesight will result from needling here.

Point Categories & Associations: Intersection-jiaohui point of the foot tai yang bladder and foot yang ming stomach channels and the governing vessel.

Location: On the tip of the nose.
Classical Location: At the very tip of the nose.
(The Great Compendium)
Local Anatomy: The lateral nasal branches of the facial artery and vein. The external nasal branch of the anterior ethmoid nerve.

Functions: Discharges heat and opens the portals; returns yang and stems counterflow.
Indications: Clouding inversion; nasal congestion; nosebleed; drinker's nose.
Supplementary Indications: Nasal polyps; copious snivel; nasal sores; excessive tearing; nasal block with dyspnea; acute infantile fright wind; clonic spasm.

Contraindications: Moxibustion is contraindicated.

Stimulation: 0.1-0.3 ″ upward oblique or perpendicular insertion.

GV-25
素髎
sù liáo
"White Bone-Hole"

Location: Below the nose, a little above the midpoint of the philtrum.
Classical Location: In the center of the trough below the nose, proximal to the nostrils. *(The Great Compendium)*
Local Anatomy: The superior labial artery and vein. The buccal branch of the facial nerve and the branch of the infraorbital nerve.

Functions: Returns inversion; clears the spirit-disposition; dispels wind pathogens; disperses heat in the interior.
Indications: Mania and withdrawal; epilepsy; infantile fright wind; stupor; clenched jaws; wryness of the eyes and mouth; facial swelling; pain and stiffness of the lumbar spinal column.

GV-26
水溝
shuǐ gōu
"Water Trough"
人中
rén zhōng
"Human Center"

Supplementary Indications: Wind strike with clenched jaws; loss of consciousness; trembling lips; fright wind; red, itchy, painful eye wind; clear, runny snivel; loss of smell; gripping pain in the heart and abdomen; qi surging into the heart and chest; inversion counterflow; inability to stand erect; wasting thirst; water swelling; headache.

Illustrative Point Combinations & Applications: GV-26 and PC-5 treat evil [ghost] madness [i.e., behaving as if one had encountered a ghost or were possessed by one]. *(Ode of Spiritual Light)*

GV-26 and BL-40 relieve acute flashes of pain in the lumbar spine. *(Song of the Jade Dragon)*

Stimulation: 0.2-0.3″ upward oblique insertion.
Moxa: 3 cones; pole 5-15 min.

Needle Sensation: Localized distention and heaviness.

Point Categories & Associations: Intersection-jiaohui point of the hand yang ming large intestine and foot yang ming stomach channels with the governing vessel.

GV-27

兌端

duì duān

"Extremity of the Mouth"

GV-27

GV-28

Figure 19.5

Location: On the anterior midline. At the junction of the philtrum and the upper lip.

Classical Location: At the peak of the upper lip. *(The Great Compendium)*

Local Anatomy: The superior labial artery and vein. The buccal branch of the facial nerve and the branch of the infraorbital nerve.

Functions: Nourishes yin and clears heat; relieves pain and quiets the spirit.

Indications: Mania and withdrawal; stiff, swollen lips; pain in the gums.

Supplementary Indications: Nasal congestion; nosebleed; mouth sores; jaundice; yellow urine; dry tongue; clenched jaws and chattering of the teeth.

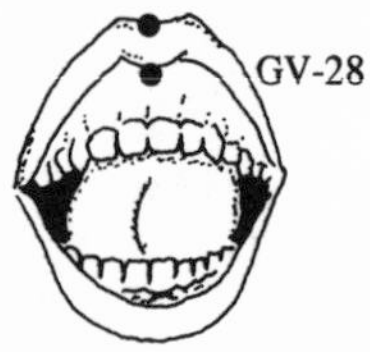

Stimulation: 0.2-0.3″ upward oblique insertion.
Moxa: 1-3 cones; pole 3-5 min.

Contraindications: This point is contraindicated for moxibustion in modern texts.

Location: Between the upper lip and the upper labial gingiva, in the frenulum of the upper lip.

Classical Location: In the cleft above the teeth.
(The Golden Mirror)

Local Anatomy: The superior labial artery and vein. The branch of the superior alveolar nerve.

Functions: Diffuses the lung and frees the portals; clears heat and drains fire; brightens the eyes and relieves itching.

Indications: Mania and withdrawal; deep-source nasal congestion; pain and swelling of the gums.

Supplementary Indications: Nasal polyp inhibiting respiration; pain along the center line of the face; clear, runny snivel and nosebleed; excessive tearing; redness, pain, and itching of the outer canthus; periodontal gan with swelling and pain; pain and bleeding of the teeth or gums; facial sores and enduring xian in children; red facial complexion; vexation.

Stimulation: 0.1-0.3 ″ upward oblique insertion or bleed with three-edged needle.

Point Categories & Associations: Intersection-jiaohui point of the conception and governing vessels and the foot yang ming stomach channel.

GV-28
齦交
yín jiāo
"Gum Intersection"

Governing Vessel			
Point	**Location**	Indications	
		Primary	**Secondary**
*GV-1	Coccyx	Hemafecia hemorrhoids	Epilepsy mania and withdrawal
GV-2	Sacrum	Menstrual disorders pain and stiffness of the lumbar spine	
*GV-3	Lumbar spine	Menstrual disorders seminal emission lumbosacral pain paralysis of the lower limbs	
*GV-4		Impotence seminal emission vaginal discharge lumbar pain	Diarrhea menstrual disorders
Coccyx to second lumbar vertebrae: Mental, genecologic, genital, and intestinal disorders			
GV-5	Lumbar spine	Diarrhea pain and stiffness of the lumbar spine	
GV-6	Thoracic spine	Diarrhea jaundice	Epilepsy
GV-7		Jaundice vomiting pain and stiffness of the lumbar spine	
GV-8		Stomach pain spinal stiffness	Epilepsy
First lumbar vertebrae to ninth thoracic vertebrae: Mental, intestinal, and stomach disorders			

Point	Location	Indications	
		Governing Vessel (continued)	
		Primary	**Secondary**
*GV-9	Thoracic spine	Jaundice cough and dyspnea	Spinal stiffness back pain
GV-10		Cough dyspnea	Clove sores
GV-11		Cough	Palpitations impaired memory
GV-12		Cough dyspnea	Epilepsy spinal stiffness back pain
GV-13		Headache	Malarial disease heat disease
*GV-14		Cough dyspnea headache stiff neck	Heat disease malarial disease epilepsy
**Seventh to first thoracic vertebrae: Mental disorders; disorders of the heart and lung, heat disease**			
*GV-15	Cervical spine	Sudden loss of voice stiff tongue with inability to speak	Epilepsy mania and withdrawal
*GV-16	Back of head	Headache stiff neck dizziness pain and swelling of the throat	Mania and withdrawal
**Neck: Mental disorders; disorders of the head and neck**			
GV-17	Back of head	Dizziness stiff neck	Epilepsy
GV-18		Headache visual dizziness	Epilepsy
GV-19		Headache dizziness	Epilepsy mania and withdrawal
*GV-20	Top of head	Headache dizziness wind-strike	Mania and withdrawal prolapse of the rectum prolapse of the uterus

		Indications	
Governing Vessel (continued)			
Point	**Location**	**Primary**	**Secondary**
GV-21	Front of head	Headache deep source nasal congestion	Epilepsy
GV-22		Headache dizziness deep source nasal congestion	Epilepsy
*GV-23		Headache deep source nasal congestion nosebleed	Mania and withdrawal
GV-24		Headache dizziness	Epilepsy
Head: Mental disorders; disorders of the head, face, and sensory organs			
*GV-25	Tip of nose	Nose disorders	Fright inversion coma
*GV-26	Philtrum	Wryness of the mouth and eyes	Epilepsy, mania and withdrawal child fright wind coma pain and stiffness of the lumbar spine
GV-27	Upper lip	Wry mouth pain and swelling of the gums	Mania and withdrawal
GV-28	Gums	Pain and swelling of the gums	Mania and withdrawal
Mouth and nose: Mental disorders; disorders of the nose, mouth, and teeth			

20. The Extraordinary Vessels

20.1 The Penetrating Vessel

Pathway: The penetrating vessel has a total of five paths. The first path starts in the lower abdomen and emerges in the qi thoroughfare, traveling up with the foot shao yin kidney channel and passing the navel to the chest area, where it disperses in the intercostal spaces.

The second path begins where the channel disperses in the chest. It runs up the throat and face, running around the lips and terminating in the nasal cavity.

The third path emerges from the qi thoroughfare in the lower abdomen at KI-11, then descends along the medial aspect of the thigh to the popliteal fossa. Continuing down along the medial margin of the tibia, it passes behind the medial malleolus before dispersing in the sole of the foot.

The fourth branch diverges from ST-30 and descends obliquely down the lower extremity to the medial malleolus. It enters the heel, crosses the tarsal bones of the foot and finally reaches the great toe.

The fifth channel separates from the main course in the pelvic cavity and runs to the spine, which it then ascends.

Basic functions:

The penetrating vessel is the sea of the major channels. It has a regulating effect on all twelve regular channels, and its main function is to regulate menstruation, for which reason it is also said, "The penetrating vessel is the sea of blood."

Main pathologic signs:

In women: gynecologic disorders, including metrorrhagia, miscarriage, menstrual block, irregular menses, scant breast milk, lower abdominal pain; and hematemesis. In men: prostatitis, urethritis, orchitis, seminal emission, impotence.

20.2 The Girdling Vessel

Pathway: Starting below the lateral tip of the tenth rib, this channel encircles the trunk like a belt, dipping down into the lower abdominal region anteriorly, and running across the lumbar region posteriorly. It intersects with three points on the foot shao yang gallbladder channel, GB-26, GB-27, and GB-28.

Basic functions:

This channel serves to bind up all the channels running up and down the trunk, thus regulating the balance between upward and downward flow of qi in the body.

Main pathologic signs:

(White) vaginal discharge, prolapse of the uterus, fullness and distention in the abdomen, limpness of the lumbar region.

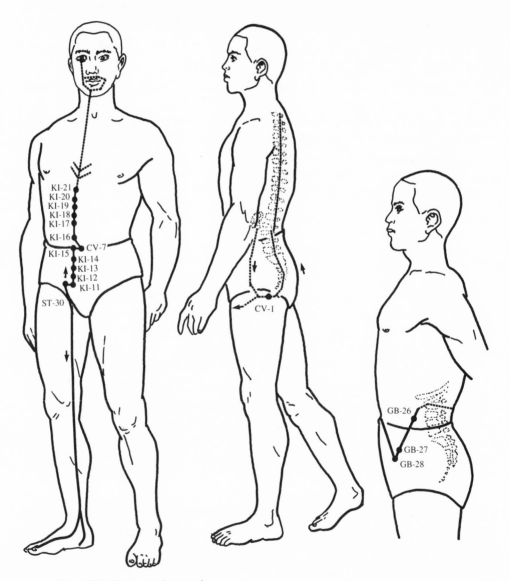

Figure 20.1 The penetrating vessel.

Figure 20.2 The girdling vessel.

20.3 Yin and Yang Motility Vessels

Pathways:

The Yin Motility Vessel: The yin motility vessel originates at KI-6 below the medial malleolus, runs up the medial aspect of the leg, penetrates the genital region and then continues internally up the abdomen and chest to emerge in the supraclavicular fossa at ST-12. It proceeds up the throat, passing in front of ST-9, then continues up the medial aspect of the cheek to the inner canthus, where it joins the foot tai yang bladder and yang motility channels to ascend over the head and enter the brain.

The Yang Motility Vessel: The yang motility vessel starts below the lateral malleolus at BL-62 and runs up the lateral aspect of the trunk, gradually curving around posteriorly to the lateral aspect of the shoulder. It crosses over the shoulder to the front of the body, then runs up the neck, over the jaw, past the corners of the mouth to the inner canthus of the eye. From here it joins with the yin motility vessel and the foot tai yang bladder channel to run up the forehead and over the lateral aspect of the head to GB-20 posterior to the mastoid process, before entering the brain at GV-16.

Basic functions:

The main physiologic functions of both the yin and yang motility channels are to control the opening and closing of the eyes, control the ascent of fluids and the descent of qi, and to regulate muscular activity in general.

Main pathologic signs:

Yang motility vessel: eye diseases, dry and itching eyes, insomnia, lack of agility, pain in the lumbar region, and spasm along the lateral aspect of the lower limb, with corresponding flaccidity along the medial aspect.

Yin motility vessel: eye diseases, heavy sensation of the eyelids or inability to open the eyes, hypersomnia, watery eyes, lower abdominal pain, pain along the waist extending into the genitals, hernia, leukorrhagia, tightness and spasms along the medial aspect of the lower limb, with corresponding flaccidity along the lateral aspect.

Regarding these latter symptoms, the ''Twenty-Ninth Perplexity'' of the *Canon of Perplexities* states, ''When the yin motility vessel is diseased, the yang vessel is relaxed and the yin vessel is tense; when the yang motility vessel is diseased, the yin vessel is relaxed and the yang vessel is tense.''

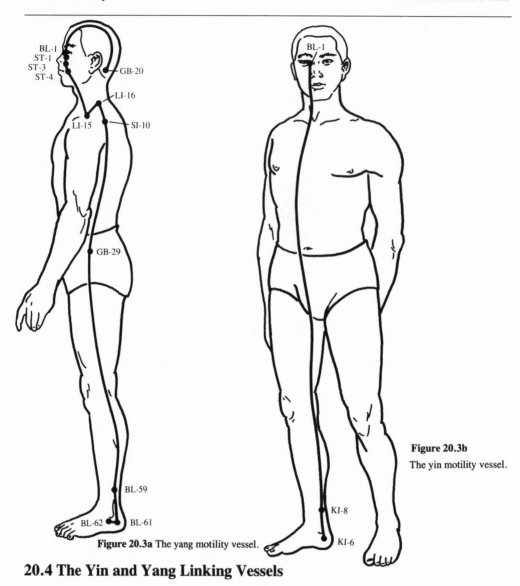

Figure 20.3a The yang motility vessel.

Figure 20.3b
The yin motility vessel.

20.4 The Yin and Yang Linking Vessels

Pathways: The yin linking vessel starts at the point KI-9 of the foot shao yin kidney channel, then runs up the medial aspect of the leg, and up the abdomen and across the chest to the throat, where it meets the conception vessel. Along its course, it intersects the foot tai yin spleen channel at SP-12, SP-13, SP-15, and SP-16. It intersects the foot jue yin liver channel at LV-14, and the conception vessel at CV-22 and CV-23.

The yang linking vessel starts below the lateral malleolus at the point BL-63 of the foot tai yang bladder channel, and runs up the leg along the path of the foot shao yang gallbladder channel. It proceeds up the posterolateral aspect of the trunk, running past the axilla, behind the shoulder, ascending the neck and crossing behind the ear to the forehead. After doubling back over the top of the head, it ends at GV-16 at the nape of the neck. Along its course, it intersects the foot shao yang gallbladder channel at GB-39, GB-21, GB-20, GB-19, GB-18, GB-17, GB-16, GB-15, GB-14, and GB-13. It intersects the hand shao yang triple burner channel at TB-15, the hand tai yang small intestine channel at SI-10, the governing vessel at GV-15 and GV-16, and the foot yang ming stomach channel at ST-8.

Basic functions:

The yin linking vessel serves to connect the flows of the yin major channels, reinforcing and balancing their respective flows, and generally regulating their activity.

The yang linking vessel serves to unite all the yang major channels, strengthening their respective flows, compensating for superabundance or insufficiency in channel circulation, and generally regulating yang channel activity.

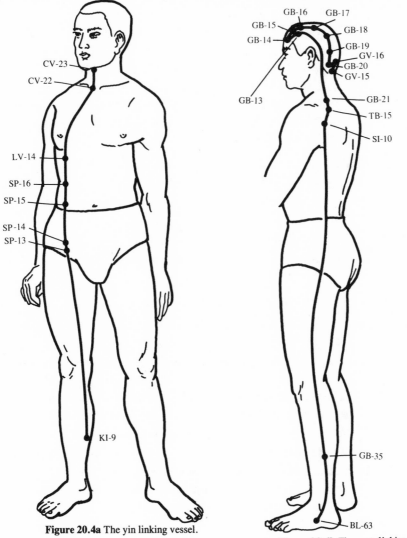

Figure 20.4a The yin linking vessel.

Figure 20.4b The yang linking vessel.

21 The Non-Channel Points

Though they are commonly used, the extra points herein listed are not part of the channel system. To encourage the systemization of nomenclature, and aid the student in cross referencing, we have adopted the extra point naming system employed by O'Connor and Bensky. Where a point listed is not included in their system, we have created an alphanumeric appellation to fit. The student may also refer to the Pinyin name of the point when attempting to cross reference sources using a unique convention.

21.1 Non-Channel Points on the Head and Neck

M-HN-1
四神聰
sì shén cōng

"Alert Spirit Quartet"

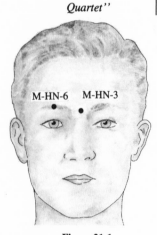

Figure 21.1

Location: One inch in front of, behind and bilateral to the GV-20.
Classical Location: One body inch from GV-20 on all four sides.
(Life-Promoting Canon of Acupuncture and Moxibustion)
Local Anatomy: Skin, superficial fascia, galea aponeurotica. The great occipital nerve, the auriculotemporal nerve, the lateral branches of the frontal nerve. The occipital artery, lateral frontal artery, and superficial temporal artery.

Functions: Courses the channels and collaterals; enhances movement of the limbs.
Indications: Wind strike hemiplegia; headache; dizziness; epilepsy; mental disorders.
Illustrative Point Combinations & Applications: Combined with KI-1 and GV-18, M-HN-1 treats wind epilepsy.
(Life-Promoting Canon)

Stimulation: 0.2-0.3 ″ transverse insertion.

M-HN-6
魚腰
yú yāo

"Fish's Lumbus"

Location: When the eyes look straight ahead, the point is directly above the pupils, in the middle of the eyebrow.
Classical Location: In the center of the eyebrows.
(The Great Compendium)
Indications: Pain, reddening and swelling of the eye; twitching of the eyelids; drooping eyelid; cloudiness of the cornea.

Supplementary Indications: Nearsightedness in young people; frontal headache.

Stimulation: 0.2ʺ transverse insertion joining BL-2 or TB-23.

Location: Midway between the medial ends of the eyebrows (the glabella).

Classical Location: In the depression between the two eyebrows. *(The Great Compendium)*

Functions: Quickens the collaterals and courses wind; quiets the spirit.

Indications: Infantile fright wind; high blood pressure; frontal headache; heavy-headedness; nosebleed; deep-source nasal congestion; insomnia.

Supplementary Indications: Headache; eye diseases; nasal congestion; postpartum blood dizziness; pregnancy epilepsy; trigeminal neuralgia.

Stimulation: 0.2-0.5ʺ transverse insertion toward GV-25 or the eyebrow; can be bled. Moxa: 3-5 cones; pole 5-10 min.

M-HN-3
印堂
yìn táng
"Hall of Impression"

Location: In the depression about 1ʺ posterior to the midpoint between the lateral end of the eyebrow and the outer canthus.

Classical Location: In the depression behind the eyebrow, at the purple vein of the temple. *(The Great Compendium)*

Functions: Courses wind and dissipates heat; clears the head and brightens the eyes.

Indications: Headache; wryness of the eyes and mouth; trigeminal neuralgia; redness and swelling of the eyes.

Supplementary Indications: Unilateral headache; dizziness; toothache; optic atrophy; retinal bleeding; facial paralysis.

Stimulation: 0.3-0.4ʺ perpendicular or backward oblique insertion; bleed with three-edged needle.

M-HN-9
太陽
tài yáng
"Tai Yang"

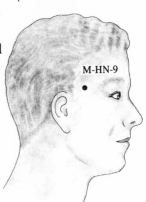

M-HN-9

Figure 21.2

M-HN-20a+b
金津　玉液

jīn jīn

yù yè

"Golden Liquid"

"Jade Humor"

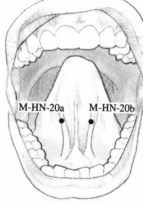

M-HN-20a   M-HN-20b

Figure 21.3

Location: At the veins on either side of the frenulum of the tongue. The left side is M-HN-20b and the right side is M-HN-20a.

Classical Location: On the underside of the tongue, at the purple vessels on either side. *(The Great Compendium)*

Indications: Painful, swollen tongue; mouth sores; throat block; vomiting; diarrhea; aphasia.

Illustrative Point Combinations & Applications: Treats wasting thirst when combined with CV-24. *(The Great Compendium)*

The patient should be asked to place her tongue tip to the roof of her mouth to expose the point.

Stimulation: Bleed with three-edged or thick gauge needle.

M-HN-10
耳尖

ěr jiān

"Tip of the Ear"

Location: On the tip of the ear.

Classical Location: On the tip of the ear. The point is located by folding the ear. *(The Great Compendium)*

Indications: Eye screens; redness, swelling and pain of the eyes; high fever.

Stimulation: 0.1-0.2″ insertion, or let three to five drops of blood. Moxa: 3-5 cones; pole 3-5 min.

N-HN-54
安眠

ān mián

"Quiet Sleep"

Location: Below the occiput on the posterior edge of the mastoid, midway between GB-20 and TB-17.

Local Anatomy: Occipital artery and vein; the minor occipital nerve and a branch of the great auricular nerve.

Indications: Insomnia; dizziness; headache; high blood pressure; mental disorders; hysteria.

Illustrative Point Combinations & Applications: Combined with points such as ST-36, SP-6, HT-7, and PC-6, M-HN-54 treats insomnia. With LI-11, GB-20, TB-20, and ST-40 it can treat dizziness.

Stimulation: 0.5-1.0 ″ perpendicular insertion.

Location: 1 ″ lateral to the posterior midline 1 ″ inferior to the posterior hairline, or 2 ″ superior to GV-14 (i.e., two-thirds of the way down from the posterior hairline to GV-14 below GB-20).
Indications: Postpartum body pain; cough; scrofula; whooping cough; sprain or spasms of the neck muscles; lung diseases.

Stimulation: 0.3-0.5 ″ perpendicular insertion.
Moxa: 7 cones; pole 5-15 min.
Needle Sensation: Sensation of pulling distention in the shoulder.

M-HN-30
百勞
bǎi láo
"Hundred
Taxations"

21.2 Non-Channel Points on the Back and Lumbar Regions

Location: On the back, 1 ″ lateral to the inferior border of the spinous process of the seventh cervical vertebra.
Indications: Cough; asthma; bronchitis; urticaria.

Stimulation: 1.0 ″ inward oblique insertion.

M-BW-1a
喘息
chuǎn xí
"Gasping"

Location: 0.5 ″ lateral to GV-14.
Indications: Asthma; pain in the shoulder and back.

Stimulation: 0.5 ″ inward oblique insertion.
Moxa: 3-5 cones; pole 10-20 min.

M-BW-1b
定喘
dìng chuǎn
"Dyspnea
Stabilizer"

Location: A series of points on both sides of the spine 0.5 ″ lateral to the lower border of each spinous process from the 1st thoracic vertebra to the 5th lumbar vertebra. These points, believed to have been used by the renowned physician Hua Tuo (208 AD) as associated-shu points, correspond in function to the bladder associated-shu points.

M-BW-35
華佗
huá tuó
"Hua Tuo's
Paravertebral Points"

Indications: Similar to those of the associated-shu points.   The paravertebral points on the upper back are indicated in disorders of the chest, heart and upper abdomen, liver, gallbladder, spleen and stomach; those in the lumbar region are used in disorders of the lower abdomen, kidney, intestines, bladder and lower extremities. (See also 4.2.12, p. 66.)

Stimulation: 0.5-1.0″ perpendicular insertion for the thoracic vertebrae. 1.5-2.0″ perpendicular insertion for the lumbar vertebrae. Moxa: 3-7 cones; pole 5-15 min.

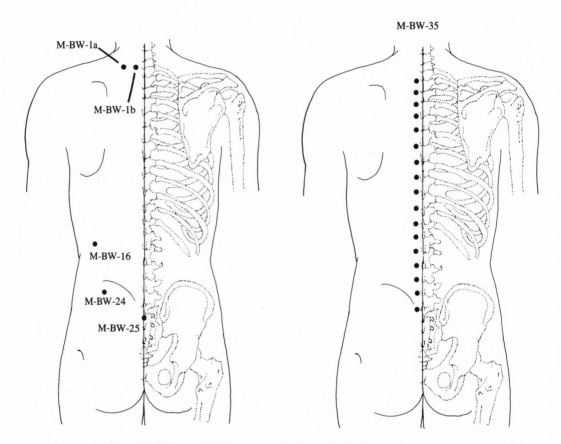

Figure 21.4 - Figure 21.5 : Non-channel points on the Back & Lumbar Region

Location: 3.5″ lateral to the lower border of the spinous process of the first lumbar vertebra.

Classical Location: Below the thirteenth vertebra, three and a half inches either side of the midline. *(The Gateway)*

Indications: Lump glomus (specifically hepatosplenomegaly); diarrhea; hernia; lumbar pain; stomach pain.

Stimulation: 0.5-0.8″ perpendicular insertion.
Moxa: 5-9 cones; pole 10-30 min.

M-BW-16
痞根
pǐ gēn
"Root of Glomus"

Location: In the depression lateral to the space between the spinous process of the 4th and 5th lumbar vertebrae. The point is located in prone posture.

Indications: Pulmonary tuberculosis; frequent urination; irregular menstruation; backache.

Stimulation: 0.5-1.5″ perpendicular insertion.
Moxa: 5-7 cones; pole 5-15 min.

M-BW-24
腰眼
yāo yǎn
"Lumbar Eye"

Location: Below the seventeenth vertebra. The lumbro-sacral joint.

Indications: Lumbar pain.

Stimulation: Intradermal needle.
Moxa: 7-15 cones; pole 10-20 min.

M-BW-25
十七椎穴
shí qī zhuī xuè
*"Seventeenth
Vertebra Point"*

21.3 Non-Channel Points on the Chest and Abdomen

Location: Make an equilateral triangle with sides of the same length as the width of the patient's mouth. Place the top vertex of the triangle at the navel. The point will be found at the lower two corners of the triangle.

Indications: Hernia.

Supplementary Indications: Shan qi; running piglet.

Stimulation: Moxa: 5-7 cones; treat disease on the right through the point on the left, and vice-versa.

M-CA-18a
臍旁
qí páng
"Beside the Navel"
臍三角灸法

M-CA-18
子宫
zǐ gōng

"Infant's Palace"

Location: 4″ below the umbilicus and 3″ either side of the mid-line.

Indications: Prolapse of the uterus; irregular menstruation; infertility; eclampsia; pain due to hernia; orchitis.

Illustrative Point Combinations & Applications: Combined with CV-3, it treats infertility, uterine bleeding, and vaginal discharge. Combined with CV-5, CV-3, and BL-23, it treats persistent uterine bleeding.

Stimulation: 0-8-1.5″ perpendicular insertion. Moxa: 5-7 cones; pole 10-15 min.

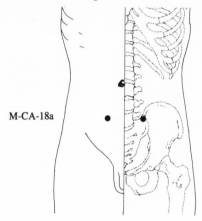

M-CA-18a

Figure 21.6

21.4 Non-Channel Points on the Upper Extremities

M-UE-1-5
十宣
shí xuān

"Ten Diffusions"

Location:

Classical Location: One point at the tip of each finger, each point being one fen from the fingernail. *(The Great Compendium)*

Indications: Acute tonsillitis; child fright wind; hypertension; wind strike; syncope due to high fever; mania and withdrawal; fright wind; vomiting; diarrhea; numbness of the fingers.

Stimulation: Bleed with three-edged needle.

Location: In the center of the palmar aspect skin creases of the proximal interphalangeal joints of the second through fifth fingers.

Classical Location: On the inner side of the middle joints of the four fingers. *(The Great Compendium)*

Indications: Infantile gan accumulation; infantile indigestion; whooping cough; roundworm.

Stimulation: Let blood and squeeze until a clear yellowish fluid appears.

M-UE-9
四縫
sì fēng
"Four Seams"

Location: On the ventral aspect of the forearm, 4″ up from the wrist crease, one point medial and one point lateral to the tendon of m. palmaris longus.

Indications: Hemorrhoids; prolapse of the rectum.

Illustrative Point Combinations & Applications: Combined with GV-20, BL-57 and GV-1, it treats prolapse of the rectum and enduring hemorrhoids. *(The Great Compendium)*

Stimulation: 0.5-1.0″ perpendicular insertion.
Moxa: 3-5 cones; pole 5-10 min.

Needle Sensation: Distention and numbness sometimes spreading toward the elbow.

M-UE-29
二白
èr bái
"Two Whites"

Location: Eight points on the dorsum of the hands between the metacarpalphalangeal joints, proximal to the web margin when a fist is made.

Classical Location: In the fork of the finger bones, four points left and right. *(The Great Compendium)*

Indications: Redness and swelling of the dorsum of the hand; spasm and contracture, or numbness of the fingers.

Supplementary Indications: Head wind; toothache; eye disease.

Stimulation: 0.3-0.5″ perpendicular insertion; bleed.

M-UE-22
八邪
bā xié
"Eight Evils"

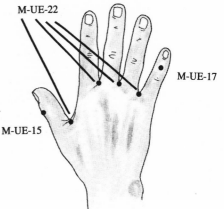

Figure 21.7

405

M-UE-15
大骨空
dà gǔ kōng

"Greater Bone Hollow"

Location: On the dorsal aspect of the thumb, in the center of the skin crease between the distal and middle phalanges.
Classical Location: Two points one on each hand, at the middle joint of the thumb, in the depression found when the thumb is flexed. *(The Great Compendium)*

Functions: Removes screens and brightens the eyes; rectifies qi.
Indications: Eye disorders; vomiting and diarrhea.

Stimulation: 0.1″ perpendicular insertion.
Moxa: 3-5 cones; pole 5-10 min.

M-UE-17
小骨空
xiǎo gǔ kōng

"Lesser Bone Hollow"

Location: On the dorsal aspect of the fifth finger, in the center of the joint between the distal and middle phalanges.
Classical Location: At the tip of the second joint of the little finger. *(Compilation of Acupuncture and Moxibustion)*

Functions: Relieves pain and brightens the eyes.
Indications: Eye disorders; deafness; pain in the hand joints.
Supplementary Indications: Ulceration of the eyelid rims and wind eye.

Stimulation: Moxa: 3-5 cones; pole 5-10 min.

M-UE-24
落枕
luò zhěn

"Crick in the Neck"

Location: On the dorsal aspect of the hand, between the second and third metacarpals about 0.5″ posterior to the metacarpo-phalangeal joint.
Indications: Inability to turn the head; crick in the neck; pain in the shoulder and arm; stomach pain.

Stimulation: 0.3-0.8″ perpendicular insertion.
Moxa: 3-5 cones; pole 10-20 min.
Needle Sensation: Distention and numbness, sometimes spreading toward the fingers.

Location: On the dorsum of the hand, 1″ distal to the wrist skin crease, one point each between the second and third, and fourth and fifth metacarpals.

Indications: Lumbar pain; acute lumbar sprain; diabetes; gynecological disorders; orchitis.

Stimulation: 0.5-1.0″ perpendicular insertion.
Moxa: 5-7 cones; pole 5-15 min.
Needle Sensation: Distention and numbness.

M-UE-19
腰痛點
yāo tòng diǎn

"Lumbar Pain Point"

Location: When the arm is abducted, the point is midway between the end of the anterior axillary fold and LI-15.

Indications: Pain in the shoulder and arm; paralysis of the upper extremities.

Stimulation: 0.6-1.0″ perpendicular insertion.
Moxa: 3-5 cones; pole 10-15 min.

Needle Sensation: Distention or numbness, sometimes spreading towards the hand.

M-UE-48
肩前
jiān qián

"Shoulder Front"

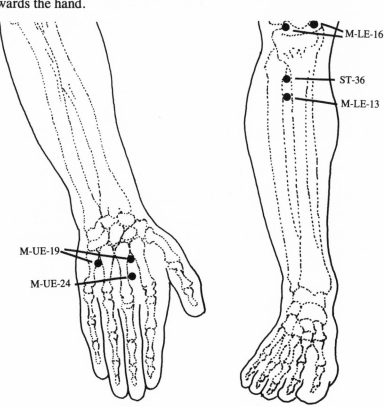

Figure 21.8 - 21.9

M-UE-46

肘尖

zhǒu jiān

"Tip of the Elbow"

Location: At the tip of the elbow, at the olecranon of the ulna.
Indications: Scrofula; yong and clove sores.

Stimulation: 0.1″ perpendicular insertion or 0.5″ transverse insertion. Moxa: 3-5 cones; pole 10-20 min.

Note: Contralateral moxibustion at this point is combined with moxibustion at GB-20.

21.5 Non-Channel Points on the Lower Extremities

M-LE-16

內膝眼

nèi xī yǎn

*"Inner Eye
of the Knee"*

Location: A pair of points in the depressions medial and lateral to the patellar ligament. The point is located with the knee flexed. The lateral point is also called ST-35.
Indications: Numbness, pain, or swelling of the knee; limpness of the lower extremities.

Stimulation: 0.5-1.0″ perpendicular insertion.
Moxa: 3-5 cones; pole 10-15 min.

M-LE-13

闌尾

lán wěi

"Appendix"

Location: At the tender point about 2″ below ST-36.
Indications: Acute and chronic appendicitis; indigestion; muscular atrophy; loss of locomotive ability of the lower extremities.

Stimulation: 0.5-1.3″ perpendicular insertion.
Needle Sensation: Arrival of qi is characterized by a painful itching sensation; the needle may be removed when the sensation subsides.

Location: At the sensitive spot about 1-2″ below GB-34.

Indications: Lateral costal pain; acute and chronic cholecystitis and cholelithiasis; biliary ascariasis; loss of locomotive ability of the lower extremities.

Stimulation: 0.5.-1.3″ perpendicular insertion.

M-LE-23

膽囊

dǎn náng

"Gallbladder Point"

Location: At the tip of the inner ankle bone.

Classical Location: At the tip of the inner ankle bone. *(The Great Compendium)*

Indications: Tonsillitis; throat bi; lochiorrhea.

Supplementary Indications: Cramp on the inner face of the leg; aching among the lower teeth.

Stimulation: 0.2″ perpendicular insertion.
Moxa: 3-7 cones; pole 5-15 min.

M-LE-17

內踝尖

nèi huái jiān

"Tip of the Inner Ankle Bone"

Location: At the tip of the outer ankle bone.

Classical Location: At the tip of the outer ankle bone. *(The Great Compendium)*

Indications: Urinary incontinence; foot qi; immobility of the toes; toothache; sore throat.

Supplementary Indications: Infantile double tongue; cramp in the outer face of the leg.

Stimulation: 0.2″ perpendicular insertion or bleed with a three-edged needle. Moxa: 3-5 cones; pole 5-10 min.

M-LE-22

外踝尖

wài huái jiān

"Tip of the Outer Ankle"

Location: Eight points, altogether located on the dorsal aspect of the feet between the toes, proximal to the web margins.

Classical Location: Eight points in the forks of the bones of the toes. *(The Great Compendium)*

Indications: Foot qi; redness and swelling of the dorsum of the foot.

Stimulation: 0.5″ upward oblique insertion; bleed.
Moxa: 5 cones.

M-LE-8

八風

bā fēng

"Eight Winds"

M-LE-18a
獨陰 (獨會)
dú yīn

"Solitary Yin"

Location: On the plantar aspect of the second toe, in the center of the distal interphalangeal skin crease.

Indications: Abdominal pain; vomiting; retention of afterbirth; hernia; irregular menstruation.

Stimulation: 0.1-0.2" perpendicular insertion.
Moxa: 3-5 cones; pole 5-10 min.

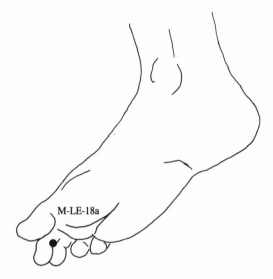

Figure 21.10

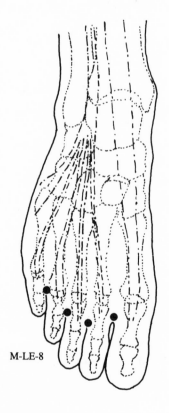

Figure 21.11

Part IV

Approaches to Point Selection & Combination

22. Selecting Points

The practitioner needs a method of choosing the best points to treat the patient at hand from the many possible choices. While there is no one method for selecting and combining points, there are several guidelines that have been developed over the ages. Below we discuss guidelines and general considerations for the selection and combination of points.

22.1 Selection of Local, Adjacent, and Distant Points

After diagnosis is completed, the practitioner must select appropriate points for the insertion of needles or application of moxibustion. In general, a combination of local points, adjacent points, and distant points are chosen.

Local points are, by definition, located at the site of the symptom or organ being treated. For this reason, any point can be employed as a local point. In this usage a point is most effective for treatment of chronic local disorders, though local points are occasionally used for acute disorders as well.

Adjacent points are those points that are near the disease site. They can replace local points for the treatment of acute disorders, or can strengthen the effects of local and distant points. Though any point can function as an adjacent point, those points that have a salient location are usually chosen.

Distant points are points far from the disease site that are related to the affected area either directly or indirectly through the channel system. GB-37, for example, treats eye disorders because the liver opens into the eyes, and the gallbladder and liver stand in internal-external relationship. ST-36 is suitable for the treatment of stomach ailments because it is a prominent point on the stomach channel, and TB-5 is especially useful for treating headaches that involve the shao yang channels of the hand and foot (gallbladder and triple burner) because it is located on the triple burner channel. The *Inner Canon* recommends treating diseases that affect the upper body with points from the lower body; lower body diseases with upper body points; diseases of the body's left side with points from the right; and diseases of the right side of the body with points from the left. In practice, distant points are considered especially useful for acute disorders, but are also suitable for more chronic ones. A strong stimulus is usually applied to these points.

The student should learn which points on the body are employed as distant points or adjacent points and which ones are applied only to treat local disorders. The chart below lists local, adjacent and distant points that are used to treat various disease sites on the body.

Choosing Local, Adjacent and Distant Points			
Affected Region	**Local Points**	**Adjacent Points**	**Distant Points**
Eyes	BL-1, TB-23	M-HN-9, GV-23, ST-2	GB-37, LV-3, SI-6
Ears	GB-2, TB-17, SI-19	GB-20, SI-17, GB-8	TB-5, GB-41, TB-3
Nose	LI-20, GV-25	M-NH-3, GV-23, BL-7	LI-3, LI-4, ST-44
Throat	CV-23	CV-22, SI-17	LI-4, LI-11, KI-6
Mouth (tongue and teeth)	ST-4, ST-6	M-HN-9, GB-20,	LI-4, HT-5, ST-44 GV-15
Lungs	BL-13, LU-1, CV-17, CV-22	GV-14, CV-12, CV-6	LU-5, LU-7, ST-40
Heart	BL-15, CV-17	CV-14, GV-11	HT-7, PC-6
Spleen & Stomach	CV-12, BL-20, BL-21	LV-13, SP-15	ST-36, SP-4, PC-6
Liver	LV-14, BL-18	CV-12, BL-20	LV-3, GB-34
Gallbladder	GB-24, BL-19	ST-21, CV-11	GB-34, GB-40, LV-3
Large Intestine	SP-15	ST-25, BL-25	LI-11, ST-37
Small Intestine	CV-4, CV-9, ST-28	BL-27	SI-4, ST-39
Kidney	BL-23, BL-52	CV-4, ST-29	SP-6, KI-3
Bladder	CV-3, BL-28	BL-23, ST-28	KI-3, KI-7
Urogenital	CV-4, ST-29, M-CA-18	BL-23, BL-32	SP-6, KI-3, LV-3
Rectum	CV-1, BL-35	BL-30, BL-34	BL-57, GV-20, M-UE-29
Lateral Costal Region	GB-26, GB-25	LV-14, SP-21	GB-38, TB-5, GB-43
Upper Abdomen	CV-12, CV-13	CV-8, ST-19	ST-36, SP-4, PC-6
Lower Back (lumbar region)	BL-23, GV-4	GB-25, GB-30	SI-6, SI-3, BL-60, BL-40
Forehead	GB-14, M-HN-9	GB-15, BL-5	LI-3, ST-43, ST-41
Vertex	GV-20, BL-7	GB-20, M-HN-9	LV-3, GB-34
Shoulder	LI-15, SI-9	LI-14	ST-38, LI-4

22.2 Selection of Points According to the Affected Channel

Once diagnosis has determined what channels are affected by a particular disease, points on those or related channels can be chosen for treatment. A majority of chosen points are on the channel of the affected organ or the channel that passes through the affected site. Points on the channel that stands in interior-exterior relationship to the affected channel, or points on the channel that communicates with the affected channel, are also commonly selected. (Communicating channels are ones that have the same name, i.e., yang ming, tai yang, etc.)

413

The chart below shows the method of selecting points according to affected channels.

Treatment According to the Channel				
Area of Body	**Region**	**Affected Channel**	**Main Points**	**Assisting Points**
Head	Occipital	BL	BL-60, BL-65	GB-20, GV-16
	Lateral	GB, TB	GB-38, TB-3	ST-8
	Vertex	GV, BL, LV	LV-3, BL-65	GV-20
	Forehead	ST	ST-44	GB-14, ST-41
	Cheek	SI	SI-3	SI-18
	Lateral to nose	ST, LI	ST-41	LI-20
	Below the chin	ST	ST-41	ST-6, ST-7
	Chin	ST, CV	ST-41	CV-24
Neck	Front	ST, CV	ST-41, CV-22	LU-7, ST-10
	Sides	LI, SI, TB	LI-4, SI-3, TB-5, GB-40	LU-7
	Back	GB, BL, GV	BL-60, GV-16	GB-20, BL-10
Back & Shoulder	Spinal Region	GV, BL	BL-60, BL-40	GV-14, GV-6, GV-4
	Lateral Regions	BL	BL-60, BL-65	BL-40, Local associated-shu points
	Shoulder (scapula)	SI	SI-3	GB-34
Chest	Axillary line	GB	GB-38	LV-3, PC-4
	Breastbone	CV, KI	CV-17, KI-3	TB-6
	Lateral to breastbone	KI	KI-3	TB-6
	Nipple line	ST	ST-40, ST-18, ST-34	SI-1, TB-6
	Lateral costal regions	LV, GB, SP	LV-3, GB-40	TB-6, PC-4, LV-2
Abdomen	Center line	CV	CV-12, CV-4	ST-36
	Nipple line	SP	SP-3, SP-6	ST-36
	Lateral regions	LV, GB	LV-3, GB-34	ST-36, LV-13
	Genital region	LV	LV-3, LV-5	CV-3, SP-6
Inner Arms	Radial aspect	LU	LU-9, LU-7	LU-5
	Center line	PC	PC-6	PC-3
	Ulnar aspect	HT	HT-5	HT-3
	Palm	HT, PC	PC-8, HT-8	PC-6
Outer Arms	Radial aspect	LI	LI-4	LI-11
	Center line	TB	TB-5	TB-10
	Ulnar aspect	SI	SI-3	SI-8
Hip Region	Anterior aspect	ST	ST-31	ST-34
	Lateral aspect	GB	GB-31	GB-30
	Posterior aspect	BL	BL-36	BL-54
Legs	Anterior aspect	ST	ST-36, ST-32	ST-40
	Posterior aspect	BL	BL-40, BL-37	GB-30, BL-36
	Medial aspect	LV, SP, KI	SP-6, LV-3, KI-3	SP-11, LV-9, KI-10
	Lateral aspect	GB	GB-34, GB-31	GB-30, GB-39

For internal disorders, determine the channel or channels involved and apply treatment directly or indirectly to those channels, selecting points that are appropriate for treatment. The following charts are included to help the practitioner proceed from diagnosis to treatment, illustrating point selection methods that combine points by channel and by disease pattern.

Lung		
Functions	**Symptoms**	**Points**
Diffuse the lung transform phlegm relieve cough calm dyspnea	Cough, dyspnea, phlegm, and thoracic distention and fullness	LU-11, LU-10, LU-9, LU-7 LU-5
Free the channels, quicken the connecting vessels	Headache	LU-7
	Hidden pulse	LU-9
Clear heat, calm pain	**Check blood loss** Expectoration of blood	LU-6, LU-10, LU-5
	Check blood loss Nosebleed	LU-11, LU-5
	Relieve pain Sore, swollen throat	LU-11, LU-10, LU-6
	Quiet and settle Mania and withdrawal	LU-11
Quicken blood, dispel stasis	Thoracic injury stasis pain	LU-7
Open the portals and revive consciousness	Shock, delirium, stroke	LU-11

Large Intestine			
Functions		**Symptoms**	**Points**
Regulate the intestines and stomach	Diarrhea or dysentery		LI-11, LI-4
	Abdominal pain		LI-4, LI-7, LI-11
	Constipation		LI-4
	Vomiting		LI-11
Drain yang ming pathogenic heat	**Lower blood pressure**	High blood pressure	LI-11, LI-15
	Staunch bleeding	Nosebleed	LI-4, L-1
	Sore throat		LI-4, LI-6, LI-7, LI-1
	Relieve pain	Toothache	LI-1, LI-4, LI-2, LI-3
		Headache	LI-4, LI-5, LI-6
	Drain fire	Fire eye	LI-1, LI-5, LI-6
		Fever without perspiration	LI-1, LI-4, LI-11
	Quiet the spirit	Hysteria	LI-4
Diffuse the lung and resolve the exterior	Common cold		LI-4, LI-11
	Relieve cough and calm gasping	Cough, gasping	LI-4, LI-1, LI-7

Stomach		
Functions	**Symptoms**	**Points**
Regulate the spleen and stomach	Stomach pain	ST-44, ST-36, ST-34
	Abdominal pain	ST-44, ST-37, ST-36
	Constipation	ST-40, ST-36, ST-25
	Vomiting	ST-44, ST-41, ST-36
	Poor digestion	ST-36, ST-25
Harmonize the qi and blood	**Rectify qi** — Cough (with phlegm) asthma	ST-40, ST-36
	Lower blood pressure — High blood pressure	ST-40, ST-36, ST-12
	Regulate menses — Irregular menstruation vaginal discharge	ST-25, ST-44, ST-36
	Regulate menses — Painful menstruation	ST-44, ST-25, ST-29
	Staunch bleeding — Nosebleed	ST-45, ST-44
	Staunch bleeding — Hemafecia	ST-25, ST-34
	Staunch bleeding — Vomiting blood	ST-36, ST-20
Clear and drain internal heat	Mastitis	ST-34, ST-18
	Relieve pain — Toothache	ST-45, ST-44, ST-6
	Relieve pain — Pain at corners of the forehead	ST-44, ST-8
	Calm and settle — Mania & withdrawal	ST-40, ST-42
	Calm and settle — Psychiatric disorders	ST-45, ST-36
	Calm and settle — Dizziness	ST-41, ST-36, ST-40
Free the channels, quicken the connecting vessels, dispel phlegm and eliminate damp	Inability to raise the arm	ST-38
	Forehead pain	ST-44
	Wry eyes and mouth	ST-36, ST-4, ST-6
Supplement and nourish	Post-partum dizziness	ST-36
	Weak constitution	ST-36

Spleen		
Functions	**Symptoms**	**Points**
Regulate the spleen and stomach	Abdominal pain and diarrhea	SP-4, SP-6, SP-9, SP-3
	Stomach pain	SP-3, SP-4, SP-8, SP-6
	Constipation	SP-3, SP-5
	Vomiting	SP-1, SP-2, SP-4
	Indigestion	SP-2, SP-4, SP-5, SP-6
Disinhibit urine and eliminate damp	Water swelling	SP-6, SP-9
	Urinary incontinence	SP-6, SP-9, SP-8
	Urinary inhibition	SP-8, SP-9
Assist the spleen to manage blood	Anemia	SP-10, SP-6
	Uterine bleeding	SP-1, SP-6, SP-8, SP-10
	Blood in the feces or urine, or nosebleed	SP-1
Free the channels and quicken the connecting vessels	Generalized body heaviness	SP-3, SP-6
	Weakness in the extremities	SP-21
	Lower extremity palsy	SP-7, SP-6
	Pain in the chest and lateral costal region	SP-21
Fortify the spleen, eliminate damp, free the channels and connecting vessels, quicken the blood and dispel stasis	Headache (phlegm-damp)	SP-4, SP-6, SP-9
	Cold-damp low back pain	SP-2, SP-9, SP-8
	Blood stasis low back pain	SP-8, SP-2, SP-10

Heart		
Functions	**Symptoms**	**Points**
Settle and quiet the spirit	Neurasthenia	HT-7, HT-6, HT-5
	Hysteria	HT-7, HT-4, HT-5
	Mania	HT-3
	Insomnia	HT-7
Drain heart fire	Steaming bone tidal fever	HT-8, HT-6
	Heat in the palms	HT-8, HT-6
Nourish the blood check blood loss	Vomiting of blood	HT-6, HT-7
	Nosebleed	HT-6, HT-7
Nourish heart yin	Night sweats	HT-6

Small Intestine		
Functions	**Symptoms**	**Points**
Drain fire	Fire eye	SI-3
	Mastitis	SI-1
	Epilepsy	SI-3, SI-7
	Hysteria	
Stop perspiration	Spontaneous sweating	SI-3
	Night sweats	
Relieve pain	Shoulder/scapula pain	SI-3, SI-9, SI-11
	Toothache	SI-18, SI-19, SI-8
	Headache	SI-1, SI-4, SI-7, SI-3
	Sore throat	SI-1
	Low back pain	SI-6, SI-4, SI-7
	Wrist pain	SI-5, SI-4
Open the portals	Tinnitus	SI-3, SI-8, SI-19
	Deafness	

Bladder			
Functions		**Symptoms**	**Points**
Clear and drain pathogenic heat	**Brighten the eyes**	Eye disorders	BL-1, BL-18, BL-2, BL-10
	Clear LV and GB heat	Hepatitis	BL-19, BL-18, BL-20
		Bitter taste	BL-19
		Cholecystitis	BL-18, BL-19
	Resolve toxins	Hemorrhoids	BL-40, BL-57
		Clove sores	BL-40
		Urticaria	BL-40
	Resolve summer heat	Summer heat strike	BL-11, BL-40
		Summer heat damage	BL-13, BL-11
Diffuse the lung, resolve exterior, relieve cough, calm dyspnea		Common cold	BL-12, BL-13
		Cough	BL-11, BL-12, BL-13, BL-43, BL-20
		Asthma	BL-11, BL-12, BL-13
		Pneumonia	BL-11, BL-12, BL-43
		Phlegm congestion	BL-20, BL-21, BL-13
		Hiccough	BL-17, BL-21
Regulate the spleen and stomach		Stomach pain	BL-18, BL-20, BL-21
		Vomiting	BL-17, BL-20, BL-21
		Esophageal constriction	BL-17, BL-21
		Diarrhea	BL-20, BL-23, BL-25
		Constipation	BL-25, BL-28
		Abdominal distention	BL-20, BL-25, BL-21, BL-22
		Indigestion	BL-21, BL-22, BL-25, BL-27
Enrich kidney yin		Night sweats	BL-17, BL-15, BL-13
		Tinnitus	BL-23, BL-62
Disinhibit water and disperse swelling		Retention of urine	BL-23, BL-32
		Inhibition of urine and stool	BL-31, BL-32, BL-33, BL-34, BL-23, BL-28
		Water swelling	BL-22, BL-20, BL-23
		Enuresis	BL-23, BL-28, BL-27, BL-39
		Inhibition of urine	BL-23, BL-22, BL-28, BL-39
Check blood loss		Nosebleed	BL-17, BL-18, BL-64, BL-66, BL-7
		Coughing blood	BL-13, BL-17
		Vomiting blood	BL-17, BL-15
		Intestinal wind	BL-20, BL-17, BL-34
		Blood in the urine	BL-17, BL-23, BL-27

Bladder continued		
Functions	**Symptoms**	**Points**
Rectify the fetus	Malposition of the fetus	BL-67
	Prolonged labor	BL-67, BL-60
Regulate the menses	Irregular menstruation	BL-33, BL-30, BL-17, BL-20
	Menstrual block	BL-20, BL-18, BL-17
	Painful menstruation	BL-23, BL-20, BL-18, BL-32
Relieve pain	Stasis low back pain	BL-23, BL-28, BL-25, BL-40, BL-57
	Vertex headache	BL-65, BL-67, BL-7
	Brow pain	BL-2, BL-67
	Toothache (upper)	BL-60
	Shoulder and scapula pain	BL-11, BL-41, BL-44
	Chest and lateral costal pain	BL-17, BL-18, BL-19
	Paralysis of the lower limbs	BL-43, BL-40, BL-60, BL-57
Quiet the spirit	Hysteria	BL-15, BL-20
	Epilepsy	BL-15, BL-62, BL-63, BL-18
	Psychiatric disorders	BL-15, BL-18, BL-2, BL-65, BL-62
	Dizziness	BL-10, BL-62, BL-7, BL-58
	Palpitations and racing heartbeat	BL-15, BL-14, BL-64
	Insomnia	BL-20, BL-17, BL-15, BL-18
	Seminal loss and impotence	BL-23, BL-52
Sober the brain and uplift yang	Stupor	BL-67
	Rectal prolapse	BL-57, BL-25

Kidney			
Functions		**Symptoms**	**Points**
Enrich kidney yin	**Ease pain**	Vertex headache	KI-1, KI-3
		Sore throat	KI-6, KI-3
		Back pain	KI-3, KI-7
		Toothache	KI-3
	Downbear fire	Bladder infections	KI-2, KI-3
		Nephritis	KI-3, KI-7
		Orchitis	KI-3, KI-8
	Check perspiration	Spontaneous sweating	KI-7, KI-2
		Night sweats	KI-7, KI-2
	Lower blood pressure	High blood pressure	KI-1, KI-3
Regulate the menses	Irregular menstruation		KI-5, KI-2, KI-6
	Uterine bleeding		KI-10
	Painful menstruation menstrual block		KI-5
	Prolonged labor		KI-6
Warm kidney yang	**Disinhibit urine**	Inhibited urine	KI-6, KI-10
		Water swelling	KI-7
	Rectify the spleen	Constipation	KI-4
	Absorb qi	Emphysema	KI-3, KI-7
		Asthma	KI-4, KI-3, KI-7
	Relieve pain	Yang vacuity headache	KI-1
		Yang vacuity low back pain	KI-3, KI-7
Promote cardiorenal interaction, settle the spirit	Hysteria		KI-1, KI-6
	Forgetfulness		KI-1
	Psychiatric disorders		KI-2, K-9
	Insomnia		KI-3

Pericardium		
Functions	**Disorders**	**Points**
Harmonize the stomach and downbear counterflow	Vomiting	PC-6, PC-8, PC-3, PC-5
	Stomach pain	PC-7, PC-6, PC-5
Drain Heart Fire	**Drain fire and quiet the spirit** — Psychiatric disorders	PC-4, PC-6, PC-7
	Hysteria	PC-4, PC-8
	Epilepsy	PC-6, PC-5
	Palpitations	PC-4, PC-7, PC-5
	Vexation	PC-6, PC-5, PC-4
	Cardiac oppression	PC-7
	Rapid heart beat	PC-4, PC-5, PC-6
	Clear heat — Halitosis	PC-7
	Heat in the palms	PC-9, PC-7, PC-5
	Fever without perspiration	PC-9, PC-7, PC-5
	Cool the blood and check blood loss — Spitting blood	PC-4
	Nosebleed	PC-4
	Vomiting blood	PC-4, PC-7
Loosen the chest and rectify qi	Asthma	PC-6
	Hiccough	PC-6

Triple Burner			
Functions		**Disorders**	**Points**
Regulate the spleen and stomach	Abdominal pain		TB-5
	Diarrhea		TB-6
	Constipation		TB-6, TB-5
	Vomiting		TB-6
Free the channels, quicken the connecting vessels, drain heat, and relieve pain	Forehead pain		TB-23, TB-5
	Toothache		TB-21, TB-17, TB-2, TB-23
	Pain in the chest and lateral costal pain		TB-6, TB-5
	Migraine headache		TB-6, TB-23, TB-3
	Sore throat		TB-3, TB-2, TB-1
	Arm pain		TB-1, TB-6, TB-5, TB-2, TB-4
	Neck and back pain		TB-3, TB-10, TB-6
Drain triple burner heat	**Brighten the eyes and open the portals**	Fire eye (conjunctivitis)	TB-2, TB-3, TB-4, TB-6
		Tinnitus deafness	TB-2, TB-3, TB-5, TB-21 TB-17
		Eye pain	TB-3, TB-6, TB-23, TB-10
	Resolve heat and eliminate vexation	Vexation	TB-1, TB-2
		Fever without perspiration	TB-1, TB-2, TB-3, TB-6
		Wasting thirst	TB-4
		Malarial disease	TB-2, TB-4, TB-5

Liver		
Functions	**Disorders**	**Points**
Course the liver and rectify qi	**Regulate the menses** — Excess menstrual flow uterine bleeding	LV-1, LV-3, LV-6, LV-5, LV-2
	Regulate the menses — Irregular menstruation	LV-5, LV-3
	Relieve pain — Painful menstruation	LV-2
	Relieve pain — Stomach pain	LV-3
	Relieve pain — Pain in the chest and lateral costal region	LV-2, LV-3, LV-13, LV-14
	Relieve pain — Shan qi	LV-1, LV-3, LV-8
	Relieve pain — Vertex headache	LV-2, LV-3
	Relieve pain — Abdominal pain	LV-3, LV-8
	Relieve pain — Genital pain or contraction	LV-2, LV-1, LV-6, LV-4, LV-8, LV-3, LV-12
	Settle and quiet — Visual dizziness	LV-2, LV-14, LV-8
	Settle and quiet — Epilepsy	LV-1, LV-2, LV-3
	Settle and quiet — Insomnia	LV-2, LV-3
	Liver-influenced digestive disorders	LV-13, LV-2, LV-3, LV-14
Quicken the blood and expel wind	Back pain	LV-5, LV-13, LV-3, LV-4, LV-2
	Wryness of the mouth and eyes (especially due to exuberant fire)	LV-2, LV-3
Drain liver and gallbladder heat	Mastitis	LV-3
	Orchitis	LV-5, LV-1
	Hepatitis	LV-4, LV-3, LV-2
	Enteritis	LV-3
	Nephritis	LV-8
	Jaundice	LV-13, LV-3, LV-4
	High blood pressure	LV-3
Regulate the waterways	Urinary inhibition	LV-5, LV-8
	Enuresis	LV-3, LV-1
Brighten the eyes	Fire eye	LV-2, LV-3
	Glaucoma	LV-3, LV-2
Disinhibit the throat	Sore throat and upper esophageal dryness	LV-3

425

Gallbladder		
Functions	**Disorders**	**Points**
Drain liver/ gallbladder heat		
	Relieve pain	
	Migraine headache	GB-20, GB-31, GB-41, GB-8, GB-5, GB-34, GB-38
	Forehead pain	GB-2, GB-14
	Pain in the chest and lateral costal region	GB-34, GB-41, GB-40, GB-44
	Toothache	GB-2, GB-3
	Sciatic pain	GB-31, GB-39, GB-30
	Back pain low back pain	GB-38, GB-39, GB-30, GB-31, GB-20
	Stop bleeding Nosebleed	GB-20, GB-39
	Quiet and settle Psychiatric diseases	GB-37, GB-43
	Visual dizziness	GB-15, GB-20, GB-16, GB-3
	Lower blood pressure High blood pressure	GB-20, GB-34
	Sharpen hearing Deafness tinnitus	GB-20, GB-43, GB-44
	Brighten the eyes Fire eye	GB-20, GB-1, GB-14, GB-16
	Eye pain (esp. outer canthus)	GB-37, GB-38, GB-44, GB-1, GB-41
	Tearing	GB-1, GB-14, GB-20, GB-43
	Optic atrophy	GB-1, GB-37, GB-20
	Hepatitis	GB-34, GB-39
	Cholecystitis	GB-34, GB-41
	Mastitis	GB-37, GB-41, GB-21
	Parotitis	GB-20
	Sinusitis	GB-20
	Tympanitis	GB-2
Regulate the menses and check vaginal discharge	Irregular menstruation	GB-26
	Vaginal discharge	GB-26
Harmonize and rectify the spleen and stomach	Vomiting	GB-24, GB-34
	Intestinal rumbling, diarrhea	GB-25
	Constipation	GB-34
	Stomach heat	GB-39
Quicken the blood and dispel stasis	Blood stasis lateral costal pain	GB-40, GB-34
	Blood stasis stomach pain	GB-24, GB-34
	Blood stasis low back pain	GB-31, GB-30

426

Conception Vessel		
Functions	**Disorders**	**Points**
Regulate the menses and check vaginal discharge	Irregular menstruation	CV-3, CV-4, CV-6
	Uterine bleeding	CV-5, CV-3, CV-4
	Painful menstruation	CV-3, CV-4
	Vaginal discharge	CV-3, CV-4, CV-6
	Menstrual block (amenorrhea)	CV-4, CV-5, CV-6
Harmonize and rectify the spleen and stomach	Indigestion	CV-12, CV-13, CV-11
	Diarrhea	CV-12, CV-5, CV-4, CV-9
	Vomiting	CV-12, CV-13, CV-11
	Constipation	CV-12, CV-6, CV-4
	Stomach pain	CV-12, CV-13, CV-15, CV-10
	Esophageal constriction	CV-17, CV-22
Downbear qi and relieve cough	Cough	CV-22, CV-17
	Asthma	CV-22, CV-17
	Hiccoughs	CV-6, CV-12
Relieve pain	Genital pain	CV-1, CV-2, CV-3, CV-4
Disinhibit water	Urinary inhibition	CV-3, CV-4, CV-9, CV-7, CV-2
	Water swelling	CV-2, CV-7, CV-9
Settle and quiet	Epilepsy	CV-14, CV-15
	Mania and withdrawal	CV-12, CV-15
	Fright palpitations	CV-14, CV-15, CV-17
Supplement the whole body	Vacuity disorders	CV-4, CV-6, CV-12
Warm the yang	Yang vacuity disorders	CV-8, CV-6, CV-4 (all moxa)

Governing Vessel		
Functions	**Disorders**	**Points**
Return the yang and stem counterflow	Prolapse of the rectum (or hemorrhoids)	GV-1, GV-20, GV-4
	Prolapse of the uterus	GV-20
	Yang vacuity headache	GV-20, GV-16, GV-23, GV-24
	Shock (clouding inversion)	GV-26, GV-20
Clear heat and resolve toxin	Clove sores (boils, etc.)	GV-10, GV-12
	Malarial disease	GV-14, GV-13
	Vacuity heat	GV-13, GV-14
	Fever	GV-14, GV-13
Quiet and settle the spirit	Epilepsy	GV-14, GV-26, GV-12, GV-4
	Mania and withdrawal	GV-23, GV-26, GV-20, GV-15
	Fright palpitations	GV-24, GV-11, GV-20
	Poor memory	GV-20, GV-11
Secure essence	Seminal loss	GV-4, GV-1
Relieve pain	Low back pain	GV-4, GV-3, GV-2
	Headache	GV-20, GV-23, GV-24
Check blood loss	Nosebleed	GV-23, GV-20, GV-16, GV-12
	Blood in the stool	GV-1, GV-4
Lower blood pressure	High blood pressure	GV-20
Nourish the blood	Anemia	GV-14, GV-9
Regulate the menses and check vaginal discharge	Irregular menstruation	GV-4, GV-3
	Vaginal discharge	GV-3, GV-4
Regulate the waterways	Incontinence	GV-4, GV-2
	Urinary inhibition	GV-4, GV-1

22.3 Selection of Points According to the Clinical Experience of Past Generations

The medical literature of China contains numerous references to points that are effective for specific diseases or regions of the body. Listed below are points that are commonly applied to specific diseases. This list is drawn mostly from the verses that were the didactic tools of acupuncturists of the Song, Yuan and Ming dynasties. These odes or verses were collected in the sixteenth century and included in acupuncture books that later became standard texts for all who studied the art.[1]

Empirically Proven Points for Specific Disorders	
Disorder	**Points**
Abdominal distention	SP-4, ST-36
Abdominal pain	SP-4, ST-34, PC-6
Abdominal water	CV-9(moxa), KI-7
Bitter taste	GB-38
Bleeding piles	M-UE-29
Chest pain & oppression	PC-6, PC-5, TB-6
Constipation	TB-6, KI-6, ST-25
Cough	LU-2, LU-3, LU-5
Diarrhea	ST-25, SP-9, ST-36, LI-11
Dizziness	GB-20, M-HN-3, GV-20, LV-3
Excessive dreaming	BL-15, HT-7, LV-3
Excessive perspiration	LI-4, KI-7
Fever	GV-14, LI-11, LI-4
Frequent urination	CV-3, KI-3, KI-7
Frozen shoulder	BL-38 joined to BL-57 (modern usage)
Gan accumulation	M-UE-9

Empirical Points for Specific Disorders (Continued)	
Disorder	**Points**
Gastric pain	CV-12, ST-34, PC-6
Gastrocnemial spasm	BL-57
General weakness	ST-36, CV-4, GV-4, CV-6
Halitosis	PC-7
Heart pain or palpitations	PC-6, PC-5, HT-6
Heel pain	PC-7, BL-40
Hoarseness	LI-18, PC-5, GV-15, LI-4
Insomnia	HT-7, SP-6, KI-3
Insufficient lactation	CV-17, SI-1
Itching	LI-11, SP-10, SP-6
Jaundice	SI-3, PC-8
Lack of pulse	LU-9, ST-12
Nasal congestion	LI-4, LI-20, LI-10
Nausea & vomiting	PC-6, CV-12
Night sweats	SI-3, HT-6, GV-14
Nosebleed	ST-44, LI-4, LU-11 (bleed), GV-20 (moxa)
Orchitis	LV-4
Pain in the lateral costal region	GB-34, TB-6
Painful urination	CV-3, LV-8
Phlegm expectoration	ST-40, LU-5, CV-12
Plum-stone qi	CV-22, PC-5, KI-6
Prolapse of the rectum	GV-20
Rectal pain	GV-1, BL-65, LU-6
Spasm	GV-1 (bleed)
Shivering	GV-14, PC-5
Somnolence	ST-36, SP-4, TB-2
Sour taste	ST-36
Uterine bleeding	LV-1 (moxa)
Vaginal itching	LV-5, LV-3
Wrist sprain	TB-5, TB-2

22.4 Selection of Points Belonging to Special Point Groups

The use of points that belong to special groups is an important aspect of point selection. It is common for every point in a prescription to be a member of a special grouping, and often the primary reason for choosing a point is because it belongs to such a grouping.

22.4.1 Application of the source-yuan points

Source-yuan points are primarily used for the treatment of diseases that affect the viscera and bowels. They are responsible for the regulation of source qi and are thus closely tied to the triple burner. Palpation of the source-yuan point of a particular channel helps identify repletion or vacuity in that channel's associated organ. The chart below outlines their clinical applications.

The Twelve Source-yuan Points	
Point	**Comments**
LU-9	Treats most lung problems. It can rectify lung qi and because it is the earth point of the metal channel it can supplement.
LI-4	Through its relationship with the triple burner, this point assists qi transformation in the whole body. It is frequently employed in the treatment of interior patterns. In addition, it can promote downbearing in the stomach and intestines.
ST-42	This point treats abdominal symptoms such as abdominal distention and nausea, and symptoms related to the stomach channel such as toothache (upper teeth) and wry eyes and mouth. It also treats heart and spirit disorders.
SP-3	This point is highly effective in rectifying spleen and stomach qi. It also treats pain and distention in the abdomen and is especially effective in combination with points such as LV-3, SP-6, ST-36, CV-12, and PC-6.
HT-7	Treats palpitations, poor memory, irritability, insomnia, visceral agitation (hysteria), and other heart-spirit related disorders.
SI-4	The small intestine manages the water aspect and is thus said to clear damp. The spleen easily suffers from damp. SI-4 is often employed in the treatment of splenic disorders because it stimulates the small intestine to drain damp.

The Twelve Source-yuan Points (Continued)	
Point	**Comments**
BL-64	Treats both vacuity and repletion in the bladder channel.
KI-3	This point enriches kidney yin and invigorates original yang.
PC-7	Treats heart disorders and is mentioned in the *Inner Canon* as the source-yuan point of the heart.
TB-4	Because both the triple burner and source-yuan points are related to the movement of source qi, the source-yuan point of the triple burner has a potent ability to regulate qi. This function is even stronger when TB-4 is combined with moxibustion at CV-12. When qi moves smoothly through the body, disease disappears.
GB-40	Treats repletion and vacuity conditions in the gallbladder channel; for example, shan qi, fullness pain in the chest and gastrointestinal spasms. It is especially effective for the treatment of pain in the instep and ankle.
LV-3	Treats liver yang headaches, fullness in the lower abdomen, penile pain, red painful eyes and other symptoms associated with the liver channel and viscera.

22.4.2 Application of connecting-luo points

The connecting-luo have two major applications as follows:

a) *Treatment of internally-externally coupled organs:* When a viscus and its related bowel are both affected by disease, it is usual to needle the connecting-luo point of the channel of the more seriously or more chronically affected organ. For example, a patient who presents with symptoms of lung and large intestine disease can be treated by either the connecting-luo point of the lung or the large intestine, depending on which organ is more seriously involved. This application includes treatment of diseases that display symptoms along the course of the channels of two organs that stand in interior-exterior relationship.

b) *Treatment of connecting vessel symptoms:* Each connecting vessel is mentioned in the *Inner Canon* as having a set of associated symptoms, which are outlined in Part III in the introductory sections of each of the 14 major channels, in the section on the connecting vessels. Note that each connecting vessel may present with symptoms of repletion as well as vacuity. The therapeutic principle is to drain repletion and supplement vacuity by employing the appropriate needle technique at the connecting-luo point.[2]

22.4.3 Applications of cleft-xi points

Clinically, cleft-xi points are commonly employed in the treatment of either stubborn or acute ailments involving the organs and channels. For example, a lung disease that presents with spitting of blood may be treated with LU-6, and acute heart and chest pain can be treated with HT-6, because these two points are the cleft-xi points of the lung and heart respectively. The effectiveness of cleft-xi points in relieving pain is evidenced by their frequent use in acupuncture anesthesia.

22.4.4 Applications of meeting-hui points

These points are employed to treat a general category of disease and are combined with others to address specific needs of the patient. For example, BL-17, the meeting-hui point of the blood, can be combined with SP-1 and LV-1 to treat metrorrhagia, and GB-34, the meeting point of the sinews, can be coupled with local points in the treatment of sprains and strains in any part of the body.

22.4.5 Applications of lower uniting-he points

The lower uniting-he points are primarily indicated for diseases of the six bowels. This therapeutic method was first mentioned in the *Essential Questions* "To treat the bowels, treat the uniting points." The following chart lists the lower uniting-he points and their major clinical uses.

Lower Uniting-He Points		
Channel	**Point**	**Symptoms Related to Home Bowel**
ST	ST-36	Poor digestion, venter pain and distention, abdominal pain, constipation, diarrhea
LI	ST-37	Intestinal yong (appendicitis), swill diarrhea
SI	ST-39	Diarrhea, abdominal pain, dysentery
GB	GB-34	Cholecystitis, bitter taste, vomiting
BL	BL-40	Urinary block, enuresis
TB	BL-39	Urinary block, enuresis

22.4.6 Applications of the command points

These points treat specific sections of the body and are appropriate for selection when the part of the body they "command" suffers from illness. ST-36 treats all abdominal disorders; BL-40 treats the back and lumbus; LU-7 treats the head and the back of the head; PC-6 treats the thoracic region; LI-4 treats the face and is of particular value for disorders in the mouth. Command points are often combined with points more specific to the disease being treated. For example, treatment of low back pain might pair BL-40, the command point of the back, with local points such as BL-23 and BL-30.

22.4.7 Applications of alarm-mu points

Alarm-mu points are generally applied in the treatment of diseases of the bowels (yang). For example, treatment of urinary disorders almost always includes the use of CV-3, the alarm-mu point of the bladder. ST-25, the alarm-mu point of the large intestine, is an excellent point for the treatment of constipation.

22.4.8 Applications of the associated-shu points

Associated-shu points are most commonly employed in the treatment of disorders involving the viscera (yin). They are also appropriate for the treatment of acute disorders. If a given organ is in a state of repletion the associated-shu point should be drained, and if the organ suffers from vacuity the point should be supplemented. By way of example, treatment of cough or dyspnea may include BL-13, the associated-shu point of the lung; and treatment of eye problems may include BL-18, the associated-shu point of the liver, because the liver opens into the eyes.

22.4.9 Applications of transporting-shu points

The transporting-shu points of the arms and legs are of particular interest because they are often chosen according to five-phase theory, or according to the relationship of the points to the celestial stems and the trigrams of *The Book of Changes*. While some five-phase applications are discussed in this text, the student should be aware that other applications exist and that point selection methods using the trigrams and celestial stems, though beyond the scope of this book, are employed by some practitioners.

a) *Employment according to the general functions of each of the five groupings:* In the *Inner Canon* it is stated that well-jing points treat diseases of the viscera; spring-ying points treat diseases that cause changes in the color of a patient's complexion; stream-shu points treat chronic diseases; river-jing points treat diseases that present with changes in the sound of the voice; and uniting-he points treat stomach diseases, or diseases that result from dietary irregularities (treatment is applied when the channels are full of blood). It also states that spring-ying and stream-shu points treat diseases that are in the channels (i.e., the exterior of the body), and uniting-he points treat diseases that are in the bowels (i.e., the interior of the body). Though not hard and fast rules, these principles should be considered when selecting points for treatment.[3]

The *Classic of Difficult Issues* relies almost exclusively on the five transporting-shu points for its method of treatment. In that classic the five transporting-shu points are given rule over the domains listed below.

Classic of Difficult Issues **Transporting-Shu Point Functions**	
Point	**Governs**
Well-jing	Fullness below the heart
Spring-ying	Body heat (fever)
Stream-shu	Bodily heaviness and joint pain
River-jing	Dyspnea, cough and alternations of cold and heat
Uniting-he	Counterflow qi and diarrhea

b) *Employment according to the seasons:* The text and commentaries of the *Classic of Difficult Issues* suggest the following: In the spring and summer months yang qi rises and the qi in the body flows on the exterior. Superficial needling is appropriate during this period, so well-jing and spring-ying points are often employed. In the fall and winter months yang qi sinks downward and the qi of the body is relatively deep. During this time it is appropriate to needle deeply, so river-jing and uniting-he points are often applied.

The above is in contradiction to the *Inner Canon* which states, ''... in winter needle the wells... in spring needle the springs... in summer needle the streams... in late summer needle the rivers... (and) in autumn needle the unions.'' This information is presented here so that the student can investigate the matter independently, and so that students realize that conflicting theories abound in Chinese medicine. Often it is the effort to reconcile seemingly conflicting theories that brings the student closer to the more abstruse meanings of Chinese medicine.

Seasonal Point Recommendations of the *Classic of Difficult Issues* and the *Inner Canon*		
Season	**Classic of Difficult Issues**	**Inner Canon**
Spring	Well-jing	Spring-ying
Summer	Spring-ying	River-jing
Fall	River-jing	Uniting-he
Winter	Uniting-he	Well-jing

c) *Employment According to Five-Phase Correspondences:* Each of the transporting-shu points has a five-phase correspondence, which differs for the yang channels and the yin channels as demonstrated in the chart below.

Five Transporting Points — Yin Channels (With the Source-Yuan Points)						
Channel	Points / Phase					
	Well-jing Wood	Spring-ying Fire	Stream-shu Earth	Source-yuan Earth	River-jing Metal	Uniting-he Water
Lung	LU-11	LU-10	LU-9	LU-9	LU-8	LU-5
Pericardium	PC-9	PC-8	PC-7	PC-7	PC-5	PC-3
Heart	HT-9	HT-8	HT-7	HT-7	HT-4	HT-3
Spleen	SP-1	SP-2	SP-3	SP-3	SP-5	SP-9
Liver	LV-1	LV-2	LV-3	LV-3	LV-4	LV-8
Kidney	KI-1	KI-2	KI-3	KI-3	KI-7	KI-10

Five Transporting Points — Yang Channels (With the Source-Yuan Points)						
Channel	Points / Phase					
	Well-jing Metal	Spring-ying Water	Stream-shu Wood	Source-yuan	River-jing Fire	Uniting-he Earth
Large Intestine	LI-1	LI-2	LI-3	LI-4	LI-5	LI-11
Triple Burner	TB-1	TB-2	TB-3	TB-4	TB-6	TB-10
Small Intestine	SI-1	SI-2	SI-3	SI-4	SI-5	SI-8
Stomach	ST-45	ST-44	ST-43	ST-42	ST-41	ST-36
Gallbladder	GB-44	GB-43	GB-41	GB-40	GB-38	GB-34
Bladder	BL-67	BL-66	BL-65	BL-64	BL-60	BL-40

436

The five-phase correspondences outlined in the preceding chart are used to treat repletion and vacuity according to the precept that vacuity is treated by supplementing the mother, and repletion is treated by draining the child. This maxim can be applied either to the affected channel or to the channels that correspond to the mother or child phase of the affected channel. Both methods of point selection are primarily used for the yin channels.

1. Mother and child treatment of the affected channel: Repletion in a given channel may be drained through the point on the affected channel that corresponds to the child phase of that channel. For example, repletion in a metal channel can be treated by applying a draining stimulation to the water point (child) on that channel. Thus a patient presenting with acute cough and dyspnea as part of a lung repletion pattern could be treated with the water point (LU-5) of the lung (metal) channel.

Vacuity in a given channel may be supplemented through the point on the affected channel that corresponds to the mother of that channel. Vacuity in a metal channel can be treated by applying a supplementing stimulation to the earth point (mother) on that channel. Therefore, a patient who has shortness of breath and copious perspiration as part of a lung vacuity pattern may be treated with the earth point of the lung channel, LU-9.

2. Treatment of the affected channel via mother and child channels: Repletion in a given channel can be treated by using a transporting-shu point on the channel corresponding to the child phase of the affected channel. This is another way of treating repletion by draining the child. For example, repletion in the liver (wood) channel may be treated by draining the heart (fire) channel. The point on the child channel that corresponds to the phase of that channel is chosen and given a draining stimulus. In this example, HT-7, the fire point of the fire (child) channel, would be drained to treat liver channel repletion. Repletion of the lung (metal) channel can be addressed by draining the water point of the kidney (water) channel, KI-10, and repletion in the heart (fire) channel can be treated with the earth point of the spleen (earth) channel, SP-3 and so on.

Vacuity in a given channel can be treated by using the transporting-shu point on the channel that corresponds to the mother phase of the affected channel. This is known as treating vacuity by supplementing the mother. For example, vacuity in the lung (metal) channel may be treated by supplementing the spleen (earth) channel. The point on the mother channel that corresponds to the phase of that channel is given a supplementing stimulus. In the example mentioned here, SP-3, the earth point of the earth channel, could be supplemented to treat lung channel vacuity. Vacuity of the heart (fire) channel can be treated by supplementation of the wood point of the wood channel, LV-1, and vacuity of the spleen (earth) channel can be addressed by employing the fire point of the fire channel, HT-8, and so on as in the chart that follows.

Use of Transporting-shu Points			
Channel	**Vacuity** / **Repletion**	**Treatment via Affected Channel**	**Treatment via Mother or Child Channel**
Lung	Vacuity	LU-9, earth of metal channel	SP-3, earth of earth channel
	Repletion	LU-5, water of metal channel	KI-10, water of water channel
Heart	Vacuity	HT-9, wood of fire channel	LV-1, wood of wood channel
	Repletion	HT-7, earth of fire channel	SP-3, earth of earth channel
Pericardium	Vacuity	PC-9, wood of fire channel	LV-1, wood of wood channel
	Repletion	PC-7, earth of fire channel	SP-3, earth of earth channel
Large Intestine	Vacuity	LI-11, earth of metal channel	ST-36, earth of earth channel
	Repletion	LI-2, water of metal channel	BL-66, water of water channel
Small Intestine	Vacuity	SI-3, wood of fire channel	GB-41, wood of wood channel
	Repletion	SI-8, earth of fire channel	ST-36, earth of earth channel
Triple Burner	Vacuity	TB-3, wood of fire channel	GB-41, wood of wood channel
	Repletion	TB-10, earth of fire channel	ST-36, earth of earth channel
Spleen	Vacuity	SP-2, fire of earth channel	HT-8, fire of fire channel
	Repletion	SP-5, metal of earth channel	LU-8, metal of metal channel
Kidney	Vacuity	KI-7, metal of water channel	LU-5, metal of metal channel
	Repletion	KI-1, wood of water channel	LI-I, wood of wood channel
Liver	Vacuity	LV-8 water of wood channel	KI-10, water of water channel
	Repletion	LV-2, fire of wood channel	HT-8, fire of fire channel
Stomach	Vacuity	ST-41, fire of earth channel	SI-5, fire of fire channel
	Repletion	ST-45, metal of earth channel	LV-1, metal of metal channel
Bladder	Vacuity	BL-67, metal of water channel	LI-1, metal of metal channel
	Repletion	BL-65, wood of water channel	GB-41, wood of wood channel
Gallbladder	Vacuity	GB-43, water of wood channel	BL-66, water of water channel
	Repletion	GB-38, fire of wood channel	SI-5, fire of fire channel

Note: When the preceding table calls for supplementation by use of a well-jing point, many practitioners substitute the uniting-he point in its place because of the difficulty of applying a supplementing stimulus to the well-jing points.

This section on the use of five-phase correspondences of the transporting-shu points is a variation of the treatment methods put forth more that 1500 years ago in the *Classic of Difficult Issues*. While modern practice makes use of some of the principles set forth in that classic, the absolute reliance on five-phase theory has been tempered by the admixture of other theories and modified to correspond with more recent clinical observations. The Chinese world view permits the simultaneous existence of seemingly conflicting theories, thus allowing for the selection of the particular theory that is best suited to cope with specific conditions. In point selection, this leaves practitioners free to choose five-phase correspondences when it seems appropriate to do so, and to ignore them when it seems to conflict with their clinical experience. For example, when five-phase theory indicates that the well-jing point of the liver channel be supplemented in order to treat a vacuity in the heart channel, some practitioners ignore this because they feel it is not possible to execute a supplementing stimulus in the shallow flesh of the well-jing point, and furthermore their clinical experience indicates to them that this point has a draining, not a supplementing, action.[4]

22.4.10 Applications of intersection-jiaohui points

When a disease affects more than one channel it is often appropriate to select an intersection-jiaohui point of the affected channels. SP-6, for example, is often used to treat disorders that affect any or all of the three leg yin channels because it is the intersection-jiaohui point of the liver, spleen, and kidney. Genitourinary disorders can be treated with point prescriptions that include CV-3 because that point is the intersection-jiaohui point of the three leg yin channels and the conception vessel, all of which are intimately connected with the genitourinary region.

If a disorder is located near an intersection-jiaohui point, then treatment of points on any of the intersecting channels may be appropriate. BL-62, for example, can treat gallbladder channel sciatic pain because GB-30 (a common site of sciatic pain) is the intersection-jiaohui point of the gallbladder and bladder channels. Point functions are often related to intersection-jiaohui points in this manner.

Intersection-jiaohui points can be employed to treat irregularities in the functions of any of the intersecting channels it unites. For example, LV-14, the intersection-jiaohui point of the spleen and liver, is often employed to treat circulatory system disorders because the spleen has the responsibility of managing the blood and the liver is responsible for storing the blood.

Although sources differ as to the exact number, there are about one hundred intersection-jiaohui points. The chart below lists the points that are commonly found in this category and asterisks (*) mark the intersections that have the most clinical significance.

Points of Intersection on the Yang Channels											
Points	GV	BL	SI	GB	TB	ST	LI	YgL	YgM	Grd	**Remarks**
CV-20	O_r	+*									
CV-24	O_r		+		+						
GV-1	O_r			+							KI
GV-13	O_r	+									
GV-14	O_r		+				+				
GV-15	O_r							+*			
GV-16	O_r							+*			
GV-17	O_r	+									
GV-26	O_r					+	+				
GV-28	O_r					+					CV
BL-1		O_r	+			+					
BL-11		O_r	+								
BL-12	+	O_r									
BL-41		O_r	+								
BL-59		O_r							+		
BL-62		O_r							+*		
BL-61		O_r							+		
BL-63		O_r						+*			
SI-10			O_r					+	+		
SI-12			O_r	+*	+*		+*				
SI-18			O_r		+						
SI-19			O_r	+*	+*						
GB-1			+	O_r	+*						
GB-3				O_r	+	+					
GB-4				O_r	+	+					
GB-5				O_r	+	+	+				
GB-6				O_r	+	+					
GB-7		+		O_r							
GB-8		+*		O_r							
GB-9		+*		O_r							
GB-10		+		O_r							
GB-11		+		O_r							
GB-12		+		O_r							
GB-13				O_r				+			

+ = Intersection O_r = Origin   * = Clinical importance

Points of Intersection on the Yang Channels										
Points	GV	BL	SI	GB	TB	ST	LI	YgL	YgM	Grd	**Remarks**
GB-14			+	O$_r$			+				
GB-15		+*		O$_r$				+			
GB-16				O$_r$				+			
GB-17				O$_r$				+			
GB-18				O$_r$				+			
GB-19				O$_r$				+			
GB-20				O$_r$				+*	+*		
GB-21				O$_r$	+*	+		+			
GB-24		+		O$_r$							
GB-26				O$_r$						+*	
GB-27				O$_r$						+*	
GB-28				O$_r$						+*	
GB-29				O$_r$					+		
GB-30		+*		O$_r$							
GB-35				O$_r$				+			
TB-13		+			O$_r$						
TB-14		+			O$_r$						
TB-15					O$_r$				+		
TB-17				+*	O$_r$						
TB-20				+	O$_r$		+				
TB-22			+	+*	O$_r$						
ST-1						O$_r$			+		CV
ST-3						O$_r$	+		+		
ST-4						O$_r$	+		+		
ST-7				+*		O$_r$					
ST-8				+*		O$_r$		+*			
ST-9				+*		O$_r$					
ST-30						O$_r$					Penetrating Ves.
LI-14		+*	+				O$_r$	+			
LI-15							O$_r$		+		
LI-16							O$_r$		+		
LI-20						+*	O$_r$				
LV-1		+*									
LV-13		+*									

+ = Intersection O$_r$ = Origin * = Clinical importance

Points of Intersection on the Yin Channels										
Points	CV	SP	LU	LV	PC	KI	HT	YinL	YinM	PenV	**Remarks**
CV-7	O$_r$									+*	GV*
CV-2	O$_r$					+*					
CV-3	O$_r$	+*			+*			+*			
CV-4	O$_r$	+*			+*			+*			
CV-7	O$_r$									+*	
CV-10	O$_r$	+*									
CV-12	O$_r$										ST*, SI*, TB*
CV-13	O$_r$										ST*, SI
CV-17	O$_r$	+*				+*					SI, TB*
CV-22	O$_r$							+			
CV-23	O$_r$							+			
CV-24	O$_r$										ST*
SP-6		O$_r$		+*		+*					
SP-12		O$_r$	+								
SP-13		O$_r$	+					+			
SP-15		O$_r$						+			
SP-16		O$_r$						+			
LU-1		+	O$_r$								
LI-13				O$_r$				+		GB*	
PC-1					O$_r$						GB
KI-6						O$_r$			+		
KI-8						O$_r$			+		
KI-9						O$_r$		+			
KI-11						O$_r$				+	
KI-12						O$_r$				+	
KI-13						O$_r$				+	
KI-14						O$_r$				+*	
KI-15						O$_r$				+*	
KI-16						O$_r$				+*	
KI-17						O$_r$				+	
KI-18						O$_r$				+	
KI-19						O$_r$				+	
KI-20						O$_r$				+	
KI-21						O$_r$				+*	
LV-14		+*		O$_r$							

+ = Intersection O$_r$ = Origin * = Clinical importance

23. General Principles of Point Combining

Acupuncture treatment utilizes a number of points in a given session. In order to maximize efficacy and minimize the number of points used, various guidelines for combining points have evolved. The major principles of point combining are outlined below.

23.1 Combining Local and Distant Points

It is common practice to choose points at or near the site of the disease and combine them with distant points that have an effect on the involved area. Headache, for example, is often treated with local points such as ST-8 and GB-20, supported by distant points such as LI-4 and ST-44. The selection of both distant and local points is determined by the nature and location of the disorder. (See the chart on page 413.)

23.2 Combining Points on the Front and the Back

Combining points on the front and back of the trunk of the body is a therapeutic principle exemplified by the dual employment of alarm-mu points and associated-shu points. Simultaneous use of these two sets of points increases the efficacy of both. Stomach pain, for example, may be treated by combining the alarm point of the stomach, CV-12, with BL-21, the associated-shu point of the stomach. The chart below lists these pairings and their scope of treatment.

Alarm-mu and Associated-shu Points			
Organ	**Associated** *shu*	**Alarm** *mu*	**Scope of Treatment**
LU	BL-13	LU-1	respiratory system disorders such as cough, dyspnea, thoracic fullness and distention
PC	BL-14	CV-17	heart diseases such as cardiac pain and palpitations
HT	BL-15	CV-14	heart and stomach disorders such as palpitations, stomach pain, and neurasthenia

Alarm-mu and Associated-shu Points (Cont.)			
Organ	Associated *shu*	Alarm *mu*	Scope of Treatment
LV	BL-18	LV-14	liver and stomach disorders such as liver region pain, vomiting and regurgitation of acid fluid
GB	BL-19	GB-24	liver and gallbladder disorders such as pain in the area of GB-24 and jaundice
SP	BL-20	LV-13	liver and spleen disorders such as enlargement or pain in either organ, abdominal pain or distention, and poor digestion
ST	BL-21	CV-12	stomach region disorders such as stomach pain or distention and lack of appetite
TB	BL-22	CV-5	water metabolism dysfunctions such as edema, ascites, and diarrhea
KI	BL-23	GB-25	kidney and genitourinary disorders, low back pain or soreness, seminal loss, and premature ejaculation
LI	BL-25	ST-25	large intestine disorders such as constipation, diarrhea, and abdominal pain
SI	BL-27	CV-4	small intestine, bladder and genitourinary disorders such as gripping intestinal pain, shan qi, enuresis, urinary block, and seminal loss
BL	BL-28	CV-3	bladder and genitourinary disorders such as enuresis, urinary block, seminal loss, and menstrual disorders

Note: Points adjacent to alarm-mu and associated-shu points have functions that are similar to those points, and may be substituted for them.

23.3 Combining Points from Yin and Yang Channels:
Dual Application of Source-yuan and Connecting-luo Points

Combining points from yin and yang channels is exemplified by, but not limited to, the application of source-yuan points and connecting-luo points. Coupling a yin channel point with one on the corresponding yang channel can increase the effectiveness of both points.

Source-yuan points and connecting-luo points are often employed together to treat diseases that affect both organs of an interior-exterior pair. The general rule is that the source point of the more seriously or more chronically involved organ is coupled with the connecting-luo point of the less involved organ. For example, severe dyspnea with mild constipation can be treated by needling the source-yuan point of the lung, LU-9, and the connecting-luo point of the large intestine, LI-6. Because the less involved channel is termed the guest, and the more involved channel is termed the host, this method of treatment is sometimes called guest-host treatment.

The following chart lists the source-yuan points and connecting-luo points of the twelve channels.

Source-Yuan — Connecting-Luo Points				
Channel		Points		Main Diseases
Host	Guest	Source-yuan	Conn-ecting-luo	
LU		LU-9		Bronchitis, sore throat, shortness of breath, copious phlegm, perspiration, heat in the palms and soles, breast pain, shoulder pain that follows the lung channel.
	LI		LI-6	
LI		LI-4		Throat and gum diseases, lymph node inflammation in the neck, mumps, sore throat, dry mouth, yellow eyes, clear nasal discharge, nosebleed, and large intestine channel shoulder pain.
	LU		LU-7	
SP		SP-3		Stiff tongue, abdominal pain, bodily weakness and heaviness, constipation, jaundice, leg pain along the spleen channel, malarial disease.
	ST		ST-40	
ST		ST-42		Nosebleed, facial numbness, stomach channel leg pain, malarial disease, abdominal distention, general weakness.
	SP		SP-4	
HT		HT-7		Heart pain, rapid heartbeat, dry mouth, yellow eyes, heart channel arm pain.
	SI		SI-7	
SI		SI-4		Submandibular swelling and pain, shoulder pain, neck pain, deafness, arm pain along the small intestine channel.
	HT		HT-5	
KI		KI-3		General weakness and lassitude, lack of appetite, decrease in visual acuity, lower back soreness, weakness in the lower extremities, grey facial color.
	BL		BL-58	
BL		BL-64		Eye pain, neck pain, pain in the back, lower back or legs, epilepsy, psychiatric disorders, nosebleed, rectal prolapse, hemorrhoids, malarial disease.
	KI		KI-4	
TB		TB-4		Deafness, sore throat, conjunctivitis, shoulder and back pain, intra-vertebral pain, constipation, urinary block, enuresis.
	PC		PC-6	
PC		PC-7		Spasms or pain in the forearm or hand, chest pain, palpitations, nausea, restlessness, heat in the palms, incessant laughter.
	TB		TB-5	
LV		LV-3		Testicular pain and swelling, shan qi pain, thoracic fullness, vomiting, abdominal pain, diarrhea, enuresis, urinary block.
	GB		GB-37	
GB		GB-40		Pain in the chest and lateral costal region, headache, eye pain, malarial disease, enlarged thyroid, swollen lymph nodes in the neck.
	LV		LV-5	

23.4 Combination of Upper Body and Lower Body Points

Points on the upper body are frequently combined with those on the lower body. This is an example of the use of the principles of yin and yang and may be applied to any relevant points in the two regions. The application of the eight confluence-jiaohui points of the extraordinary vessels is a unique example.

The confluence-jiaohui points can be employed singly or in pairs to treat diseases associated with the extraordinary vessels. The chart below outlines the treatment scope of each pair of confluence-jiaohui points.

The Confluence-Jiaohui Points of the Eight Extraordinary Vessels		
Confluence Point	**Extraordinary Vessel**	**Regions of Effect**
PC-6 SP-4	Yin linking Penetrating	Heart, stomach, and chest
TB-5 GB-41	Yang linking girdling	Outer canthus, area behind the ear, shoulder, neck (front)
LU-7 KI-6	conception Yin motility	Diaphragm, throat, lung
SI-3 BL-62	Governing vessel Yang motility	Inner canthus, neck (front and back), ear, shoulder Small intestine and bladder

23.5 Dual Application of Cleft-xi Points and Meeting-hui Points

In practice, meeting-hui points are often combined with cleft-xi points. For example, an acute case of coughing up of blood may be treated by combining BL-17, the meeting-hui point of the blood, with LU-6, the cleft-xi point of the lung, and acute stomach pain may be alleviated by use of the cleft-xi point of the stomach, ST-34, and the meeting-hui point of the bowels, CV-12.

24. General Therapeutic Principles

24.1 Treatment of Root and Branches

Root and branches are relative terms that represent various aspects of the disease condition. These terms differ in meaning according to context. Root can refer to the body's correct qi in which case branches refer to a pathogen. If root refers to an enduring condition, branches refer to a more recent disease, and if root is a reference to an interior disease then branches is a reference to an exterior one. Because patients often present with complex disease patterns it is important to determine treatment priorities. Root and branches provide guidelines for determining symptoms that must be attended to first and symptoms that can wait.

24.1.1 Treatment of the root

When treating a patient whose source qi is debilitated or one who has suffered from an enduring disease, it is imperative to first restore the strength of the correct qi and treat any lingering disease before directing attention toward disorders of recent onset. This principle holds true for conditions where the acute disease is not of a serious nature, and is termed *treating the root before the branch*.

24.1.2 Treatment of the branches

When the correct is not debilitated and a patient suffering from an enduring disorder contracts a relatively serious acute disease, it is best to treat the acute disease first and any longstanding disorders second. This order of treatment is termed *treating the branch before the root*. In addition, symptomatic treatment is appropriate in the following situations:

• Branch treatment is fitting when the root is clearly determinable but the acute condition is serious enough to demand immediate attention. Acute appendicitis is an example of this.

• If the patient suffers from an acute and painful disorder one may apply symptomatic treatment before a thorough investigation of the disease root is deemed practical. Acute abdominal pain, severe headache, shock (clouding inversion) and trauma are cases where this principle applies.

• Symptomatic treatment is suitable in instances where a patient presents with a single symptom that does not appear to have any root cause. If, for example, a patient who has no other symptoms and a normal pulse and tongue complains of insomnia, it may be appropriate to use points such as N-HN-54 and N-LE-50, which are points for the symptomatic relief of insomnia.

24.1.3 Simultaneous treatment of root and branches

In general, it is considered best to direct treatment at the root, but formularies often contain points that also treat the branches. For example, a patient suffering from debilitation of kidney water and hyperactivity of liver yang who presents with low back pain, seminal loss, spiritual lassitude, headache, and dizziness, as well as spiritual disquietude and insomnia, may require points to enrich kidney water and calm liver yang to treat the root of the disease. The addition of one or two spirit-quieting points such as HT-7 will treat the branch.

Simultaneous treatment of root and branches is the most common form of treatment. The practitioner can keep the number of points used to a minimum by employing ones that address both the root and branches of a disease. LI-4, for example, is an excellent point for treatment of headache due to exogenous contraction, because it not only addresses the root (by resolving the exterior), but is also an excellent point for the symptomatic relief of headache.

24.2 Additional Considerations of Point Combining

When treating diseases that affect the head, trunk, internal organs or both sides of the body, it is common to treat bilaterally corresponding points. For example, nausea can be treated by needling PC-6 on both arms.

Practitioners generally choose points that address the underlying disharmony and then add points to relieve particular symptoms. The above description of simultaneous treatment of branch and root provides a good example.

Use of the same points for each treatment should be avoided, as repeatedly employing the same points reduces their efficacy. Adjacent points and other points of similar function should be substituted to maximize effectiveness.

Point formularies should be as concise as possible, varying according to the disorder being treated. The following types of point formularies provide a guideline in this regard.

• *Major formularies* contain a large number of points (10-15 needles), and use thick-gauged needles in order to produce a strong stimulus. This type of prescription treats serious disorders such as wind strike, high fever, and tetany.

• *Minor formularies* contain few points and use thin needles to produce a mild stimulus. This is suitable for disorders of recent onset, mild disorders and for persons of weak constitution.

• *Moderate formularies* are suitable for disorders that require long-term treatment. Generally, a light stimulus is sought and the needles are retained for 20 to 30 minutes.

• *Emergency prescriptions* contain a small number of carefully chosen points that are given a strong stimulus. This type of prescription is used to treat acute, serious conditions such as inversion patterns (shock or syncope), fright spasm, and cholera.

• *Single-point prescription* refers to the use of a single point to relieve a particular discomfort. Needling LI-4 to relieve toothache, or PC-6 to ease stomach pain are examples of this type of treatment. Strong stimulation and needle retention characterize the single-point prescription.

It is usually necessary to modify or combine the above prescriptions to fit the situation at hand.

Section Notes

[1]These books are *The Great Compendium of Acupuncture and Moxibustion*, and *The Glorious Anthology of Acupuncture*.

[2] According to the *Spiritual Axis,* it is useful to bleed connecting vessels (i.e., the blood connecting vessels) when those vessels exhibit symptoms of repletion and qi counterflow.

[3]According to the *Classic of Difficult Issues* the reasoning for the assignment of a point category to its area of governance lies in five-phase theory. The well-jing points govern fullness below the heart because these points are associated with the wood phase (in regard to the viscera), and the liver channel, which is also associated with wood, penetrates the diaphragm and disperses over the chest area. The spring-ying points govern body heat because they are associated with the fire phase, and heart fire that overcomes the lung produces fever. The stream-shu points can treat bodily heaviness and joint pain, because these symptoms are signs of disease in the earth phase, and these points are associated with the earth phase. The river-jing points belong to metal (lungs) and thus are employed in the treatment of cough and alternation of cold and heat. The uniting-he points are associated with water and the kidney. The kidney and the penetrating vessel are intimately connected so that an insufficiency in the former results in counterflow qi in the latter. Kidney insufficiency also can result in diarrhea (the kidney opens at the two yins); thus counterflow qi and diarrhea can be treated through uniting-he points.

[4]*The Classic of Difficult Issues* style of point selection is more complex than the system mentioned here. The student is referred to Paul Unschuld's translation, *Medicine in China: The Nan-Ching Classic of Difficult Issues* for further elaboration.

Glossary of Terms

Glossary of Terms

accumulation 積 *jī*: See *concretions and gatherings*.

assisting bone 輔骨 *fǔ gǔ*: Radius; fibula.

bi 痹 *bì*: A generic term denoting conditions attributable to pathogenic qi that causes blockage in the limbs, trunk, or in the organs or channels. Bi patterns are generally the result of a combination of wind, cold, and damp pathogens invading the exterior channels and joints, giving rise to articular or muscular pain, severe swelling, and leaden heaviness. Synonym: Obturation.

binding depression of liver qi 肝氣鬱結 *gān qì yù jié*: Impairment of hepatic free coursing and upbearing effusion due to anger, annoyance, and general emotional disturbance. The main general signs are distention and fullness or scurrying pain in the lateral costal region, usually emotion-related. Globus hystericus may occur when liver qi ascends counterflow. Pain in the venter, vomiting of sour fluid, and poor appetite are observed when liver qi invades the stomach, affecting gastric harmony and downbearing. Binding depression of liver qi may cause qi stagnation and blood stasis. In such cases, there is stabbing pain in the lateral costal region, with the possibility of formation of concretions and gatherings. Menstrual disorders, neurosis, hepatocystic disease, hepatosplenomegaly, and indigestion are often related to binding depression of liver qi.

blood ejection 吐血 *tù xuè*: Vomiting or expectoration of blood.

boost 益 *yì*: See *supplementation*.

bowstring and elusive masses 痃癖 *xián pì*: Bowstring masses are elongated masses lateral to the navel; elusive masses are ones located in the lateral costal region that occur intermittently with pain and at other times are not detectable by palpation. The two are usually referred to together.

branching fullness 支滿 *zhī mǎn*: This term describes the feeling of distention and fullness that usually occurs in the thoracic or diaphragmatic region and can branch out to the lateral costal region. The word *zhī*, here rendered as branching, can be a description of the nature of the fullness or an indirect reference to the thoracic or diaphragmatic region, or can imply the upward lift caused by the fullness.

brighten the eyes 明目 *míng mù*: Enhance visual acuity, or otherwise benefit the eyes.

calm 平 *píng*: To reduce (liver yang, dyspnea). Liver calming is a method of treating ascending liver yang that is appropriate regardless of the cause. It is often seen in combination with extinguishing liver wind because ascending liver yang and liver wind frequently coexist. The Chinese character means peace, tranquility, and evenness, and expresses both the ability of certain points to settle liver yang and the patient's resultant calm and tranquility.

clear 清 *qīng*: Clearing is used to describe the function of ridding the body of heat. Heat can be cleared from the heart (which actually means the pericardium), lung, intestines, gallbladder, construction aspect, qi aspect, or blood aspect. The method of clearing heat is often combined with exterior resolution in exterior heat patterns. Draining is similar in meaning to clearing, but describes the elimination of heat, fire, and damp-heat in the lower burner, or fire and heat in the organs that manifest in upper-body heat signs. In the eight methods of treatment, clearage is a generic term that includes clearing heat, draining fire, cooling the blood, resolving (heat) toxin, and dispelling summerheat.

clonic spasm 瘛瘲 *chì zòng*: A spasm in which rigidity of the muscles is followed immediately by relaxation.

clouding inversion 昏厥 *hūn jué*: Clouding of the consciousness in inversion patterns.

clove sore 疔瘡 *dīng chuāng*: Any small, hard, deep-rooted pyogenic lesion. The name derives from the fact that it is shaped like a nail or clove.

cold malaria 寒瘧 *hán nüè*: Malaria resulting from the contraction of wind-cold when there is deeplying cold in the inner body. It is characterized by chills more pronounced than fever with episodes occurring daily or every other day.

completion bone 完骨 *wán gǔ*: The mastoid process of the occipital bone.

concretion 癥 *zhēng*: See *concretions and gatherings*.

concretions and gatherings 癥瘕積聚 *zhēng jiǎ jī jù*: The collective term for concretions *(zhēng)*, conglomerations *(jiǎ)*, accumulations *(jī)*, and gatherings *(jù)*, all four of which refer to abdominal masses associated with pain and distention. Concretions and accumulations are masses of definite form and fixed location, associated with pain of fixed location. They stem from disease in the viscera and at blood level. Conglomerations and gatherings are masses of indefinite form, which gather and dissipate at irregular intervals and are attended by pain of unfixed location. They are attributed to disease in the bowels and at qi level. Accumulations and gatherings chiefly occur in the middle burner. Concretions and conglomerations chiefly occur in the lower burner, and in many cases are the result of gynecological disorders. In general, concretions and gatherings arise when emotional depression or intemperate eating causes damage to the liver and spleen. The resultant organ disharmony leads to obstruction and stagnation of qi, which in turn causes static blood to collect gradually in the inner body. Most often the root cause is insufficiency of correct qi.

conglomeration 瘕 *jiǎ*: See *concretions and gatherings*.

cool 涼 *liáng*: See *drainage*.

correct qi 正氣 *zhèng qì*: That which maintains the normal functioning of the human body and seeks to re-establish it when pathogenic qi is present.

counterflow 逆 *nì*: Flow counter to the normal direction. See *inversion*.

course 疏 *shū*: To enhance flow (of qi, especially depressed liver qi); eliminate (pathogens such as wind in the exterior); to free (the exterior or channels from pathogens such as wind). Coursing the liver is the method used to restore hepatic free coursing, applied to binding depression of liver qi. The Chinese ideogram means to dredge or comb, and open or well-spaced. See also *soothe*.

crick in the neck 落枕 *luò zhěn*: Stiffness of the neck that frequently results from sleeping in the wrong posture or exposure to a draft.

dai yang 戴陽 *dài yáng*: [*dài*, to wear on the head; to look upwards] A disease pattern characterized by tidal flushing of the cheeks and attributable to upfloating of vacuous yang. It is a pattern of true cold in the lower body and false heat in the upper body. The tidal flushing is characterized by pale red patches, giving the cheeks the appearance of having been dabbed with rouge. The patches often constantly change location. Other symptoms include counterflow frigidity of the lower limbs and long micturition with clear urine. False heat signs include nosebleed and bleeding gums, and a painful swollen throat. The pulse is large and floating, but feeble and vacuous. In serious cases it is faint and fine, verging on expiry.

deathlike inversion 屍厥 *shī jué*: Clouding inversion and inversion cold in the limbs giving the patient a deathlike appearance. Though unconscious, the patient has a pulse beat.

deep-source nasal congestion 鼻淵 *bí yuān*: Nasal congestion with thick, turbid, malodorous mucus, sometimes accompanied by soreness in area of the nose located between the eyes. It is caused by contraction of wind-cold that affects the brain and the presence of heat in the gallbladder channel.

depression 鬱 *yù*: Reduction of normal activity characterized by unvented stagnation. In physiology, depression refers either to binding depression of qi dynamic or to flow stoppage due to congestion. The term also describes inhibition of normal emotional responses, expressing itself in the form of melancholy, oppression, frustration and irascibility. Though often associated with psychosomatic disorders, this term bears broader connotations in Chinese medicine than it does in Western psychology.

desertion 脫 *tuō*: Patterns of critical depletion of yin, yang, qi, or blood, mainly characterized by pearly sweat, inversion frigidity of the limbs, gaping mouth and closed eyes, limp, open hands and enuresis, and fine pulse verging on expiry.

detriment 損 *sǔn*: Loss or damage (to blood, fluids, organs etc.)

diarrhea 泄瀉 *xiè xiè*: Any deviation from established bowel rhythm characterized by increased frequency of the stool. Diarrhea is classified in three distinct ways: a) according to cause or pathomechanism, e.g., summerheat diarrhea, digestate damage diarrhea, cold diarrhea, heat diarrhea, and vacuity diarrhea; b) according to the associated morbid organ, e.g., splenic diarrhea, gastric diarrhea, small intestine diarrhea, large intestine diarrhea, and kidney diarrhea; c) according to signs, e.g., daybreak diarrhea, enduring diarrhea, efflux diarrhea, outpour diarrhea, swill diarrhea, clear-food diarrhea, duck-stool diarrhea. These categories are not mutually exclusive. Digestate damage diarrhea, for example, is the result of damage to the digestive system by ingested food, as opposed to pre-existing dysfunction. It may therefore include certain forms of gastric, large intestine, and small intestine diarrhea, but excludes large intestine diarrhea due to lung qi vacuity (these two organs standing in exterior-interior relationship). Association between causes and form of diarrhea is variable. For example, daybreak diarrhea is always a form of kidney diarrhea, while thin-stool diarrhea may form part of either heat or cold patterns.

diffuse 宣 *xuān*: To promote the smooth flow of qi, especially that of the lung. ''Diffusing the lung'' means promoting the normal diffusion of lung qi.

diminished qi 少氣 *shǎo qì*: Feeble speech, together with weak, short rapid, distressed breathing; mainly attributable to visceral qi vacuity, especially of center and pulmorenal qi.

disinhibit 利 *lì*: To promote fluency, movement, or activity. The Chinese ideogram was originally a pictorial representation. The left-hand portion represents a grain stock heavy with seed, and the right side is a symbolic depiction of a knife blade. A sharp knife cutting the grain, speedily bringing the benefit of the harvest. In its modern usage, the character retains the meaning of sharpness, favorability, profit and benefit. In Chinese medicine, the meaning is to promote favorable movement, which we render as disinhibit. In other words, forms of treatment that address inhibited flow of qi, blood or fluids, or inhibited physical movement are described as disinhibiting. Substances that are commonly disinhibited are urine, damp, qi and water, and regions that commonly require disinhibition are the throat, the large intestine and joints. Disinhibit is similar to "move" and "free," the difference being in usage. Moving is primarily used in regard to the hampered flow of qi or water. Freeing (or unblocking) usually describes the promotion of free flow of qi, the menses, stool, breast milk or the waterways. *Lì* is often rendered by other writers as benefit or promote.

dispel 祛 *qū*: See *drainage*.

disperse 消 *xiāo*: See *drainage*.

dissipate 散 *sàn*: See *drainage*.

dizziness 眩暈 *xuàn yūn*: Any form of dizziness, including what Western medicine classes as true vertigo and lightheadedness.

dormant papules 癮疹 *yǐn zhěn*: Remittent outthrust of faint papules in changing locations; includes what Western medicine terms urticaria.

drainage 瀉 *xiè*: 1) Elimination, specifically of fire (the form of heat that is active and rising in nature) and lower burner damp-heat. 2) A strong stimulus applied in acupuncture to eliminate repletion. Words of similar meaning include: *dispel*: destroy or drive out (pathogens from the body); *eliminate*: destroy (pathogens, especially phlegm or damp); *expel*: remove (parasites from the body); *disperse*: break up or cause to disappear (glomus, phlegm and digestate accumulations, and swellings); *dissipate*: eliminate (cold) or whittle away (stasis nodules and binds); *dry*: eliminate (damp by using dry, bitter agents); *disinhibit*: promote the free movement (of fluids, qi or blood through parts of the body), or the elimination (of damp, water qi); *resolve*: eliminate (pathogens, especially those affecting the exterior), or free (parts of the body from pathogens); *clear*: Eliminate (heat); *cool*: remove heat (from the blood aspect).

crane's knee wind 鶴膝風 *hè xī fēng*: Painful swelling of the knee joint with emaciation of the lower leg, due to depletion of kidney yin and invasion by cold-damp; in most cases it develops from articular wind.

dysentery 痢 *lì*: 1) Diarrhea. 2) Dysenteric disease.

dysenteric disease 痢疾 *lì jí*: Diarrhea with either pus or mucus (white dysentery) or blood (red dysentery) in the stool, accompanied by abdominal pain and tenesmus; usually occurs in hot weather.

ejection 吐 *tù*: 1) The spontaneous expulsion of matter from the digestive tract through the mouth. 2) Induced expulsion of matter from the digestive tract, throat, or lungs through the mouth.

eliminate 除 *chú*: See *drainage*.

emolliate the liver 柔肝 *róu gān*: The method of treating liver yin vacuity (or insufficiency of liver blood), characterized by loss of visual acuity, dry eyes, night blindness, periodic mental dizziness and tinnitus, and pale nails, or poor sleep, excessive dreaming, dry mouth with lack of fluid, and a fine, weak pulse. Since the liver is the unyielding viscus and relies on the blood for nourishment, liver yin vacuity is often treated with points that nourish the blood.

engender 生 *shēng*: See *supplementation*.

enrich 滋 *zī*: See *supplementation*.

esophageal constriction 噎膈 *yē gé*: Constriction of the esophagus characterized by a sensation of blockage when swallowing, and/or blockage at the diaphragm preventing the downflow of digesta. Upper esophageal constriction may occur alone, although it usually portends the development of the dual condition. Causes include damage to the spleen by excessive preoccupation, excessive consumption of tobacco and alcohol, qi stagnation and heat depression, hard foodstuffs, and phlegm-rheum and blood stasis.

evil 邪 *xié*: See *pathogen*.

expel 驅 *qū*: See *drainage*.

eye gan 眼疳 *yǎn gān*: Ulceration of the eyelids.

eye screen 目翳 *mù yì*: Any visible visual impediment in the eyeball.

fire 火 *huǒ*: 1) In physiology, a transmutation of yang qi explained as a vital force, e.g., imperial fire, ministerial fire, and lesser fire. 2) A type of pathogen that manifests in signs classified under heat among the eight parameters and includes the following forms: a) One of the six environmental excesses; b) The product of the transformation of yang qi due to emotional disturbance (affect damage) or the action of exterior pathogens as they interiorize. c) Vacuity fire resulting from depletion of yin humor and yin yang imbalance in the organs giving rise to heat signs, particularly in the upper body. See *heat*.

foot qi 脚氣 *jiǎo qì*: A disease characterized by numbness of the legs, water swelling, and heart disease. Serious cases are marked by abstraction of spirit-disposition, and deranged speech. Different forms include damp foot qi, cold-damp foot qi, and phlegm-damp foot qi. Foot qi corresponds in Western medicine largely to beriberi, which is attributed to vitamin B1 deficiency.

fortify 健 *jiàn*: See *supplementation*.

fright epilepsy 驚癇 *jīng xián*: 1) Epilepsy caused by fright. 2) Fright wind (in Tang and Song medical records).

fright palpitation 驚悸 *jīng jì*: Heart palpitations brought on by fright. The causes are similar to those of general palpitation but are most frequently seen in patients who suffer from constitutional heart qi vacuity. Factors such as insufficiency of heart blood, detriment to kidney yin, blood stasis, internal collection of water-rheum and phlegm-fire must also be considered as possible causes.

fright wind 驚風 *jīng fēng*: Disease occurring in infants and children, characterized by convulsive spasm and loss of consciousness. Synonym: infantile convulsions.

fulminant clouding 暴昏 *bào hūn*: Sudden stupor or loss of consciousness.

gan 疳 *gan*: 1) Indented mucosal ulceration, often accompanied by putrefacion of the flesh and mild suppuration, e.g., periodontal gan, which refers to ulceration of the gums. 2) Gan accumulation.

gan accumulation 疳積 *gān jī*: A pediatric disease caused by splenogastric vacuity. Signs include yellow complexion, emaciation, dry hair, abdominal distention with visible superficial veins, and loss of essence-spirit vitality. It corresponds to child malnutrition as well as some parasitic and debilitating diseases in Western medicine.

gastric reflux 反胃 *fǎn wèi*: A pattern characterized by distention and fullness after eating, the vomiting in the evening of food ingested in the morning, or the vomiting in the morning of food ingested the previous evening, untransformed food in the vomitus, spiritual fatigue, and lack of bodily strength. Its principal cause is splenogastric vacuity cold, but it may also occur when congealed damp-heat stagnation leads to impairment of gastric harmony and downbearing.

gathering 聚 *jù*: See *concretions and gatherings*.

ghost talk 鬼言 *guǐ yán*: Speaking as if possessed.

glans penis 陰頭 *yīn tóu*: The cap-shaped expansion that forms the head of the penis. Synonym: balanus.

glomus 痞 *pǐ*: The sensation of a lump, generally of limited size, in the abdominothoracic cavity. Also called focal distention. When palpable, it is referred to as lump glomus. In texts that predate *A Treatise on Cold Damage,* glomus denoted what was later termed lump glomus.

goose foot wind 鵝掌風 *é zhǎng fēng*: Xian of the hand caused by wind toxin or damp invading the skin. In the initial stages, it is characterized by small vesicles and itching. Later, white skin sheds. When it persists for long periods, the skin becomes thick and rough and tends to crack, especially in winter.

gu 蠱 *gǔ*: Disease caused by parasites and characterized by drumlike abdominal distention. See Unschuld, *Medicine in China*, pp. 46-50.

harmonize 和 *hé*: To coordinate (one organ with another or with the body as a whole). Gastric harmonization and hepatic harmonization are the two most common forms of single organ harmonization, and hepatogastric, hepatosplenic, splenogastric, and gastrointestinal harmonizations are the most frequently encountered methods of harmonizing two organs. In addition, construction and defense, yin and yang, and qi and blood are subject to harmonization. Shao yang disease is one that is located between the exterior and interior of the body, and treatment of this condition is known as harmonization of the shao yang.

heat 熱 *rè*: 1) One of the eight parameters. 2) Any pathogen manifesting in signs classified as heat among the eight parameters (the environmental excesses fire and summerheat, and fire or heat as the result of vacuity or the product of transformation of interiorizing pathogens or yang qi due to affect damage). 3) Fever or subjective sensations of heat that may or may not be classified as heat among the eight parameters. See *fire*.

heat malaria 熱瘧 *rè nüè*: Malarial disease characterized by pronounced fever and mild chills.

hemilateral wind 偏風 *piān fēng*: Hemiplegia.

increase 增 *zēng*: See *supplementation*.

infantile disruption 小兒客忤 *xiǎo ér kè wǔ*: Crying, fright, disquietude, or even digestive irregularities in infants precipitated by seeing a stranger or being exposed to unfamiliar surroundings or circumstances.

intestinal pi 腸澼 (澼) *cháng pì*: 1) Dysenteric disease (ancient name). 2) Bloody stool due to intestinal stasis.

intestinal wind 腸風 *cháng fēng*: 1) Bleeding hemorrhoids. 2) Bloody stool due to disharmony of qi and blood that results from wind-cold and heat toxin contending in the large intestine. 3) Wind dysentery. 4) A condition in which fresh red blood is discharged from the anus prior to evacuation.

inversion 厥 *jué*: The disruption of qi dynamic chiefly associated with clouding inversion (i.e., loss of consciousness) and inversion frigidity of the limbs (severe cold in the limbs associated with desertion patterns), in which adequate supplies of qi and blood fail to reach the head and extremities. Inversion patterns are those characterized by these symptoms. For example, cold inversion refers to a pattern characterized by clouding inversion and inversion frigidity of the limbs, attributed to yang qi vacuity. Blood inversion refers to patterns caused by blood disease (vacuity or repletion) and characterized by the two symptoms of inversion. The notion of inversion is closely associated with that of counterflow. Inversion frigidity of the limbs and counterflow frigidity of the limbs are identical in meaning. However, counterflow is otherwise associated with disruption of the qi dynamic of organs such as the liver, stomach and lung. Both the ideograms for *jué* and *nì* carry connotations of adversity; *jué* has connotations of disruption, breaking off, and finality. The ideogram *jué* is that occurring in the term jué yīn channel, interestingly rendered by Porkert as yin flectens and by Bensky and O'Connor as Absolute Yin.

invigorate 壯 *zhuàng*: See *supplementation*.

jie 疥 *jiè*: A lesion most commonly occurring between the fingers of the hand and characterized by an insufferable penetrating, prickly itching sensation, which can lead to suppuration when scratched.

ju 疽 *jū*: A deep, inflammatory, pyogenic lesion of the flesh identified by a broad, low elevation.

kui shan 㿗疝 *kuí shàn*: 1) Pain, swelling, hardening or numbness of the scrotum 2) Swelling and suppuration of the male or female external genitals.

lateral costal region 脅 *xié*: The sides of the ribcage, or hypochondriac region.

malign blood 惡血 *è xuè*: Extravasated blood that accumulates and necrotizes in the tissues surrounding blood vessels.

mania and withdrawal 癲狂 *diān kuáng*: Mania and withdrawal are forms of mental derangement. Mania denotes states of excitement characterized by noisy, unruly, and even aggressive behavior, offensive speech, constant singing and laughter, irascibility, and inability to remain tidily dressed. This is a repletion pattern of the heart spirit straying outwards owing to hyperactivity of yang qi. Withdrawal refers to mental depression, indifference, deranged speech, taciturnity, and obliviousness of hunger or satiety. It is a vacuity pattern caused by binding of depressed qi and phlegm or cardiosplenic repletion.

mania evil 狂邪 *kuáng xié*: Pathogen giving rise to mania.

moisten 潤 *rùn*: See *supplementation*.

nourish 養 *yǎng*: See *supplementation*.

origin 元 *yuán*: The foundation of health; original qi; specifically, the lower origin, which refers to the kidney.

pathogen 邪 *xié*: Any harmful influence opposing correct qi. Synonym: evil.

periodontal gan 牙疳 *yá gān*: Swelling, reddening, and ulceration of the gums, usually caused by wind-heat.

qi lump 氣塊 *qì kuài*: Any lump caused by stagnation of qi.

quicken 活 *huó*: To increase activity, to enliven. Moving the blood is often referred to as quickening the blood. The connecting vessels can also be quickened. This latter usage of the word implies an unblocking of the vessels and promotion of the flow of qi and blood within them.

quiet 安 *ān*: To reduce movement or activity. Disquietude of the spirit is treated by quieting. The ideogram is a pictorial representation of a woman covered by a roof (a woman at home). It connotes security, peace, calm, and quiet. Spiritual disquietude can be the result of various disharmonies and thus quieting is often combined with other therapeutic methods such as qi supplementation, heat draining, heart nourishing, phlegm abduction, or promotion of cardiorenal interaction. Fetal disquietude manifests as excessive fetal movement or tendency to miscarry and is treated by quieting the fetus. Sometimes gastric harmonization or hepatogastric harmonization is referred to as quieting the center.

rectify 理 *lǐ*: To correct, set right. Most often this term is applied to blood stasis or qi stagnation or counterflow, where it denotes moving qi, quickening the blood, resolving depressed qi, downbearing counterflow, or dispelling stasis. In its most general meaning rectifying qi or blood can include supplementing qi and the blood, cooling the blood, and staunching blood loss. Rectify can also be used in regard to the spleen, in which case it means the rectifying of spleen qi. Center rectification is a method that includes warming the center and dispelling cold in the treatment of splenogastric vacuity cold patterns.

regulate 調 *tiáo*: To restore normal functioning. Regulate is primarily used to describe treatment of irregular menstruation or counterflow qi. These two therapeutic methods are called regulating the menses and regulating qi respectively. Regulating the menses is wider in scope than disinhibiting the menses, and qi regulation is similar to qi rectification except that the former is limited to the regulation of the quality and direction of flow.

resolve 解 *jiě*: To terminate (disease patterns), eliminate (pathogens), or free (parts of the body from pathogens). The Chinese ideogram consists of an animal horn 角 , a knife 刀 , and a bovine 牛 Its original meaning may have been a knife that was made from bovine horn, or the act of separating the bovine from its horn. Its adopted meaning in everyday Chinese is to separate, untie, liberate, relieve, and dispel. In Chinese medicine, it is commonly found in the following phrases: resolve the exterior (liberate it from a pathogen); resolve the muscles (liberate them from a pathogen); resolve toxin (dispel); resolve depression (relieve, dispel); and allay thirst (relieve).

return 回 *huí*: See *supplementation*.

running piglet 奔豚 *bēn tún*: A sensation of qi rising from the lower abdomen to the chest and throat accompanied by gripping abdominal pain, thoracic oppression, rapid breathing, dizziness, palpitation, and vexation. This pattern is considered to be one of the five accumulations and is a result of an upsurging of kidney qi or counterflow rising of liver fire.

saber and pearl-string lumps 馬刀俠癭 *mǎ dāo xiá yǐng*: Scrofulous lumps. Saber lumps are scrofula occurring in a configuration that looks like the shape of a saber, while pearl-string lumps that occur on the neck give the appearance of a pearl necklace.

settle 鎮 *zhèn*: To calm; in herbology, to calm (the spirit) with heavy settling agents.

sha 痧 *shā*: A summertime febrile disease characterized by a papular outthrust. When the sha is in the skin and qi aspect, there are faint red speckles, like a measles rash (red sha); when it brews in the blood aspect, the whole body is painfully swollen and distended, and there are blackish patches (black sha). Synonyms: Sha qi, sha distention.

shan 疝 *shàn*: Any of various diseases characterized by pain or swelling of the abdomen or scrotum, including hernia.

shan qi 疝氣 *shàn qì*: 1) Shan. 2) Hernia. *Shàn qì* now translates the Western medical term hernia, and is most commonly used in this sense in modern texts.

sinew 筋 *jīn*: 1) Any palpable muscle mass or tendon. 2) Visible blood vessel. 3) The aspect of the muscles governed by the liver (muscle power).

sinew gathering 宗筋 *zōng jīn*: 1) The gathering point of the three yin and three yang channel sinews at the pubic region. 2) The penis.

somnolence 嗜睡 *shì shuì*: Drowsiness and excessive sleep.

soothe 舒 *shū*: To relax. Soothing the sinews is a general term that means to relax the sinews when they are tensed and heal them when they are damaged. Soothing the liver is synonymous with coursing the liver. The Chinese equivalents of soothe and course are pronounced the same and overlap in meaning.

spirit-disposition 神志 *shén zhì*: The spirit, will, and emotion; roughly equivalent to consciousness.

stomachache 胃痛 *wèi tòng*: Gastric pain.

strangury 淋 *lín*: Disease characterized by urinary frequency and urgency and difficult voiding, as well as dribbling incontinence; includes stone (calculous) strangury (which also includes sabulous strangury), qi strangury, blood strangury, unctuous strangury, and taxation strangury, known collectively as the five stranguries.

straw shoe wind 草鞋風 *cǎo xié fēng*: Itching, pain and sores that begin in the upper thigh and can spread down to the feet. This typically follows the kidney channel and results from damp-heat pouring down into the legs.

supplementation 補 *bǔ*: The method of increasing or strengthening any element of the body. The original meaning of the Chinese ideogram is to patch or make up, and this meaning is reflected in Chinese medicine. Like a patch, supplementation is applied to the aspect of the body that needs it. Yin, yang, qi and blood may all be supplemented; the organs that most commonly receive supplementation are the spleen and kidney. Because supplementation is often associated with qi, the term is frequently seen together with the word boost. Terms of similar meaning, but more specific usage include: *nourish:* to supplement (heart, stomach, kidney, and liver, in particular their yin aspect); *enrich:* to nourish and moisten (yin, especially kidney or liver yin); *increase:* to supplement (fluids to treat patterns including dry stool); *engender:* to supplement (fluids lost through disease); *moisten:* to eliminate dryness (especially of the lung or large intestine); *boost:* to supplement (qi, spleen, and occasionally yin); *strengthen:* to supplement (yin, especially kidney yin); *invigorate:* to supplement (yang, especially kidney yang); *emolliate:* to supplement (liver blood); *return:* to supplement (deserting yang); *fortify:* to strengthen (splenogastric function).

sweat macule 汗斑 *hàn bān*: White and purple macules occurring in patients suffering from accumulated heat in the organs on contraction of wind-damp, which enters through the pores and causes qi and blood to stagnate, blocking the pores. They appear on the neck and trunk, growing larger and larger to eventually coalesce. They may become itchy if they persist.

taxation 勞 *láo*: 1) Severe, usually gradual detriment to the viscera. The five taxations are cardiac, hepatic, splenic, pulmonary, and renal taxation. 2) Taxation fatigue, denoting fatigue due to overexertion.

thoracic oppression 胸悶 *xiōng mèn*: Discomfort and vexation in the chest caused by damp-heat or phlegm-damp obstructing the central burner and inhibiting qi.

throat bi 喉痹 *hóu bì*: Swelling, pain and a sensation of blockage in the throat that hinders swallowing and results from localized blockage of qi and blood. Causes include wind-heat, wind-cold and yin vacuity.

throat moth 乳鵝 *rǔ é*: Painful, hot, red swellings in the throat. Western equivalent: tonsillitis.

throughflux diarrhea 洞瀉 *dòng xiè*: Diarrhea due to indigestion; refers specifically to: a) a form of cold diarrhea characterized by evacuation shortly after eating, or b) soft stool diarrhea.

tidal fever 潮熱 *cháo rè*: Fever, sometimes only felt subjectively, occurring at regular intervals, usually in the afternoon or evening; may form part of both vacuity and repletion patterns.

transform 化 *huà*: To eliminate gradually (phlegm, damp, or rheum by promoting their reabsorption by the body or rendering them more easily expectorated).

two yin 二陰 *èr yin*: Anus and genitals.

untransformed digestate 完谷不化 *wán gǔ bú huà*: Partially digested food in the stool due to impaired digestion.

vaginal protrusion 陰挺 *yīn tíng*: Prolapse of the uterus, or swelling of the vaginal wall.

vexation 煩 *fán*: A feeling of solicitude that is often associated with heat (either repletion or vacuity) and the heart. It implies less activity than agitation, which is often paired with it. *Fan* is often rendered by other writers as irritability, uneasiness, or restlessness.

visceral agitation 臟燥 *zàng zào*: A paroxysmal mental disorder most prevalent in women; heralded by melancholy and depression, illusions, emotionalism, and increased or diminished sensitivity. Attacks are characterized by vexation and oppression, rashness and impatience, sighing for no apparent reason, and sadness with an urge to weep. In serious cases, there may be convulsive spasms, which, unlike those occurring in epilepsy, are accompanied by a white complexion or complete loss of consciousness. Cardiohepatic blood vacuity and emotional depression constitute the prime causes.

visceral bi 臟痺 *zàng bì*: Forms of bi disease that develop when sinew bi, vessel bi, bone bi, and skin bi etc., due to repeated contraction of cold, wind and damp, affect the associated viscus. They may also be caused by qi and blood vacuity, essence depletion, or non-movement of yang qi permitting pathogenic qi to enter and gather in the chest and abdomen.

vulpine shan 狐疝 *hú shàn*: Protrusion of the small intestine into the scrotum. The intestine retracts periodically of its own accord, and can be drawn back in by the patient himself in lying posture. The name derives from the sly, unpredictable way in which the intestine slides in and out of the scrotum, resembling the way in which a fox slips in and out of its lair.

wasting thirst 消渴 *xiāo kě*: 1) Generally denotes diseases characterized by thirst, increased fluid intake, and polyuria, and categorized as upper burner, middle burner, and lower burner wasting thirst, depending on the operant pathomechanism; Western medical correspondences include diabetes insipidus and hypoadrenocorticism. 2) Specifically denotes a disease characterized by increased intake of both fluids and solids, maciations, polyuria, and glycosuria and broadly corresponding to diabetes melitus in Western medicine. Pathomechanisms include: a) accumulated heat in the the middle burner occurring in patients fond of alcohol and sweet, fatty foods; b) fire formation following depression of physiologic activity due to dispositional excess; c) wearing of kidney essence due to excessive sexual activity, causing frenetic vacuity fire. All three pathomechanisms involve the mutual exacerbation of yin vacuity and dryness heat scorching kidney yin essence and the fluids of the lung and stomach. Yin vacuity is primarily associated with the kidney, and according to the principle that detriment to yin affects yang, kidney yang vacuity is also observed in enduring cases.

water gu 水蠱 *shuǐ gǔ*: Disease characterized by abdominal distention which gurgles when the patient moves. Synonym: water drum distention. See Paul Unschuld, *Medicine in China, a History of Ideas* pp. 46-50.

water qi 水氣 *shuǐ qì*: Pathologic excesses of water in the body and diseases provoked by them. The main cause is impairment of movement and transformation of water due to splenorenal yang vacuity.

water swelling 水腫 *shuǐ zhǒng*: Edema due to organic dysfunction (spleen, kidney, lung).

wind papules 風疹 *fēng zhěn*: A disease common among children, caused by the invasion of wind-heat, which becomes depressed in the lung and effuses through the skin. The eruption, often accompanied by a mild cough, reaches completion within roughly twenty-four hours, and abates within two to three days. The papules dry and scale as they disappear.

wind strike 中風 *zhòng fēng*: 1) Disease characterized by sudden loss of consciousness, hemiplegia, or wry mouth, and impeded speech; occurs under the following circumstances: a) when depletion of yin-essence or sudden anger causes hyperactivity of liver yang, which stirs liver wind; b) when, owing to a predilection for rich, fatty foods, phlegm heat congests in the inner body and transforms into wind; c) when vacuity of qi and blood give rise to vacuity wind; d) when a patient suffering from inner-body vacuity suddenly contracts exogenous wind. Distinction is made between connecting-vessel strike, channel strike, bowel strike, and visceral strike (in ascending order of severity). Correspondences in Western medicine include cerebral hemorrhage, cerebral embolism, and cerebral thrombosis, as well as a number of diseases of the brain and cranial nerves. Patterns including initial-stage fever invariably correspond to cerebrovascular disease. 2) Exogenous wind contraction, characterized by fever, headache, and a moderate floating pulse (*Treatise on Cold Damage*).

wind taxation 風勞 *fēng láo*: Taxation resulting from enduring wind patterns.

withrawal 癲 *diān*: See *mania and withdrawal*.

xian 癬 *xiǎn*: Skin disease characterized by elevation of the skin, serous discharge, scaling, and itching; often associated with damp.

yong 癰 *yōng*: A pyogenic inflammatory lesion of the skin and subcutaneous tissue. Yong result when channel blockage gives rise to congealing and stagnation of qi and blood. Channel blockage can occur when damp-heat and fire toxin resulting from excessive consumption of rich foods become depressed in the inner body, or when toxin is contracted through unclean wounds. Yong start with swelling and redness; then pus begins to form, and the skin becomes redder, forming a head that produces a rippling sensation under pressure. The healing process begins after the head bursts. There are internal and external yong.

Bibliography of Chinese Language Books

針灸大成校釋		啓業書局	台北 1987
中國針灸學概要		啓業書局	台北 1982
論經絡學說的理論及臨床運用	管遵惠編	雲南人民出版社	雲南 1984
三百種醫籍錄		啓業書局	台北 1986
針灸歌賦校釋	范土生著	山西科學教育出版社	山西 1987
針灸治療學	范 銘著	文源書局	台北 1982
針灸配穴		啓業書局	台北 1983
針灸學	上海中醫學院編	人民衛生出版社	北京 1974
黃帝內經		聯國風出版社	台北 1984
傷寒論新註	承澹盦著	文光圖書公司	台北 1979
新針灸臨床治療學	馬康慈編	衆文圖書公司	台北 1983
臨床內外科針灸學	針灸研究中心編	武陵出版社	台北 1984
針灸聚英	（明）高 武著	武陵出版社	台北 1983
醫宗金鑒	（明）張介賓著	新文豐出版社	台北 1984
簡明中醫字典		貴州人民出版社	貴州 1985
中醫難字典	李 戎編	四川科學技術出版社	成都 1986
中醫學基礎	上海中醫學院編	人民衛生出版社	北京 1984
中國醫學大辭典	謝利恆編	商務印書館	香港 1974
中國大辭典		啓業書局	台北 1983
中醫詞典	徐元貞等編	河南科學技術出版社	河南 1982
針灸經穴學	楊維傑編著	樂群出版公司	台北 1979
經絡學	李 鼎編著	上海科學技術出版社	1984

Chinese Language Books Cited in the Text

1. 銅人針灸腧穴圖經　　　王惟一

Bronze Statue Illustrated Canon of Acupuncture Points (Bronze Statue). Wang Wei-Yi, 1026.

2. 針灸集成　　　廖潤鴻

Compilation of Acupuncture and Moxibustion. Liao Run-Hong, 1874.

3. 難經　　　漢

The Classic of Difficulties. Anon., Han Dynasty.

4. 醫學入門　　　李梴

The Gateway to Medicine (The Gateway). Li Yan, 1575.

5. 針灸聚英　　　高武

The Glorious Anthology of Acupuncture (The Glorious Anthology). Gao Wu, 1529.

6. 醫宗金鑒　　　吳謙

The Golden Mirror of Medicine (The Golden Mirror). Wu Qian, 1742.

7. 針灸大成　　　楊繼洲

The Great Compendium of Acupuncture and Moxibustion (The Great Compendium). Yang Ji-Zhou, 1601.

8. 類經圖翼　　　張介賓

Illustrated Supplement to the Differentiated Canon (Illustrated Supplement). Zhang Jie-Bin, 1624.

9. 內經

The Inner Canon (consisting of *The Spiritual Axis* and *The Essential Questions*.) Anon., 100 B.C.

10. 針灸資生經　　　王執中

The Life-Promoting Canon of Acupuncture and Moxibustion (Life-Promoting Canon). Wang Zhi-Zhong, 1220.

11. 萬病回春　　　龔廷賢

Recovery from the Myriad Illnesses. Gong Ting-Xian, 1587.

12. 神農經　　　秦漢

The Shen Nong Canon. Anon., Qin-Han Dynasty.

13. 素 問

Spiritual Axis. See *The Inner Canon.*

14. 針灸甲乙經   皇甫謐

The Systemized Canon of Acupuncture (The Systemized Canon). Huang Pu-Mi, 282 A.D.

15. 太平聖惠方   王懷隱

Taiping Sagacious Remedies. Wang Huai-Yin, 987.

16. 千 金 方   孫思邈

The Thousand Gold Piece Prescriptions. Sun-Si Miao, 625.

17. 傷 寒 論   張仲景

Treatise on Cold Damage. Zhang Zhong-Jing, 200 A.D.

Chinese Language Odes and Songs Cited in the Text

1. 攔 江 賦   針灸聚英

Ode of the Dammed River. First recorded in *The Glorious Anthology of Acupuncture,* 1529.

2. 標 幽 賦   針灸指南

Ode to Elucidate Mysteries. First recorded in *Guide to Acupuncture and Moxibustion,* 1241.

3. 百 症 賦   針灸聚英

Ode of a Hundred Patterns. First recorded in *The Glorious Anthology of Acupuncture,* 1529.

4. 玉 龍 賦   針灸聚英

Ode of the Jade Dragon. First recorded in *The Glorious Anthology of Acupuncture,* 1529.

5. 靈 光 賦   針灸大全

Ode of Spiritual Light. First recorded in *The Complete Book of Acupuncture and Moxibustion,* 1439.

6. 席 紅 賦   針灸大全

Ode of Xi Hong. First recorded in *The Complete Book of Acupuncture and Moxibustion,* 1439.

7. 天星秘訣

The Secrets of the Celestial Star. n.d.

8. 勝 玉 歌　　　針灸大成

Song More Precious than Jade. First recorded in *The Great Compendium of Acupuncture and Moxibustion,* 1601.

9. 天元太乙歌　　針灸聚英

Song of Celestial Origin and Supreme Unity (Song of Supreme Unity). First recorded in *The Glorious Anthology of Acupuncture,* 1529.

10. 玉 龍 歌　　扁鵲神應針灸玉龍經（元）

Song of the Jade Dragon. First recorded in *Bian Que's Jade Canon Spiritual Guide to Acupuncture and Moxibustion,* Yuan dynasty.

11. 肘 後 歌　　　針灸聚英

Song to Keep Up Your Sleeve. First recorded in *The Glorious Anthology of Acupuncture,* 1529.

12. 馬丹陽天星十二穴歌　　扁鵲神應針灸玉龍歌（元）

Song of Ma Dan Yang's Twelve Celestial Star Points. First recorded in *Bian Que's Jade Dragon Canon Spiritual Guide to Acupuncture and Moxibustion,* Yuan dynasty.

13. 行針指要歌　　針灸聚英

Song of Needle Practice. First recorded in *The Glorious Anthology of Acupuncture,* 1529.

14. 回陽九針歌　　針灸聚英

Song of the Nine Needles for Returning Yang. First recorded in *The Glorious Anthology of Acupuncture,* 1529.

15. 雜病穴法歌　　醫學入門

Song of Point Applications for Miscellaneous Disease. First recorded in *The Gateway to Medicine,* 1557.

Bibliography of English Language Books

1. Beijing College of Traditional Chinese Medicine, et al. *Essentials of Chinese Acupuncture*. Beijing: Foreign Languages Press, 1980.

2. Berkow, Robert, ed. *The Merck Manual*. 13th ed. Rahway, NJ: Merck, Sharp and Dohme Research Labs, 1977.

3. Friel, John P., ed. *Dorland's Illustrated Medical Dictionary*. 26th ed. Philadelphia: W.B. Saunders, 1981.

4. O'Connor, J. and Dan Bensky, trans. *Acupuncture, a Comprehensive Text*. Chicago: Eastland Press, 1981.

5. Unschuld, Paul U. *Medicine in China: History of Ideas*. Berkeley: University of California Press, 1985.

6. ———. *Medicine in China: Nan Jing Classic of Difficult Issues*. Berkeley: University of California Press, 1986.

7. Williams, P. and Roger Warwick, eds. *Gray's Anatomy*. 36th ed. London: Churchill Livingstone, 1980.

8. Wiseman, N. and Andrew Ellis, trans. *Fundamentals of Chinese Medicine*. Brookline, MA: Paradigm Publications, 1985.

Index

This index is arranged to facilitate the selection and application of points. The first section follows the outline of *Part IV, Approaches to Point Selection and Combination*. Page references are listed for each of the methods and summary tables detailed in the text. The second section contains all the primary indications of every point. The final section lists a page reference for every point.

Proceeding from a Chinese medical diagnosis and/or a symptom assessment, you may determine which regions or channels are most indicated. The channel assessment allows determination of which function and symptom set is most worthy of research. This, in turn, will provide you with a list of points closely associated with the condition. Other points related to the primary indications may be researched through the *Indications Index*. Point group applications and combinations will be presented at the page references given.

Treatment References			
Method		**Text**	**Tables**
Local, adjacent and distant points		412-413	413
Selection according to affected channel	communications	36-37	32-39
	general	43	32-34, 57-58, 414
	abdomen	52	413-414
	head & face	43	413-414
	neck & throat	47	413-414
	shoulder & scapula	48	413-414
	trunk	49	413-414
	diurnal qi flow	37	38
	interior-exterior	35	38
Method		**Indications**	**Functions**
Selection by functions & symptoms	general	58	58
	bladder	237-242	420
	conception vessel	366-368	427
	gallbladder	327-330	426
	governing vessel	390-392	428
	heart	172	419
	kidney	263-265	422
	large intestine	107-108	416
	liver	343-344	425
	lung	88	415
	pericardium	276	423
	small intestine	189-190	419
	spleen	161-162	418
	stomach	140-143	417
	triple burner	294-295	424
Selection by clinical experience		429	429-430

Method		By Group	In Combination
Selection by point groups	source-yuan points	60, 431, 436	445
	confluence-jiaohui points	62	446
	connecting-luo points	61, 432	445
	cleft-xi points	61, 433	
	meeting-hui points	62, 433	
	lower uniting-he points	62, 433	
	the command points	63, 434	
	alarm-mu points	434	443-444
	the associated-shu points	434	443-444
	transporting-shu points	65, 434, 436, 438	
	five-phase correspondences	436, 438	
	intersection-jiaohui points	439-443	
Other point applications	a-shi points	67	
	cutaneous regions, the twelve	41	
	ghost points, the thirteen	67	
	guest-host treatment	445	
	heavenly star points of Ma Dan Yang	67	
	Hua Tuo's paravertebral points	66	
	nine needles for returning yang	66	
	seasonal point selection	436	

Indications Index

—• A •—

abdominal distention: 124, 127, 133, 136, 148-149, 151-154, 208-209, 212, 225-227, 251, 257, 259, 314, 342, 355-356; [and fullness]: 139; [and pain]: 125

abdominal fullness: 257

abdominal pain: 98, 100, 127, 129, 135, 150, 153, 156, 158, 205, 220, 225, 257-260, 350-351, 354, 410; [and constipation]: 283; [and distention]: 138, 211

abdominal pain or distention: 134

abdominal pain, vomiting and diarrhea: 99

abdominal swelling: 341

abdominothoracic distention and fullness: 323

aching and pain in the lower leg: 337

aching in the shoulder and upper arm: 99

aching knee and tibia: 133

aching of the hand and arm: 97

aching of the shoulder and arm: 97

aching shoulder and arm: 98

acid regurgitation: 313

acute and chronic appendicitis: 408

acute and chronic cholecystitis and cholelithiasis: 409

acute lumbar sprain: 407

acute tonsillitis: 404

adiaphoretic heat diseases: 149

amenorrhea: 350

ankle pain: 151

aphasia: 400

arm pain: 288

asthma: 80-83, 85, 104, 121-123, 135, 160, 203, 205, 221-223, 249, 260-263, 401

atony, bi and numbness of the lower limbs: 318-319

atony of the lower extremities: 134, 137, 232, 251

atony or bi of the lower extremities: 135

atrophy, bi and impeded bending and stretching of the lower limbs: 130

axillary pain: 322, 324

axillary swelling: 272, 325

—• B •—

back pain: 208, 226-228 [and stiffness of the neck]: 377

backache: 224, 403; [and weakness of the knee]: 210; [referring to the testicles]: 135

beriberi: 130

bi and atony of the lower limbs: 317

bi pain in the lower limbs: 233

bi pain in the lumbus and thigh: 317

biliary ascariasis: 409

bitter taste in the mouth: 207, 319

blood ejection: 203-206, 222

blurred vision: 180, 196

borborygmi: 97, 127, 133-134, 150-151, 225, 259, 314, 354-355; [and abdominal pain]: 97

breast yong: 122-123, 133

bronchitis: 401

—• C •—

cardiac pain: 169, 171, 203, 205, 269-275, 377

cardiothoracic pain: 358-359

chest and back pain: 376

chest pain: 135, 170, 360-362

child fright wind: 404

clenched jaws: 84, 116-117, 290, 304, 387 clouded vision: 94, 210, 250, 289; [cloudiness of the cornea]: 398

471

clouding inversion: 87, 93, 171, 177, 247, 275, 387

clove sores: 271, 377-378

cold and pain in the elbow and arm: 166

cold in the lower leg and foot: 139

cold knees: 130

color blindness: 195

common cold: 379

constipation: 127, 133, 136, 149, 151, 157-158, 211, 213, 216-217, 226, 229, 256-258, 283, 351, 371

convulsive spasm: 167, 335

copious phlegm: 135

cough: 80-83, 85-86, 104, 120-123, 159-160, 200, 203-205, 221-223, 260-263, 269, 361-363, 376-379, 401; [and asthma]: 84, 186; [cough counterflow and asthma]: 87; [cough, dyspnea]: 122; [coughing of blood]: 82, 248-249

crick in the neck: 406

—• D •—

deafness: 97, 118, 178, 188, 210, 249, 281-285, 290, 292, 300, 302, 305-306, 406; [and tinnitus]: 186-187

deep source nasal congestion: 198, 310-311, 385-386, 389, 399

diabetes: 407

diarrhea: 127, 133-134, 150-151, 154, 157, 208, 211-213, 217, 224-225, 248, 251-252, 255-257, 260, 314, 341, 349-351, 356, 371, 373, 375, 400, 403-404; [and dysentery]: 138, 209

difficult delivery: 231, 236, 312; [labor]: 151

difficult evacuation: 247

difficult ingestion: 205, 224-225; [in swallowing]: 364

distention and fullness in the chest: 359; [and lateral costal region]: 160, 261-262, 320

distention of the lateral costal region: 121, 335

dizziness: 119, 133, 135-136, 168, 196, 198-199, 232, 247, 289, 335, 381, 383, 385, 400

drinker's nose: 387

drooling: 116, 365

drooping eyelid: 398

dry, sore throat: 250

dry tongue: 247

dysentery: 95, 100, 127, 133-134, 149-150, 153, 157-158, 208, 213-214, 217; [dysenteric disease]: 355-356

dyspnea: 119-120, 360-363, 376-379

—• E •—

ear pain: 291, 306; [with purulent discharge]: 118

eclampsia: 404

eczema: 155

edema: 127, 138, 153, 210, 227, 251, 350-351, 354-355

enuresis: 151, 155, 170, 210, 213, 334-335, 347-351

epigastric pain: 226

epilepsy: 133, 135, 178, 182, 196-197, 204, 206, 232-234, 250, 272, 274, 284, 286, 305, 307, 335, 357-359, 379-382, 385-387, 398; [epilepsy patterns]: 335, 372, 375-376, 378

eructation: 224

esophageal constriction: 358-359

evacuative difficulty: 252

excessive dreaming: 148, 326

expectoration of blood: 85-86

extremities: 131, 322

eye disorders: 406

eye pain: 94, 118, 196, 199, 236, 300, 321, 386

eye screens: 177, 179, 400

—• F •—

facial itching: 106

facial pain: 114

facial paralysis: 84

facial swelling: 97, 106, 289, 365, 387

fever: 86, 200-201

flowery vision: 247

foot qi: 133-134, 149, 323, 409

frequent urination: 403

fright inversion: 275

fright mania: 339

fright palpitations: 169, 204, 273, 377, 386

fright wind: 148, 404

frontal headache: 308, 399; [vertical headache]: 196

fullness: 342; [in the chest]: 80

—• G •—

gastric reflux: 208, 357, 359; [and acid regurgitation]: 356, 358

generalized heaviness: 149

generalized pain: 160

genital itch: 248, 250, 318, 339, 347-348, 353

genital pain: 151, 154, 339, 348

glomus: 156

goiter: 287

goose foot wind: 274

gynecological disorders: 407

—• H •—

halitosis: 274

headache: 95-97, 118, 135-136, 178-179, 196-201, 230-232, 234-236, 280-281, 283, 287, 290-291, 293, 300, 302-303, 305-311, 335, 378, 381-383, 385-386, 399-400; [and heavy-headedness]: 292; [and pain in the neck: 306; [and stiffness of the neck]: 84; [at the top of the head]: 385; [dizziness]: 398

heat disease: 87, 93-94, 100, 138-139, 171, 177-181, 270, 272, 280-281, 283, 311, 325-326, 378-379

heat in the palm: 169-170, 275

heat in the soles of the feet: 236, 247

heaviness of the shoulder: 288

heavy-headedness: 230, 399

hemafecia: 217, 371

hematuria: 213

hemiplegia: 134, 220, 317-319, 323, 381

hemorrhoids: 217, 228-229, 371-372, 405

hernia: 127-129, 151, 156-157, 214-216, 250, 254, 315, 334-337, 341, 348-351, 353, 403, 410

hiccough: 205, 313, 342, 360, 363

high blood pressure: 399-400

high fever: 400

hypertension: 404
hypertonicity and pain in the elbow and arm: 82, 101
hypertonicity of the elbow: 167, 181, 272; [and arm]:
    167; [arm, and fingers]: 178
hypertonicity of the fingers: 95, 170
hypertonicity of the jaws: 292
hypertonicity of the lumbar region and back: 229
hypertonicity of the popliteal sinews: 218, 220, 319
hypertonicity of the shoulder and arm: 231
hypertonicity of the shoulder and back: 221
hysteria: 400

—• I •—

immobility of the toes: 409
impaired memory: 377
impotence: 210, 217, 227, 249, 254, 348, 372-373
inability to bend and stretch the fingers: 281
inability to move the arm: 312
inability to turn the head: 406
incessant diarrhea: 354
incessant menorrhagia: 335
increased dreaming: 139
indigestion: 126, 133, 408
infantile epilepsy: 231
infantile fright wind: 247, 335, 387, 399; [convulsions]:
    233
infantile gan accumulation: 405
infantile indigestion: 405
infertility: 404
inhibited bending and stretching of the arm: 283
inhibited bending and stretching of the leg: 132
inhibited defecation and urination: 215
inhibited movement of the hip joint: 220
inhibited opening and closing of the jaws: 118
inhibited urination: 128, 151, 153, 170, 216-217, 219,
    227, 247, 249-250, 337, 339-340; [or incontinence]:
    154
insomnia: 151, 169, 232, 249-250, 306, 335, 386,
    399-400
intestinal rumbling: 354
intestinal yong: 134
inversion cold and numbness in the thigh and knee: 152
irregular menstruation: 127, 151, 155, 210, 215-216,
    248-250, 252, 255-256, 315, 337, 339-340, 347-348,
    351, 353, 372-373, 403-404, 410
itching of the canthus: 195
itchy skin: 170

—• J •—

jaundice: 154, 179, 206-208, 225, 313, 375-376

—• K •—

knee pain: 154, 320-321

—• L •—

lactation insufficiency: 360
lateral costal distention: 269
lateral costal pain: 166, 283, 313, 319, 323, 326, 409
limp, weak limbs: 160

limpness of the lower extremities: 408
lochiorrhea: 409
loss of appetite: 355
loss of locomotive ability of the lower limbs: 136, 151,
    216, 220, 228, 321, 324, 371, 408, 409
loss of locomotive power, pain, and swelling of lower
    extremities: 135
loss of visual acuity: 300
loss of voice: 104, 247
lower abdominal distention: 340; [and fullness]: 128
lower abdominal pain: 157, 217, 256, 316, 339, 348-
    349; [and distention]: 213
lower intestinal distention and fullness: 219
lumbar and hip pain: 315-317
lumbar and lateral costal pain: 314-315
lumbar pain: 211-212, 215-217, 220, 229-231, 233,
    249, 341, 373, 375, 403, 407
lumbosacral pain: 228, 230; [referring to the lower
    abdomen]: 339
lump glomus: 226; [specifically hepatosplenomegaly]:
    403
lung diseases: 401

—• M •—

malarial disease: 178, 272, 281-282, 322, 324,
    378-379
malposition of the fetus: 236
mammary yong: 122, 131, 135, 159, 261, 312
mania and withdrawal: 87, 126, 139, 148, 169, 171,
    181, 199, 206, 232, 234, 253, 272-274, 347, 358-
    359, 365, 380-383, 386-389, 404
menalgia: 349
menstrual block: 95, 129, 151, 155
menstrual disorders: 129, 153, 349
menstrual pain: 250
mental disorders: 398, 400
metrorrhagia: 148, 151, 155, 252, 254, 256, 334-335,
    337, 348, 351, 353
mouth sores: 274, 400
mumps: 117
muscular atrophy: 408

—• N •—

nasal congestion: 105-106, 196-200, 230, 236, 308,
    383, 387
nausea: 358
night blindness: 114, 195, 206, 321
night sweating: 169, 178, 203, 205, 222
non-conception: 151
nosebleed: 81, 87, 94-95, 97, 105-106, 115, 138-139,
    196, 198, 206, 230-231, 235-236, 271, 310, 380-
    381, 386-387, 399
numbness of the arm: 167; [and elbow]: 221; [fingers]:
    93, 178, 404; [gluteal region]: 218; [hand and arm]:
    98; [lower leg]: 319
numbness, pain, or swelling of the knee: 408

—• O •—

occipital headache: 380

orchitis: 404, 407

—• P •—

pain and cramp in the legs: 229

pain and distention [in the lateral costal region]: 158-159; [of the breast]: 321, 324-325

pain and heaviness of the shoulder and back: 283

pain and hypertonicity [elbow and arm]: 272; [of the fingers]: 87; [of the leg and foot]: 219

pain and inhibited movement of the hand and arm: 182

pain and lack of strength in the shoulder and arm: 183

pain and numbness [in the upper limbs]: 184; [of the knee]: 132

pain and paralysis of the lower limbs: 228

pain and rigidity of the neck: 186

pain and stiffness [root of the tongue]: 151; [back]: 223-224, 227; [back and spinal column]: 377; [the neck]: 287-288, 306, 310-311, 381; [lumbar spinal column]: 209, 213-214, 372-373, 378, 387

pain and swelling [of the anus]: 347; [axillary region]: 269; [external genitalia]: 129; [external malleolus]: 324; [eyes]: 195, 293; [gums]: 389; [knee]: 131, 319; [testicles]: 252

pain due to hernia: 404

pain, hypertonicity, and numbness of the elbow and arm: 100

pain in [the anterior chest, back, shoulder blade]: 269; [arm]: 95, 272, 284, 287; [preventing bending and stretching]: 103; [hand]: 281; [lateral aspect of the arm]: 180; [axillary and lateral costal region]: 167; [back and lumbus]: 201, 234

pain in the cheek: 283; [and submandibular region]: 325; [chest]: 85, 262-263; [chest and lateral costal region]: 160, 171, 208, 224, 273, 321-322, 341-342; [and wrist]: 85; [shoulder, and arm]: 81; [shoulder and back]: 80; [elbow and arm]: 83, 98, 100, 270, 281; [external genitalia]: 341; [external malleolus]: 233, 335; [fingers]: 181, 283;[forearm]: 285; [genitals]: 254-255; [genital region]: 336; [gums]: 388; [hand joints]: 406; [heel]: 231-232, 249; [inside of thigh]: 155; [knee and medial aspect]: 339; [knee and thigh]: 323; [medial knee]: 254, 338

pain in the lateral costal region: 169, 179, 206-207, 269, 324-325, 335; [neck]: 321, 324; [neck, shoulder]: 286; [leg]: 340; [lower leg]: 229; [lower leg and knee]: 253; [lower back and hip joint]: 215; [lumbar, sacral, gluteal and femoral regions]: 217; [lumbar and iliac region]: 130; [lumbar spine]: 371-372; [lumbus and leg]: 232, 234; [lumbus and thigh]: 218; [medial aspect of the arm]: 81-82; [nape]: 182; [outer canthus]: 302-303, 308, 322, 324-325

pain in the region of the heart: 167; [and ribs]: 166; [shoulder and arm]: 102, 406-407; [shoulder and back]: 221, 311, 401; [shoulder, arm, and elbow]: 180; [shoulder blade]: 182, 184, 200; [shoulder blade and the lateroposterior aspect]: 183; [spine and back]: 206; [superciliary ridge]: 196; [supraclavicular fossa]: 120, 322; [temporal region]: 304; [thigh]: 130; [umbilical region]: 157; [upper limbs]: 284; [venter]: 208, 226, 258, 375; [pain in the wrist]: 96, 180; [and arm]: 168

pain, reddening and swelling of the eye: 398

pain swelling of the dorsum of the foot: 324

painful menstruation, menstrual block and other menstrual disorders: 349

painful, red eyes: 114, 256, 309, 311, 325; [and swelling]: 95-96

painful stiffness of the neck: 117

painful swelling of the dorsum of the foot: 138, 248 [of the groin]: 155; [tongue]: 400

palpitations: 85, 170-171, 270-273, 358; [and racing of the heart]: 168

paralysis: 230, 317 [due to wind strike]:133; [lower extremities]: 130-131; [upper extremities]: 98-100, 102, 407

periumbilical pain: 353

poor appetite: 124-125, 153

poor memory: 169, 204, 222

postpartum abdominal pain: 256, 258

postpartum body pain: 401

postpartum hemorrhage: 349-351, 353

premature ejaculation: 128

prolapse of the rectum: 354, 371, 383, 405

prolapse of the uterus: 129, 151, 248, 250, 252, 316, 334, 339, 348-349, 404

prolonged labor: 95

pulmonary tuberculosis: 207, 221-222, 403

purulent discharge from the ear: 188, 292

—• Q •—

qi goiter: 104

—• R •—

racing of the heart: 169

red facial complexion: 119

red, swollen, painful eyes: 335

reddening and swelling dorsum of the foot: 325

reddening of the eyes: 178, 206, 280-281; [and swelling]: 196, 291, 399; [and tearing]: 300; [and pain]: 196

redness and swelling of the dorsum of the foot: 137

redness and swelling of the dorsum of the hand: 405

redness and swelling of the dorsum of the foot: 409

redness and swelling of the external malleolus: 230

redness and swelling of the eyes: 399

redness and swelling of fingers & backs of hands: 94

retching: 272; [of blood]: 271

retention of afterbirth: 410

rigidity of the neck: 185, 200

roundworm: 405

rumbling intestines: 151, 208-209, 211, 251; [and abdominal pain]: 98, 138; [and diarrhea]: 125

—• S •—

scant breast milk: 123, 159, 177

scant metrorrhagia: 349-350

scrofula: 101-102, 166-167, 401, 408

scrofulous lumps: 100, 102, 104, 286, 322

seminal emission: 128, 151, 153-154, 210, 213, 215, 222, 227, 248-249, 254-255, 336, 339, 347-349, 372-373 sensation of the throat being obstructed: 187

shoulder pain: 103, 134; [and arm pain]: 166, 286-288; [and back pain]: 185-186, 200, 223, 312

sluggish tongue and drooling: 364

sore throat: 82-86, 247, 249, 409; [and swollen]: 87, 93-97, 100, 104, 119-120, 135, 168, 177, 186-187, 280-281, 363, 381

spasm and contracture, or numbness of the fingers: 405

splenogastric vacuity diarrhea: 373

spontaneous or night sweating: 251

sprain or spasms of the neck muscles: 401

steaming bone tidal fever: 203, 379

stiff neck: 178-179, 181, 200-201, 231, 234-235, 289, 312

stiff, swollen lips: 388

stiff tongue: 280; [preventing speech]: 168, 364

stiffness and pain in the [lumbar region]: 219, 249; [neck]: 221; [shoulder blade]: 184

stiffness of the neck: 221, 379-382

stiffness of the spinal column: 373, 375-376, 378

stomach pain: 124-126, 131, 133, 149-150, 270, 272-273, 355-357, 376, 403, 406

stupor: 387

subglossal swelling: 364

sudden loss of hearing: 289

sudden loss of voice: 167-168, 283-285, 363-364, 380

summerheat strike: 275

sweating or absence of it in heat diseases: 95

swelling of the axillary region: 313; [cheek]: 116-117, 182, 187, 290, 306; [and submandibular region]: 304; [face]: 95, 138-139; [gums]: 305, 365; [head and face]: 136; [lips and cheek]: 115; [neck and submandibular region]: 180; [submandibular region]: 93; [thighs]: 251

syncope due to high fever: 404

—• T •—

tearing on exposure to wind: 114, 118, 195-196, 308

tension and stiffness of the spinal column: 379

thin stool: 125; [with untransformed digestate]: 151

thoracic and lateral costal pain: 324

thoracic fullness: 81-82; [and distention]: 121

thoracic oppression: 203, 269

thoracic pain: 123; [and distention]: 122, 159

throat bi: 409

throat block: 400

tidal fever: 82, 205, 207

tinnitus: 118, 188, 199, 210, 281, 283, 290-292, 300, 302, 305-306, 325-326, 383

tonsillitis: 409

toothache: 93-94, 96, 115-118, 138-139, 187, 249, 285, 291-292, 300, 302, 306, 365, 409

trembling hands: 167, 270

trembling of the arm: 270

trigeminal neuralgia: 399

twitching of the eyelids: 114-116, 187, 196, 293, 308, 398

—• U •—

unilateral headache: 286, 302-304, 309, 322, 326

untransformed digestate: 208-209, 222, 259, 341, 355-356; [in the stool]: 158

urinary block: 348

urinary frequency: 249-250, 348-349

urinary incontinence: 409

urinary stoppage: 128, 155-156, 213, 254, 335-336, 339, 347-350

urinary tract pain: 335

urticaria: 401

—• V •—

vaginal discharge: 151, 210, 215-217, 255, 315-316, 348-351, 353, 373

vaginal protrusion: 215

vertex headache: 247

vexation: 126, 169, 204, 280; [and agitation]: 270, 272; [and oppression]: 275

visual dizziness: 118, 196-197, 206, 230-231, 234-235, 293, 302, 307-309, 311, 324-326, 335, 381-383, 385-386

vomiting: 100, 124-126, 133, 150, 203, 205, 208-209, 224-225, 257-260, 270, 272-274, 283, 313, 341-342, 355-358, 400, 404, 410; [and acid eructation]: 324; [and diarrhea]: 149, 220, 406; [jaundice]: 319

—• W •—

water swelling: 97, 125, 133, 154, 208-209

weakness and atony of the lower extremities: 320

weakness of the legs: 230

weakness of the wrist: 84

whooping cough: 401, 405

wind damage; cough: 201

wind papules: 100, 102

wind strike: 312, 383, 404; [desertion patterns]: 351, 354; [hemiplegia]: 398; [with loss of speech]: 381; [with stiffness of the tongue]: 380

withdrawal patterns: 136

wrist pain; arm and shoulder pain: 282

wryness of the eyes and mouth: 84, 95, 114-115, 118, 187, 290, 302, 306, 365, 387, 399

wryness of the mouth: 105-106, 116-117, 137-139, 335

—• Y •—

yellowing of the eyes: 169, 187

yellowing of the sclera: 166

yong and clove sores: 408

Point Index

Point	Page	Point	Page	Point	Page	Point	Page
BL-1:	195	BL-51:	226	GB-10:	305	GV-16:	380
BL-2:	195	BL-52:	227	GB-11:	306	GV-17:	381
BL-3:	196	BL-53:	227	GB-12:	306	GV-18:	382
BL-4:	196	BL-54:	228	GB-13:	307	GV-19:	382
BL-5:	197	BL-55:	228	GB-14:	307	GV-20:	383
BL-6:	197	BL-56:	229	GB-15:	308	GV-21:	384
BL-7:	198	BL-57:	229	GB-16:	309	GV-22:	385
BL-8:	199	BL-58:	230	GB-17:	309	GV-23:	385
BL-9:	199	BL-59:	230	GB-18:	310	GV-24:	386
BL-10:	199	BL-60:	231	GB-19:	310	GV-25:	387
BL-11:	200	BL-61:	232	GB-20:	311	GV-26:	387
BL-12:	201	BL-62:	232	GB-21:	312	GV-27:	388
BL-13:	202	BL-63:	233	GB-22:	312	GV-28:	389
BL-14:	203	BL-64:	233	GB-23:	313	HT-1:	166
BL-15:	204	BL-65:	234	GB-24:	313	HT-2:	166
BL-16:	205	BL-66:	235	GB-25:	314	HT-3:	167
BL-17:	205	BL-67:	236	GB-26:	315	HT-4:	167
BL-18:	206	CV-1:	347	GB-27:	315	HT-5:	168
BL-19:	207	CV-2:	347	GB-28:	316	HT-6:	168
BL-20:	207	CV-3:	348	GB-29:	316	HT-7:	169
BL-21:	208	CV-4:	349	GB-30:	317	HT-8:	170
BL-22:	209	CV-5:	350	GB-31:	318	HT-9:	171
BL-23:	210	CV-6:	351	GB-32:	318	KI-1:	247
BL-24:	211	CV-7:	353	GB-33:	319	KI-2:	247
BL-25:	211	CV-8:	353	GB-34:	319	KI-3:	248
BL-26:	212	CV-9:	354	GB-35:	320	KI-4:	249
BL-27:	212	CV-10:	355	GB-36:	321	KI-5:	250
BL-28:	213	CV-11:	355	GB-37:	321	KI-6:	250
BL-29:	214	CV-12:	356	GB-38:	322	KI-7:	251
BL-30:	214	CV-13:	357	GB-39:	323	KI-8:	252
BL-31:	215	CV-14:	358	GB-40:	323	KI-9:	253
BL-32:	215	CV-15:	358	GB-41:	324	KI-10:	253
BL-33:	216	CV-16:	359	GB-42:	325	KI-11:	254
BL-34:	216	CV-17:	360	GB-43:	325	KI-12:	255
BL-35:	217	CV-18:	360	GB-44:	326	KI-13:	255
BL-36:	217	CV-19:	361	GV-1:	371	KI-14:	256
BL-37:	218	CV-20:	361	GV-2:	371	KI-15:	256
BL-38:	218	CV-21:	362	GV-3:	372	KI-16:	257
BL-39:	219	CV-22:	363	GV-4:	372	KI-17:	257
BL-40:	219	CV-23:	364	GV-5:	373	KI-18:	258
BL-41:	220	CV-24:	365	GV-6:	375	KI-19:	258
BL-42:	221	GB-1:	300	GV-7:	375	KI-20:	259
BL-43:	222	GB-2:	300	GV-8:	376	KI-21:	260
BL-44:	222	GB-3:	301	GV-9:	376	KI-22:	260
BL-45:	223	GB-4:	302	GV-10:	377	KI-23:	261
BL-46:	223	GB-5:	303	GV-11:	377	KI-24:	261
BL-47:	224	GB-6:	303	GV-12:	378	KI-25:	262
BL-48:	224	GB-7:	304	GV-13:	378	KI-26:	262
BL-49:	225	GB-8:	304	GV-14:	379	KI-27:	263
BL-50:	226	GB-9:	305	GV-15:	380	LI-1:	93

Point	Page	Point	Page	Point	Page	Point	Page
LI-2:	93	M-CA-18a:	403	SI-15:	186	ST-25:	126
LI-3:	94	M-CA-18:	404	SI-16:	186	ST-26:	127
LI-4:	95	M-HN-1:	398	SI-17:	187	ST-27:	127
LI-5:	96	M-HN-3:	399	SI-18:	187	ST-28:	128
LI-6:	96	M-HN-6:	398	SI-19:	188	ST-29:	128
LI-7:	97	M-HN-9:	399	SP-1:	148	ST-30:	129
LI-8:	98	M-HN-10:	400	SP-2:	148	ST-31:	129
LI-9:	98	M-HN-20a+b:	400	SP-3:	149	ST-32:	130
LI-10:	99	M-HN-30:	401	SP-4:	150	ST-33:	130
LI-11:	99	M-LE-8:	409	SP-5:	150	ST-34:	131
LI-12:	100	M-LE-13:	408	SP-6:	151	ST-35:	132
LI-13:	101	M-LE-16:	408	SP-7:	152	ST-36:	132
LI-14:	101	M-LE-17:	409	SP-8:	153	ST-37:	134
LI-15:	102	M-LE-18a:	410	SP-9:	153	ST-38:	134
LI-16:	103	M-LE-22:	409	SP-10:	154	ST-39:	135
LI-17:	104	M-LE-23:	409	SP-11:	155	ST-40:	135
LI-18:	104	M-UE-1-5:	404	SP-12:	156	ST-41:	136
LI-19:	105	M-UE-9:	405	SP-13:	156	ST-42:	137
LI-20:	106	M-UE-15:	406	SP-14:	157	ST-43:	137
LU-1:	80	M-UE-17:	406	SP-15:	157	ST-44:	138
LU-2:	80	M-UE-19:	407	SP-16:	158	ST-45:	139
LU-3:	81	M-UE-22:	405	SP-17:	158	TB-1:	280
LU-4:	82	M-UE-24:	406	SP-18:	159	TB-2:	280
LU-5:	82	M-UE-29:	405	SP-19:	159	TB-3:	281
LU-6:	83	M-UE-46:	408	SP-20:	160	TB-4:	282
LU-7:	84	M-UE-48:	407	SP-21:	160	TB-5:	282
LU-8:	85	N-HN-54:	400	ST-1:	114	TB-6:	283
LU-9:	85	PC-1:	269	ST-2:	114	TB-7:	284
LU-10:	86	PC-2:	269	ST-3:	115	TB-8:	284
LU-11:	87	PC-3:	270	ST-4:	115	TB-9:	285
LV-1:	334	PC-4:	271	ST-5:	116	TB-10:	285
LV-2:	334	PC-5:	271	ST-6:	117	TB-11:	286
LV-3:	335	PC-6:	272	ST-7:	117	TB-12:	287
LV-4:	336	PC-7:	273	ST-8:	118	TB-13:	287
LV-5:	337	PC-8:	274	ST-9:	119	TB-14:	288
LV-6:	337	PC-9:	275	ST-10:	119	TB-15:	288
LV-7:	338	SI-1:	177	ST-11:	120	TB-16:	289
LV-8:	338	SI-2:	177	ST-12:	120	TB-17:	289
LV-9:	339	SI-3:	178	ST-13:	121	TB-18:	290
LV-10:	340	SI-4:	179	ST-14:	121	TB-19:	291
LV-11:	340	SI-5:	179	ST-15:	122	TB-20:	291
LV-12:	341	SI-6:	180	ST-16:	122	TB-21:	292
LV-13:	341	SI-7:	181	ST-17:	123	TB-22:	292
LV-14:	342	SI-8:	181	ST-18:	123	TB-23:	293
M-BW-1a:	401	SI-9:	182	ST-19:	124		
M-BW-1b:	401	SI-10:	182	ST-20:	124		
M-BW-16:	403	SI-11:	183	ST-21:	125		
M-BW-24:	403	SI-12:	184	ST-22:	125		
M-BW-25:	403	SI-13:	184	ST-23:	126		
M-BW-35:	401	SI-14:	185	ST-24:	126		

25. Simplified Channel Pathways

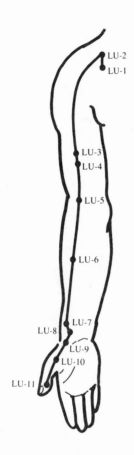

Figure 25.1: Simplified Lung Channel Pathway

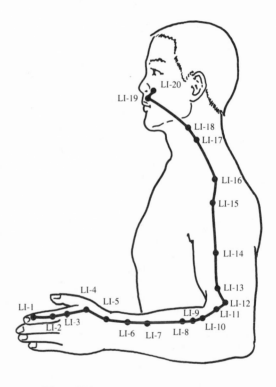

Figure 25.2: Simplified Large Intestine Channel Pathway

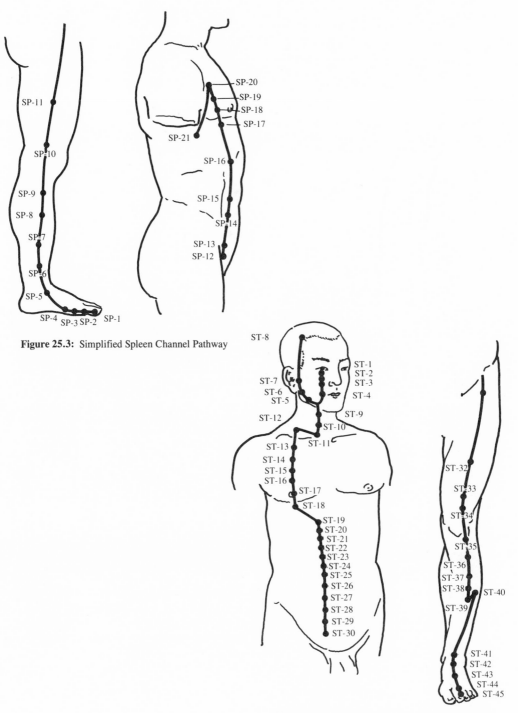

Figure 25.3: Simplified Spleen Channel Pathway

Figure 25.4: Simplified Stomach Channel Pathway

479

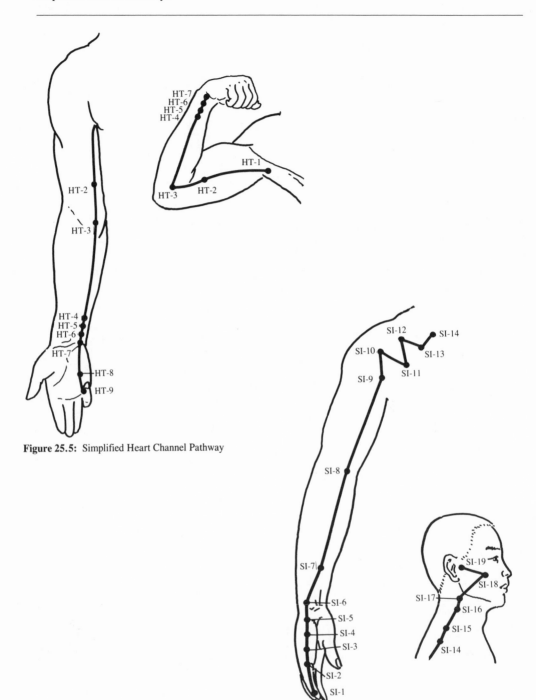

Figure 25.5: Simplified Heart Channel Pathway

Figure 25.6: Simplified Small Intestine Channel Pathway

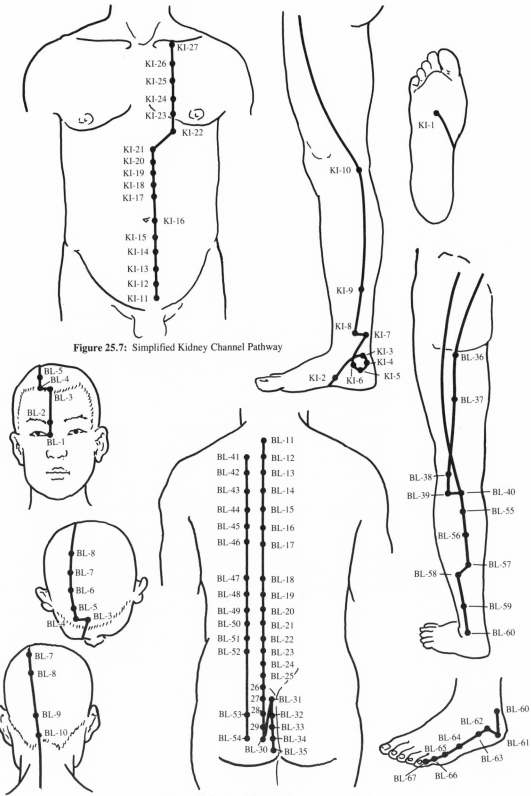

Figure 25.7: Simplified Kidney Channel Pathway

Figure 25.8: Simplified Bladder Channel Pathway

481

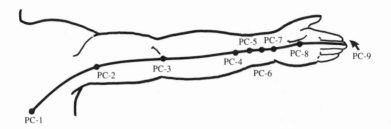

Figure 25.9: Simplified Pericardium Channel Pathway

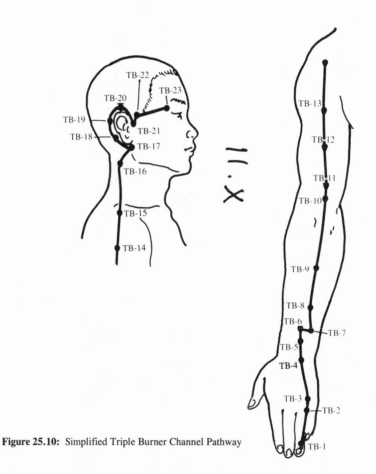

Figure 25.10: Simplified Triple Burner Channel Pathway

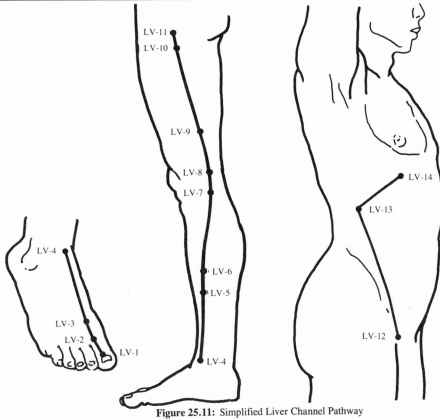

Figure 25.11: Simplified Liver Channel Pathway

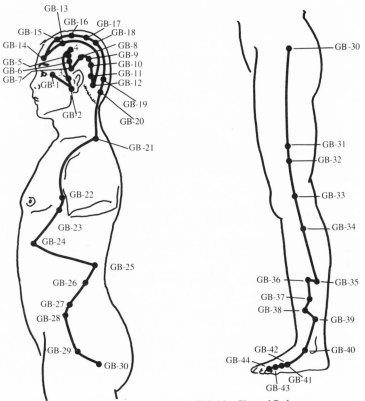

Figure 25.12: Simplified Gallbladder Channel Pathway

483

Figure 25.13: Simplified Conception Vessel Pathway

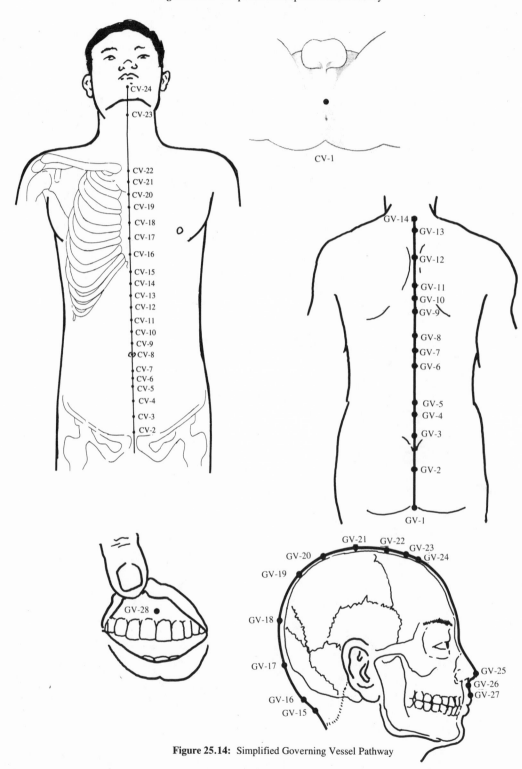

Figure 25.14: Simplified Governing Vessel Pathway